The

Economics

of

Health Care

Finance and Delivery

Seymour E. Harris

Littauer Professor of Political Economy, Emeritus
Harvard University

and Professor of Economics and Medical Economics
University of California, San Diego

McCutchan Publishing Corporation
2526 Grove Street
Berkeley, California 94704

Library of Congress Catalog Card Number 73-17612
ISBN 0-8211-0725-9

Printed in the United States of America

For
Dorothy

Contents

Acknowledgments

My greatest debt is to Myrtle Williams. Without her help I could not have written this book. She contributed so much under the most adverse conditions. Zipporah Collins was a superb editor. Dan Williamson was a productive research assistant. Elizabeth Burford and Jane Nizyborski typed more than one version of this long book. They also achieved the almost impossible: reading my very bad script and then typing with accuracy.

Ida Merriam, Assistant Commissioner of Social Security, kindly put much material at my disposal. More important, the vast, high-quality output of her Office of Research and Statistics contributed much to this book. William Behn and Judith Carnoy greatly improved the organization of this material and generally were most helpful in cutting unnecessary redundancies. Judith Carnoy also prepared the index.

As I finish my fifty-one volumes in fifty-one years, I should also apologize to those who are rightfully annoyed with compulsive writers. I promise this is my last.

Seymour E. Harris

Introduction

Costs of medical care can be measured in various ways. *Direct* costs are payments for various services, such as those provided by physicians and hospitals. By 1971, direct costs amounted to $75 billion, a rise from a few billion dollars in 1929. A more comprehensive measure includes *indirect* costs also. These measure the impact of illness and premature death on the economy. Such a comprehensive indicator may show that costs come to $200 billion or more. This enormous total becomes further inflated as expenditures reflect rising incomes. A third measure estimates the lifetime health care expenditures of a current generation of members of the labor market. Here again the costs may well reach $200 billion or $300 billion.

These are large sums. But costs are not the only relevant figures. The analyst must measure these estimates against the rise of income. Incomes compounded at 5 percent would rise in ten years by 63 percent; in twenty-five years they would increase by 238 percent; and in fifty years they would rise by 1,047 percent! Past experience with increases in prices and productivity shows that a 5 percent annual rise is not unreasonable. Gross national product, another indicator of income, is expected to escalate to about $1,300 billion. While wages and prices increase, another element that accounts for rising expenditures is "real" improvements in medical care. Still another factor to consider is the gain made against illness and premature death through investment in education, sanitation, housing, and the like, as alternatives to spending on medical care.

Expenditures on medical care are disproportionately consumed in rising prices and incomes for purveyors, with adverse effects on the quality and quantity of services. Yet over a period of forty-six years the proportion of gross national product allocated to medical care expenditures roughly doubled. How much the prices of medical services have risen is a matter of dispute. Index numbers have not always been properly weighted, and different techniques yield different results. Although it is widely believed that the burden of financing medical care continues to increase, this is not a sustainable position. Per capita disposable income, a helpful guide of capacity, has increased considerably more than the cost of living.

Medical markets are highly inflationary in part because gains in productivity are slow and inadequate compared to rising costs. Hence a potent anti-inflationary measure would be increased productivity.

One approach to increase productivity is through recourse to less costly alternatives: use of nursing homes rather than hospitals; generic drugs rather than brand names; physician assistants rather than physicians; and large hospitals rather than small.

Productivity suffers when there are wastes, inefficiencies, or even corruption. It is difficult to justify the fact that Americans undergo twice as much surgery in relation to their population as the people of England and Wales. It is difficult to justify a 75 percent drop in surgery when prior approval of operations by a medical board is introduced. It is difficult to justify the numerous facilities for specialized treatments located within 100 miles of a major treatment center such as Massachusetts General Hospital.

Deterioration of quality is another defect of modern medicine. Unfortunately, we do not have adequate measures of quality. Nevertheless, it is evident—particularly in recent Medi-Cal experiences—that as costs are reduced, quality tends to deteriorate. Price trends are concealed by practices in ghetto areas, where physicians' visits consume only five minutes apiece, and fifty to one hundred visits are made in a day.

Where prices rise excessively, the solution is to increase supply and to reduce demand. This is the obvious therapy for the physician market. But even if the number of doctors grows, there are problems of distribution: the poor do not get a fair share. Despite very large advances in physicians' incomes, the number of doctors is still inadequate. Shortages of hospital beds can be treated by increasing supplies; but federal aid under the Hill-Burton Act failed to put them where they were most needed.

Insurance coverage has expanded at a reasonable rate in recent years. It has clearly improved the competitive position of low-income people. But it has excessively favored services tied to hospitals and has wasted resources by creating the financing for overutilization of health care facilities. Blue Cross and Blue Shield have lost ground as the independent insurance companies, emphasizing experience rate-making, gained enrollees. The independents improved reimbursement methods, experimented, and favored benefits unpopular with the Blues.

Large monopoly elements are found in medical care markets. In drugs, for example, we find concentration among a few large companies, wide variations in prices, and heavy outlays for promotion, which typify monopoly organizations. In the market for physicians, there is little competition. Each doctor offers a practice differentiated by type of service and location. Hospitals also operate in a far from competitive market. The doctor and the hospital decide on entry. Nursing homes are in short supply, given the unusual rise in demand for extended care services. Their profits are large and their services inadequate. Conflicts of interests are troublesome: doctors who control pharmacies and nursing homes cooperate in giving unnecessary services. These monopolistic trends raise prices and profits and reduce services.

In the current markets, general practitioners are in short supply. In a generation, the excess income of specialists over general practitioners dropped from 80 percent to 20 percent, a result of large increases in the numbers of specialists and substantial reductions in the general practitioner population.

In the last generation, the emphasis has been on finding funds to finance medical care. But of late the stress has shifted to improving the planning, administration, and supplies of personnel, institutions, and equipment, and to improving the health care delivery system.

The delivery system especially needs to give more help to the poor and avoid requiring heavy outlays by them through coinsurance, deductibles, premiums, and other payments. These out-of-pocket expenses are much more burdensome for low-income groups than for others.

Reasonable and customary payments to physicians are attractive to doctors but their precise values are unknown. Cost reimbursements to hospitals raise serious problems in eliminating incentives for efficient operation. Fortunately, this reimbursement approach is not as widely used as is generally assumed.

An important advance in financing health care could be made through greater use of postpayment rather than prepayment. Insurance is a costly manner of financing. A serious illness comes on the average every ten to fifteen years. By the time the insured receives a substantial benefit, he has used up a large part of his insurance premium. Insurance is financed out of low current income, whereas credit is financed out of the rising future income. In twenty-five or fifty years, vast increases of income occur, so that the burden of credit proportionately declines. Yet only a very small part of the $600 billion of available credit is currently used for medical bills.

Dissatisfaction with benefits, distribution, prices, and the inadequacy of insurance have greatly increased public enthusiasm for national health insurance. There is now widespread support for some form of national program, particularly if payments are to be based on ability to pay, in contrast to the current programs where financing is placed disproportionately on those with low incomes.

Acceptance of national health insurance awaits agreement on numerous issues by the supporters. Who is to control the program? How comprehensive will the benefits be? Who is to be covered? How is the program to be financed? How much will the government contribute? These will be answered in the near future.

PART I

Issues, Costs, and Expenditures

1

Major Issues

Over the last forty years, the emphasis in the health care policy has been on obtaining adequate funds to finance medical care. Health expenditures in the United States increased from a few billion dollars in 1929 to $83 billion in 1972. To an extent, this vast increase in outlays marked efforts on the part of government and others to ensure individual access to medical care, manifesting the view that adequate medical care is a right that should be available to all. The increases in expenditures also reflected the fact that medical care was plainly more expensive than it had been in the past. The growth of services was not at all commensurate with the increased flow of cash. One significant result, from a policy perspective, was a renewed demand for greater efficiency in the delivery of services.

But the shifting face of the medical care crisis reveals more than a change in emphasis from finance to delivery. The issues of finance and delivery are intertwined in the structure of medical markets. To describe the operation of medical markets adequately we need answers to many questions. Who pays and who receives medical care? How do the cost, quality, and accessibility of medical care vary according to the individual's income class, sex, and race? Who provides health services and for what compensation? What are the patterns of delivery, and what are the incentives for efficient provision of quality care? Moreover, these questions must be asked in a normative sense—who should pay for and who should receive medical care; how should services be provided and under what system of incentives and compensation? This chapter examines some of the major issues in the economics of health care as they arise from this perspective.

Medical Care Markets

It appears that a dual system of health care exists today: good and sometimes luxurious care is available to the affluent while fragmented, mediocre care is provided for the majority in sometimes uncomfortable and humiliating circumstances. Disparities in care are in part the result of federal programs and a system of taxation that force the middle class to finance care for the poor and elderly, while they must frequently forgo these services themselves. Lower-middle-class Americans are precariously situated just one illness or accident removed from poverty. This situation is related both to monopolistic features of the market for medical care, which bid up the price and restrict and differentiate the service, and to significant inequalities in the distribution of income among Americans.

Monopolistic Features of Medical Care Markets

Elements of monopoly are to be found in most markets for medical care. Monopoly power affords control over resources to the parties who exercise that power. It enables them to raise the price of services and diminish their availability, whereas such control of the situation would not obtain in a competitive market. The almost uncontrollable rise of prices and costs, the unusually high profit rates of pharmaceutical companies and hospital suppliers, and the excessive physician incomes seen today are related to these monopoly forces. Paired with a situation where people of varied economic means have unequal abilities to purchase medical services, it is assured that medical needs will go unmet.

Possibly the most glaring example of the consequence of monopoly power in medical care markets is to be found in the drug industry. Profits in drugs have been as high as those in any other industry in the United States since World War II. For example, between 1954 and 1966, the drug and medicine industry had the nation's highest industrywide profit rate: 18.5 percent. Next came the motor vehicle industry at 17 percent and the computing machines industry at 15.5 percent.[1] Drug profits cannot be justified by the risk of obsolescence of a line of drugs. Control of the drug industry is concentrated in relatively few companies, and these firms have exceptionally high profit rates. Patents having a life of seventeen years help protect monopolistic features of the drug industry.

Sale prices for the same or comparable drugs may vary ten to twenty times from minimum to maximum, and yet the high-priced drugs seem to be free of competition from the low-priced drugs. Drugs are sold at different prices to manufacturers, retailers, and the government, and prices vary greatly depending on the country of residence of the consumer. Excessive recourse to differentiation of drug prices brings small numbers of units and high unit costs. Sellers have not succeeded in justifying large price differentials on the basis of quality differentials. The high prices of drugs are especially unwelcome because insurance coverage of drug costs is limited, and the most vulnerable groups, e.g., the old, who spend disproportionate amounts on drugs, suffer appreciably.

Hospitals also manifest monopoly elements. For example, they charge less than cost for room and board and more than cost for ancillary services. This would be impossible in a competitive pricing situation. Monopoly aspects also prevail in the markets for equipment and hospital supplies.[2]

Hospitals indulge in only restricted competition for patients. More typically, exclusionary principles are applied that reflect the hospital affiliations of physicians. Individual consumers have financial and geographic access to certain physicians and thereby particular hospitals. Public hospitals are becoming the hospitals of last resort for the poor. Low-income patients rely on emergency rooms for primary care—an expensive and inappropriate use of such services. The less expensive forms of care, such as outpatient services, are frequently provided in only fragmentary fashion. The teaching and research priorities of the better hospitals affiliated with medical schools can make these facilities unavailable for routine hospital care, even to residents of their local communities.

The extent to which noneconomic considerations determine hospital size also points to monopolistic features. There are too many small hospitals, because too many communities of moderate size have built hospitals at high unit costs. The large hospitals, despite their economies of scale, tend to be high cost. The reason given is that they assume disproportionate responsibilities for high-cost procedures.

Nursing home residents are also victims of monopolistic forces, especially with the large expansion and overcapitalization of these facilities in recent years. These institutions then assess heavy capital charges on consumers of their services.

Confronted with the large and growing demand for medical services and a relatively small increase in the supply of physicians, doctors have restricted their services by increasing their fees or cutting down on their output. The decision to reduce visits or time is indicative of monopolistic elements in the market for physician services. Under pure competition, a rise in prices would result, rather than a reduction of services. In ghettos the practice tends to be to reduce the quality of services—e.g., spending 2½ minutes per visit and increasing the number of visits substantially produce a large rise in income. This is in fact a disguised increase in prices.

Fee-splitting and conflicts of interest (such as ownership of pharmacies and nursing homes by physicians) also signify an absence of price competition. Health professionals in nonprofit enterprises are frequently allied with companies that supply services on a profit-making basis (drug companies, hospital supply companies, hospital construction firms, and commercial insurance companies).

Physicians have moved in several regions to foreclose expansion of prepaid group practice because it would replace fee-for-service arrangements. Foundations for medical care have been established that are designed to keep control over fees and medical knowledge in the hands of doctors. These foundations further aim to undertake self-regulation of physicians' performances, excluding the government and consumers from such review.[3]

Shortages of Physicians

Where shortages or bottlenecks occur in a *competitive* market, the remedy is generally to increase the payments for a given service in the short term, thereby encouraging a larger supply in the future. A shortage of physicians has been identified as such for over a decade. Physicians have an average income in excess of $40,000.[4] That level of compensation should be enough to attract qualified personnel. Yet most experts still find that serious shortages of physicians are troubling the nation.

There are roughly 350,000 physicians now licensed in the United States, but only 200,000 are practicing. The other 150,000 are performing teaching, research, or administrative tasks or are retired. The Bureau of Labor Statistics projects an annual need of 22,000 new physicians during the 1970s. Medical schools are now graduating slightly more than half that number (12,000) per year, while an equal number of applicants are turned away from American schools each year. The introduction of national health insurance and health maintenance organizations would further compound the shortages by widening the base and extending the coverage of medical care.

Not only have American medical markets failed to respond to the increased demand for physicians, but the burden has also been placed on less-developed nations. The United States siphons off physicians trained abroad at the expense of foreign interests.[5] Iran, for example, produces 600 medical graduates a year. Approximately 100 members of each graduating class of the past decade are now in the United States. South Korea has about 13,000 doctors to serve its entire population, yet there are 2,000 Korean medical graduates in the United States. India lost over 800 physicians to the United States in 1971, equivalent in number to the combined graduating classes of eight American medical schools. In fact a twofold drain on physicians from other countries occurs, since a significant number of premedical students in the United States who are passed over in the competition for a place in medical schools here go abroad for medical training only to return home to practice medicine.

The cost of a medical education in the United States runs to $100,000 on the average. At this rate, the United States is a net debtor-nation in medical personnel by a substantial margin. We receive services from abroad without paying the commensurate cost. One out of every five physicians now practicing in the United States (63,391 out of 334,028 in 1970) received his or her training outside the United States and Canada. Over half the net increase in licensed physicians in 1971 was comprised of foreign-trained physicians.[6] The 4,300 foreign medical graduates licensed in the United States in 1971 are equivalent to the output of forty-three of our average-size medical schools. If these doctors were unavailable, American citizens would have to bear the cost of building and staffing the necessary medical schools. Capital costs could run to $4 billion and annual training expenses to $430 million. This latter figure may be compared to the roughly $600 million in after-tax profits garnered by the drug industry each year, or the $400 million in after-tax profits going to hospital suppliers, or the $200 million in profits claimed by proprietary hospitals and nursing homes.[7]

Instead of depending on the training of more doctors, the physician shortage could be treated in part through a rise of productivity, as Dr. Rashi Fein has argued. But it is not easy to increase productivity, nor is the government justified in measuring gains in productivity solely by the number of visits achieved. The rise in visits should also be tied to increased inputs of capital and labor.[8]

A potentially significant approach to the shortage of physicians is to find lower-cost substitutes, such as greater use of technology, capital, drugs, assistant physicians, and technical personnel (including more highly trained nurses). A substitute for the physician is also found in greater knowledge about medical care on the part of the consumer.

The allied health professions, once highly touted as a way to ease the demands on physicians, exhibit further monopolistic features of the medical market. Because physicians' prerogatives are closely guarded, the most productive division of tasks between physicians and others on routine procedures has not been accomplished. In consequence, members of the allied health professions frequently find themselves in redundant positions, since their skills are not fully employed, and this adds further to medical care costs. In the second place, exclusionary rules, erected in the name of quality care, raise the prices of services and lower their availability. As quality control replaces price control of a service (whether the service is health care, education, or another field), poor people face more limited choices and receive more inferior service. Monopolistic features of the market facilitate the displacement of price control by quality control in fields where professional standards can be invoked.

Maldistribution of Physicians

The problems raised by a shortage of physicians are compounded for many poor and rural Americans by the maldistribution of physicians from region to region and by field of specialization. Increasing the number of physicians alone would not alleviate the shortage of physicians faced by rural communities, transitory populations such as migrant farmworkers, or groups served by inner-city hospitals and clinics, since these populations are situated in locations that are considered undesirable by medical practitioners. Regional group medical practices may be the answer in some rural areas. However, the policy objective should not be to equalize physician-population ratio, but rather to distribute physicians according to the particular health needs of the population, taking account of its economic circumstances, the health hazards it faces, and its age distribution.

Part of the shortage of physicians is attributable to the fact that doctors have assumed added responsibilities in administration and have entered research and teaching in greater numbers. Relatively fewer physicians are preparing to deliver primary care today as family doctors, internists, or pediatricians. In the last generation, the rise of medical specialists and the decline of the general practitioner, both absolutely and relatively, have greatly changed the health care system. As more and more doctors become specialists, serious shortages emerge in primary care practice.[9] Reflecting both increased supplies in the specialties and increased demand for GPs, the excess income of specialists over GPs dropped from 80 percent to 20 percent in one period.

Apparently doctors do not choose their specialty primarily according to expected income or anticipated rise of income. This may suggest that they are not as materialistic as they are at times held to be, or that, at high levels of income, the choice of type of work carries more weight than the gain in income to be realized in one type as opposed to another.[10]

Monopoly power in medical care markets thus enables providers to raise the prices of services and restrict their availability. The shortage of medical personnel bestows a monopoly power on physicians that permits them to act as price-discriminating monopolists in charging patients who pay fees out of pocket. Further, consumer ignorance about the price and quality of medical services discourages competitive forces from pushing down prices.[11]

Inflation in Medical Costs

There have been vast increases in the outlays for health services over the past several decades. From 1950 to 1972 the medical care bill rose from 4.6 to 7.6 percent of GNP. That seems like a reasonable increase if it represents improved social welfare, but there are still large gaps in benefits, and the quality of health care is often below an acceptable level. The increased outlay reflects not only an increase in the services provided but also a dramatic inflation in the prices of these services.

Per capita expenditures on all health services and supplies from 1929 to 1971 rose from $27.77 to $346.57, a rise of twelve times, while per capita expenditures on hospital care rose from $5.36 to $134.21, a rise of twenty-five times. In this period, the cost of living rose one and a third times, and the population increased by 70 percent. Per capita disposable income (after-tax income), which is a measure of capacity to pay, rose four times as much as the cost of living, or 5.3 times.[12] Figure 1.1 shows the relative movement of medical care prices and the consumer price index between 1959 and 1970.

The increasing price of medical care has outpaced the consumer's ability to pay for health services. The purchaser of hospital care in particular is burdened since the price of hospital care has risen more rapidly than the general price index. It has also outpaced the increase in workers' earnings (see figure 1.2). Most bills for hospital services are not paid out of pocket by the consumer but are met by third-party reimbursement mechanisms such as Blue Cross. Typically hospitals are reimbursed by these third parties on the basis of their costs, and thus their incentive to keep costs down is limited. Mr. Leonard Woodcock of the United Auto Workers union presented a study on health expenditures for a typical family to the Senate Finance Committee. Assuming no catastrophic illness, a family with earnings of $7,000 would spend $1,759 per year.[13] The auto workers and other unionists sponsored a national health insurance plan that would "embrace the entire range of personal health services—including care for the prevention and early detection of disease, the treatment of illness and physical rehabilitation. There would be no restrictions on needed services, no cut-off points, no coinsurance, no deductibles, and no waiting periods."[14]

In light of the soaring costs of medical care, it is not surprising that in the early 1970s even strong proponents of national health insurance were concerned over the failure to control the rise of expenditures for medical care. Professor I. S. Falk, a leading expert on medical economics, referred to the "idiocy of signed blank check reimbursement of practitioners and full cost reimbursement of institutions guaranteed under recently enacted public programs without feasible and institutional controls."[15]

FIGURE 1.1   Quarterly Index of Consumer and Medical Care Prices, 1959-70

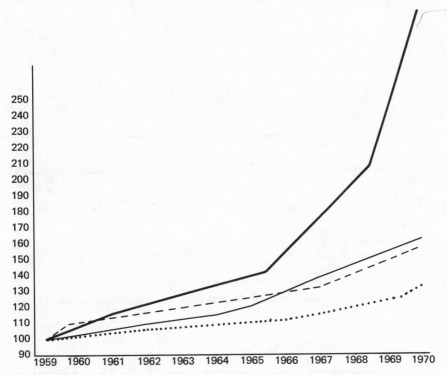

Index: 1957-59=100

—————— Hospital Daily Service Charges
——————— Physicians' Fees
– – – – – All Medical Care Items
••••••••• CPI, All Items

A comparison of the rise of outlays and the rise of available services at a given level of quality has been a cause of unhappiness to those who want a genuinely comprehensive medical care program. It is not surprising that the Committee on National Health Insurance (Committee of 100) could find possible savings of $14 billion (23 percent) in the operation of our medical care program.[16] Inefficiency in the operation and utilization of hospitals is a primary point of concern.

Excessive surgery is one common source of wasted resources.[17] The committee estimated, partly on the basis of Dr. J. Bunker's

FIGURE 1.2   Comparison of Increases in Hospital Costs and Workers' Earnings, 1959-69

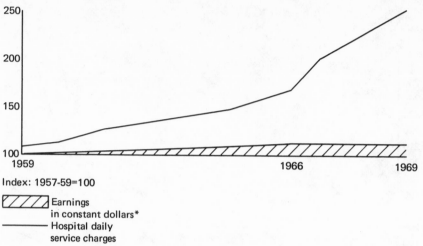

Index: 1957-59=100

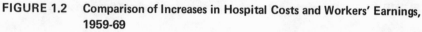 Earnings
              in constant dollars*
              ———— Hospital daily
              service charges

Sources: Social Security Administration and Bureau of Labor Statistics

*Average weekly take-home pay, after federal taxes, of nonsupervisory worker in private employment.

revealing comparison of the amount of surgery in the United Kingdom and the United States, that we could reduce operations here by 25 percent.[18] Recourse to surgery was twice as great in the United States as in England in relation to population. A Columbia University study revealed that the introduction of a prior approval cut down one category of surgery by 75 percent.

Fear of the impact of a continued rise in expenditures has affected policy in some respects. Increasing attention is being paid to economizing on outlays. There is more emphasis on choosing the least costly alternatives for medical care, such as extended care facilities instead of hospitals, and there is more reluctance to reimburse on the basis of a fee per service, as favored by physicians, or to guarantee costs for institutional reimbursement. Greater recourse to preventive medicine, including education and multiphasic screening, would also reduce total costs to the individual and society. Greater dependence on comprehensive prepaid group insurance could cut direct outlays.

Physicians would then be compensated on a capitation rather than a fee-for-service basis. Under capitation programs, a fixed sum is received by the physician or medical group for provision of health care to an individual or group over a period of one year, irrespective of the services rendered. As economies are realized, they accrue to the provider of the services.

It could be argued that, while expenditures on medical care are indeed rising, personal income is also rising, so that the ability to meet increased medical costs is keeping pace. On the basis of past trends, it is estimated that income on a per capita or per family basis should rise about 2½ times in twenty-five years and 10½ times in fifty years.[19] Thus, one could say that the $100 per day hospital bill today—or a $1,000 per day hospital bill in the year 2020—is not out of line with income trends.

This ignores two important facts, however. For one, substantial inefficiencies in the provision of hospital care exist, and there are alternative claims on the dollars that could be saved. In the second place, while average family income may increase over time, the distribution is uneven, and, as a result, certain families may have much less ability to pay. Even if the difference in the relative income shares of the richest 20 percent of all families and the poorest 20 percent declines over time, the *absolute* difference in the average income of these two groups can be increasing. This has in fact occurred: between 1947 and 1969 the absolute difference in the average income of these two quintiles increased from $10,565 to $19,071 (in 1969 dollars).[20]

Postpayment for Health Care

Medical care is financed primarily through taxation and insurance, and to a lesser extent from direct out-of-pocket expenditures. The exchange involved is either prepayment (taxes and insurance) or direct payment upon receipt of services. Postpayment—financing medical care through credit—has not been used extensively in the United States. While consumer debt and credit finance are substantial, private enterprise has not exploited credit for medical care, and consumers have not expressed great interest in this method of financing.

Today, credit finances the purchase of many durable as well as nondurable goods. Most frequently these are financed by use of credit cards. In each instance, the family can plan the expenditure for each item so that the cost of the items purchased, including finance charges, fits within the family budget.[21]

Spending on medical care, however, differs from these purchases. Some families spend a large fraction of their income on it while others are graced with good health and spend relatively little. For example, a study of federal employees in 1969 showed that over half of the families of four spent less than $260 on medical care (including both out-of-pocket expenditures and payments by insurance companies), while 10 percent of the families of four spent more than $1,500, and 5 percent spent more than $2,600.[22] Families whose medical care costs ran over $2,600 in one year spent a much greater proportion of family income on health care than those spending less than $260. For a family of the working poor with no medical insurance, medical expenses can use between 20 percent and 40 percent of income.

Whatever the circumstances, the decision to purchase essential medical care on credit is a decision made *after* receipt of the service. It thus reflects the options of distributing the cost of services received over time, not a decision that is integral to the purchase of the service itself. The decision to purchase a freezer, for example, is not forced upon the consumer so that he or she is left with the dilemma of how to finance it. Rather, the price, including finance charges, the use value of the item, and the preferences of the consumer figure in the purchase decision. Some nonessential medical care can be deferred or forgone, and thus is comparable to such a purchase, but most health care is not.

An advantage of credit financing in inflationary periods is that, with credit terms fixed, rising income over time reduces the burden of financing medical care.[23] But, like holders of mortgage debts, who benefit as property owners from inflation of prices and income, medical debtors would suffer equally as consumers on payment for goods and services and short-term credit. And credit finance is both harder to obtain and more costly for the poor credit risk in our society.

An important factor working against postpayment for medical care is that individuals cannot schedule an illness as they can other purchases. A major illness at age fifty-five or sixty cannot easily be financed by a long-term loan. Income at that stage of life usually will not be rising, and the illness may be so disabling that it impairs the individual's earning capacity. Financial institutions view such people as poor credit risks.

If medical care expenses from an illness total less than the cost of premiums for full coverage insurance for the period since the last major illness, credit finance does become attractive. But the uncertainty about spending for medical care and the associated financial risk are exactly what encourage people to seek medical insurance coverage. Deductibles, coinsurance, and limits on insurance coverage do reduce the attractiveness of medical insurance, however, and may force consumers to use credit financing if it is available.

Credit financing of medical care *is* advantageous for postpayment of a short-term debt incurred for a minor disorder. The prospect of requiring credit financing, like the need for direct payment, may discourage a person from using medical procedures that may be unnecessary. However, the poor and near poor are the ones most likely to be discouraged from seeking "unnecessary" care; they are also the ones most likely to lose tragically if a minor illness becomes more acute, because their employment is generally insecure (their employers are less tolerant of any prolonged absence from the job); and they are ultimately the ones who bear the cost of most short-term credit financing through credit cards, since the well-to-do can meet payment within thirty days and avoid interest charges, while the poor pay interest rates designed to finance the credit card system for all users.[24]

Since the income gap between the rich and the poor is increasing over time, even with a growing gross national product, the credit position of the poor is unlikely to improve in absolute terms without federal assistance. The opportunity for postpayment by the poor is thereby diminished. The poor and the medically indigent do not now fare well under our system of financing of medical care, and it seems reasonable to expect that federal intervention in capital markets to improve access to and terms of credit would be a mixed blessing.

A credit finance plan proposed by Martin S. Feldstein does include government-guaranteed, low-interest loans to help consumers pay medical bills.[25] The maximum amount to be financed by credit is limited to a proportion of the individual's or family's income (here 10 percent), with the balance subsidized by a form of catastrophic illness coverage. However, the plan is regressive, because it places a greater burden on low-income families. Making all initial payments out-of-pocket heavily discourages the poor from seeking medical care. One of the purposes is to make the consumer cost-conscious, but there is no provision to encourage providers, who have more control over costs, to be cost-conscious. For full coverage insurance (including dental care and drugs, as well as hospitalization and physicians' service), premiums averaged over $1,000 in 1973 for a family of four.[26]

With coverage under Social Security (OASDHI) increasing in terms of both numbers of people and benefits paid, part of the rising surplus of this trust fund could be used to finance health benefits through a program for extending credit. Other trust funds, such as private pension funds, have proved to be important sources of capital in the financial markets, and theoretically money from these funds could be put to use by members of the pension plan to finance programs such as health services. Such funds, with their rising surplus (due to the growing number of people paying into the fund with claims deferred), offer a more important source of capital than growing personal income to finance medical care under private credit arrangements.

Insurance

Medical care expenses are the single largest cause of personal bankruptcy in the United States. Medical insurance is our main mechanism at present for reducing the financial risk associated with spending for medical care. The demand for health insurance is created by the uncertainty surrounding family medical care spending. As medical knowledge and services expanded in the first half of this century, and the cost of medical care rose sharply, families found themselves without the means to pay for medical care that was now considered essential. At the same time, the extended family was declining, so that relatives no longer were available to help out when extended illness or disability arose.

Another important impetus for hospital insurance plans came during the depression years when hospitals were unable to cover their bad debts. Insurance companies, pooling the finances and risks of many families, could charge premiums equal to the mean insured risk plus administrative charges, advertising costs, and a return to their capital investors. By paying this premium, an individual family could avoid heavy financial burdens if serious illness or injury occurred. And hospitals were assured of payment for their services, even when expenses mounted. Economists generally agree that insurance is needed most for catastrophic illnesses—those incurring extraordinarily high medical expenses.[27]

Despite its contribution, private insurance pays only about one-third of the average family's medical bills. Most enrollees do not have full coverage, so they must pay a deductible amount, such as $50 per year, before any benefits are received under the insurance. Then, many policies have a coinsurance provision, whereby the enrollee pays part of the bill and the insurance company the rest—often 20 percent and 80 percent respectively. And finally, coverage is limited to only certain expenses and services by most policies. For example, drugs, dental care, and psychiatric treatment are often excluded, so that an enrollee requiring these must pay the full cost himself.

More than 20 percent of the civilian population (37 million people) have no medical insurance whatsoever. Some could afford to buy insurance but prefer to take their chances on being able to pay out of pocket for any health care they may need. Most of those who are uncovered, however, are poorer individuals and families who have to spend their income for the immediate necessities of life. These people also have a greater risk of illness and less ability to pay for care. They are further discouraged from buying insurance by the deductibles, coinsurance, and limited coverage of health care policies.[28]

The inequities in present insurance coverage point to the conclusion that either adequate medical care should be made a right of every citizen, financed out of public revenues, or the burden of health costs should be spread progressively according to family income.[29]

Table 1.3 shows the relation between health insurance coverage and income for 1970. For families with incomes under $3,000, 39.9 percent were covered by hospital insurance and 36.7 percent by surgical insurance. The corresponding statistics for families with incomes of $10,000 or more are 90.1 percent and 88.3 percent. Table 1.4 illustrates in greater detail the unevenness of insurance coverage. Items such as drugs prove particularly costly for the aged. The financial dilemma of low-income families is clear. Those who cannot afford a $10 to $15 fee for a physician's office visit are discouraged from seeking medical care.

TABLE 1.3   Health Insurance Coverage by Income Level, 1970

Income Level	Percentage of Population Under 65 Covered	
	Hospital Insurance	Surgical Insurance
Under $3,000	39.3	36.7
$3,000-$4,999	53.1	50.2
$5,000-$6,999	74.5	71.8
$7,000-$9,999	84.3	81.9
$10,000 or more	90.1	88.3

Source: HEW, Social Security Administration, *Medical Care Expenditures, Prices, and Costs: Background Book* (September 1973), p. 83.

Health Maintenance Organizations

In the last few years, there has been much discussion of health maintenance organizations and of capitation fees to cover all medical services. The proponents of these plans say they do not seek to fix fees for doctors; what they want is single agreed per capita fees rather than a fixed fee for each service.

Dr. H. F. Newman, director of the Group Health Cooperative in Puget Sound, Washington, concluded that prepaid group practice plans have been able to supply care for a substantially lower dollar

TABLE 1.4   Gaps in Private Health Insurance Coverage, 1971

Type of Care	Population under 65 with Coverage		Population under 65 without Coverage	
	Number (Millions)	Percentage	Number (Millions)	Percentage
Hospital care	147.3	79.8	37.4	20.2
Surgical services	142.8	77.3	41.9	22.7
In-hospital visits	140.7	76.2	44.0	23.8
X-ray and laboratory exams	137.5	74.4	47.2	25.6
Office and home visits	91.5	49.5	93.2	50.5
Dental care	15.2	8.2	169.5	91.8
Prescription drugs	103.7	56.1	81.0	43.9
Nursing home care	33.4	18.1	151.3	81.9
Private duty nursing	101.4	54.9	83.3	45.1
Visiting nurse service	106.2	57.5	78.5	42.5

Source: HEW, Social Security Administration, *Medical Care Expenditures, Prices, and Costs: Background Book* (September 1973), p. 82.

outlay than the predominant fee-for-service system. He noted that the Puget Sound program offered a comprehensive package of services for approximately two-thirds of what it would cost elsewhere in the nation. "Measuring annual hospital days per 1000 persons covered, those under prepaid group practice plans in six major areas of the country were hospitalized about half as much as those covered under other forms of insurance."

In 1966, federal employees enrolled in prepaid group practice plans underwent half as many appendectomies, one-fourth as many tonsillectomies and adenoidectomies, and half as many female surgical operations as those under fee-for-service health care plans.[30]

In California the health maintenance organization approach received increased attention when the state Medicaid administration considered signing contracts with nine or more prepaid medical groups to provide health services to subsidized enrollees for a monthly per capita fee. As these agreements became more popular, they lost some of their glamour. In some cases excessive payments, inefficiencies, and even fraud have come to light. An especially troublesome difficulty is how to maintain quality standards when reimbursement is based on the number of enrollees.

President Nixon in 1971 praised prepaid group practice plans for providing strong financial incentives for better preventive care and more efficient medical care. He proposed this system as the wave of medicine's future, but his administration has not provided substantial sums for health maintenance organizations.[31]

Despite rising interest in these organizations, apparently only 8 million people were enrolled in them in a recent year. The health maintenance organization concept appeals to young doctors, but most physicians are not ready to abandon the fee-for-service reimbursement system, which yields them large returns. The Nixon administration stressed the possibility that medical care providers would not cooperate if they were denied their usual fees.

Federal Health Programs

Medicare and Medicaid

By any account, passage of Medicare and Medicaid marked significant points in the history of health care costs. The costs of medical care, particularly the prices of physicians' services and hospital care, have risen dramatically since then. The rate of inflation in the medical care sector was approximately three times that of all items in the economy as measured by the consumer price index (see table 1.5). The need for cost-control measures is apparent from this alone. A number of regulatory measures have been proposed to control costs while providing incentives to the providers of services to experiment with new modes of delivery, primarily health maintenance organizations.[32]

The federal government's role in the finance of medical care grew with the expansion of Medicare and Medicaid. Between 1966 and 1972, the portion of the medical care dollar coming from public funds rose from 25.7 percent to 39.4 percent. The possible effects of the two programs on the price of hospital care had not been foreseen in 1966.[33] The use of cost-plus reimbursement of hospital expenses and health insurance coverage that encouraged utilization of hospitals both contributed significantly to the rise of hospital care prices.

The increasing wages of hospital workers, who were historically underpaid, does not explain all of the increase in payroll expenses in the period following enactment of Medicare (see table 1.6). Much of the growth in payroll expenses was due to an increase in the number of hospital employees. The number of employees per patient in community hospitals increased from 2.46 to 2.92 between 1966 and 1970.[34] Improvements in service (i.e., increased inputs of capital and labor) and increases in wages and prices account more or less

TABLE 1.5   Increases in Medical Care Costs and All Consumer Price Index Items, 1955-72

Year	Percentage of Increase		
	All Items	Medical Care	Semiprivate Room
1955	2.2	3.8	6.9
1960	2.0	4.1	6.3
1965	1.3	2.5	5.8
1967	2.9	7.1	19.8
1969	5.4	6.8	13.4
1970	5.9	6.3	12.9
1971	4.3	6.5	12.2
1972	3.3	3.2	6.6

Source: Cost of Living Council, "Control of Hospital Costs under the Economic Stabilization Program," *Federal Register*, January 24, 1974, p. 2693.

TABLE 1.6   Percentage Increases in Hospital Expenses, 1960-71

	Percentage Increase	
Expense Item	Pre-Medicare (1960-65)	Post-Medicare (1966-71)
Total expense	10.2	17.0
Payroll expense	10.1	15.9
Nonpayroll expense	10.4	18.6
Personnel	5.1	5.6
Average salary	4.7	9.8
Increase in plant assets	8.0	9.1

Source: Cost of Living Council, "Control of Hospital Costs under the Economic Stabilization Program," *Federal Register,* January 24, 1974, p. 2694.

equally for the total rise in expenses per patient day in recent years (see table 1.7). How to control capital expenditures is a controversial issue in the discussion of cost controls generally.

Inflation in the cost of medical care along with reductions in the amount and scope of benefits under Medicare and Medicaid have brought out-of-pocket expenses by the poor and elderly up to about the same proportion of their income as they paid for health care before these federal programs. In 1967, persons over sixty-five paid 8.1 percent of their income for medical services. This proportion

TABLE 1.7   Increase of Hospital Services Compared with Increases in Wages and Prices, 1951-72

	Average Annual Percentage Increase					
Cost Factor	1951-60	1960-65	1965-67	1967-69	1969-71	1971-72
Total increase	7.5	6.7	10.3	13.8	14.8	14.0
Increase in wages and prices	3.8	3.5	4.1	8.0	8.2	6.2
Wages	5.2	4.7	4.7	9.9	10.0	8.1
Prices	1.5	1.3	2.9	4.8	5.1	3.3
Improvement in services	3.7	3.2	6.2	5.8	6.6	7.8
Labor	3.1	1.7	3.8	2.8	3.7	3.0
Other	4.6	5.6	9.6	9.8	10.3	14.2
Percentage of total increase due to						
Wages and prices	50.0	51.5	39.7	58.2	55.3	44.2
Improved services	50.0	48.5	60.3	41.8	44.7	55.8

Source: HEW, Social Security Administration, *Medical Care Expenditures, Prices, and Costs: Background Book* (September 1973), p. 40.

fell to 6.3 percent in 1968 and 1969 but rose again to 8.0 percent in 1972.

Table 1.8 shows the distribution of benefits under current federal health programs. As expected, Medicare and Medicaid payments benefit primarily the poor while the federal tax system subsidizes the purchase of private health insurance for higher-income people.

One improvement in Medicare was an amendment on October 30, 1972, to cover certain catastrophic illnesses. It extended federal payment to persons under sixty-five, their spouses, and their dependent children if they had a chronic kidney disease requiring hemodialysis or a renal transplant (both very costly treatments).

Effects of Nixon's Economic Stabilization Program

The Economic Stabilization Program put into operation by the Nixon administration in August 1971 has provided experience by which to judge the efficacy of alternative means of federal control of health costs. Its final incarnation in Phase IV focused on controlling hospital revenues on a per admission basis.[35] Despite disagreement about the form cost controls should take, there is substantial support for some action in this area.[36]

In the period under the Economic Stabilization Program there was a substantial reduction in hospital expenses per patient-day and per admission (see table 1.9).[37] Likewise, while physicians' fees continued to rise, the annual rate of increase fell from 7.4 percent before the

TABLE 1.8   Distribution of Benefits under Federal Programs by Income and Age, 1970

		Program			Age Group	
Income	Total Federal Benefits	Medicare Payments	Federal Medicaid Payments	Federal Tax Subsidies	Under 65	65 and Over
Total amount of benefits (millions)	$14,224	$7,494	$2,930	$3,800	$4,994	$9,230
Under $5,000	45%	54%	67%	13%	28%	54%
$5,000 to $9,999	28%	26%	24%	31%	32%	26%
$10,000 to $14,999	16%	14%	5%	26%	21%	13%
$15,000 or more	11%	7%	4%	30%	19%	7%

Source: K. Davis, "Financing Medical Services: The Federal Role," in U.S. Congress, Joint Economic Committee, *Hearings on Medical Policies and Costs* (May 15, 1973), p. 70.

TABLE 1.9   Increase in Hospital Expenses, 1963-73

Period		Percentage Increase		
	Expense per Patient-Day	Expense per Admission	Ratio of Wages and Prices to Expense per Patient-Day	Ratio of Wages and Prices to Expense per Admission
Before Medicare (1963-65)	7.5	8.2	3.0	3.7
After Medicare (1966-69)	12.2	14.4	7.2	9.0
Before Economic Stabilization Program (1969-71)	13.9	11.6	5.1	2.3
Phase II (1972-73)	10.4	8.9	4.2	2.8
Phase III (1973-74, projected)	9.0	7.4	2.9	1.9

Source: Cost of Living Council, "Control of Hospital Costs under the Economic Stabilization Program," *Federal Register,* January 24, 1974, p. 2694.

stabilization program to 2.4 percent during Phase II. Physicians' incomes rose more rapidly than physicians' fees, however, indicating that doctors were providing more service in the same number of hours of work per week. This could result from improved productivity or from declining quality of care.

One hopeful sign from the point of view of cost control is the decline in the length of the average hospital stay since 1969 (see table 1.10). As one consequence, hospital services are being used more intensively. The occupancy rate is also declining, which means higher costs per patient-day, as fixed costs are spread over relatively fewer patient-days. This could lead to pressure for marginal admissions and prolonged stays. The drop in the occupancy rate indicates the need for a moratorium on hospital bed construction in many areas of the country.

TABLE 1.10   Hospitals, Beds, Size, and Utilization, 1965-72

Year	Hospitals	Beds (Thousands)	Average Bed Size	Average Length of Stay (Days)	Occupancy Rate
1965	5,736	741	129	7.8	76.0
1968	5,820	806	138	8.4	78.2
1970	5,859	848	145	8.2	78.0
1972	5,843	884	151	7.9	75.2

Source: Cost of Living Council, "Control of Hospital Costs under the Economic Stabilization Program," *Federal Register,* January 24, 1974, p. 2696.

National Health Insurance

A program of national health insurance has been under discussion in the United States for many years, but a variety of obstacles prevented its enactment. In the early 1970s, numerous plans were proposed by congressmen and administration leaders, differing in the benefits to be covered, the amounts to be spent, the manner of financing, the contribution of government (especially at the federal level), the degree of free choice allowed to patients, doctors, and other participants, the degree of control by government and private insurance companies, the time at which the program should be initiated, and the degree of centralization.

Fundamental clashes in ideology were expressed in the plans proposed by Senator Long, Senator Kennedy, and President Nixon. Long's proposal was a minimal program to provide catastrophic illness insurance under federal auspices. Nixon put forth a program offering family health insurance for low-income families—partly financed by the government—to replace Medicaid, catastrophic insurance for middle-income families, with federal aid, encouragement to health maintenance organizations to develop and expand, and a system of incentives to employers to increase the health care benefits they provided.[38] Kennedy offered a comprehensive, cradle-to-grave health care program, financed and controlled by the government, replacing both Medicare and Medicaid, and providing for full coverage, no deductibles, no coinsurance, and compulsory enrollment. The Nixon proposal was attacked as being too complicated, being regressive in its sources of finance, and offering better benefits to the well-to-do than to the poor. Kennedy's bill was accused of being too expensive.[39] Senator Kennedy responded that his opponents were not allowing for the savings that would accrue when his comprehensive plan replaced all or parts of many existing programs.

In 1974, President Nixon and Senator Long submitted considerably liberalized versions of their proposals, providing more benefits for the poor and equalizing the effects of the programs on different income groups. Senator Kennedy then drastically altered his proposal as well, offering a much more limited and conservative program of benefits, with deductibles and coinsurance provisions similar to Nixon's, and allowing private insurance companies to play a substantial role. Most observers now feel that some national health insurance legislation will be passed in 1975. The three major proposals under consideration by Congress are:

(1) The Long-Ribicoff Catastrophic Health Insurance and Medical Assistance Reform Act, which provides insurance coverage for catastrophic illness, a federalized health insurance program for the poor, and voluntary guidelines for private insurance coverage for the health care of the rest of the population.

(2) The Nixon Comprehensive Health Insurance Plan, which enables all individuals and families to purchase private health insurance policies on a voluntary basis and favors the creation of health maintenance organizations.

(3) The Kennedy-Mills National Health Insurance Program, which requires all people to have health insurance, unless they are covered by Medicare, and provides the same benefits and government aid to the poor as the Nixon proposal.

None of the three proposals restructures the health care delivery system in a fundamental way. All continue to rely on private health insurance carriers, private providers of health services and supplies, and private academic institutions for the training of medical personnel.

How much national health insurance will cost is a matter of some debate. In the past, actual expenditures have considerably exceeded estimates, sometimes by vast amounts. For example, estimates made in 1965 of the cost of benefits paid for services by extended care facilities for 1967 were only a tenth of the actual costs two years later (see table 1.11).

In 1969, a comprehensive national health insurance program was estimated to cost a total of $35.8 billion, with $20.5 billion to come from new payroll taxes and $15.3 billion from the federal government.

TABLE 1.11   Estimated and Actual Costs of Extended Care Benefits, 1967

	Cost per Day	Days per Beneficiary	Cost per Beneficiary per Year
1965 estimate of 1967 costs	$11	0.16	$ 1.80
1967 actual costs	18	1.00	18.00

Source: U.S. Senate, Committee on Finance, *Hearings on Medicare and Medicaid* (1969), p. 23.

Of the federal share, $10.0 billion was expected to come from savings in programs now underway that would be supplanted, and only $5.3 billion in additional general revenues would be required.

As prices of medical services have risen, estimated expenditures have escalated. Even assuming that expenditures were kept down to 7 percent of gross national product, the direct costs of national health insurance would have reached at least $90 billion by 1973. The financial burden is reduced when financing comes mainly from federal tax revenues (which are tied progressively to income), Social Security funds, and private insurance. Payroll taxes, on the other hand, hit those in the low-income brackets especially hard.

Economies could be effected to keep costs of a national health insurance system down. At Senate hearings in 1970, it was estimated that wastes of about $14 billion could be eliminated from present programs. Changing from fee-for-service reimbursement to comprehensive prepayment group insurance is expected to result in further savings, although there is disagreement on how much these would amount to. In contrast, Medicare and Medicaid underwrite costs that are largely determined by the providers of medical services themselves. One expert commented that under this system, the provider is treated more generously than the consumer. Dr. Fred Anderson advised the Senate Committee on Labor and Public Welfare, "Congress ought to think twice before subsidizing a health insurance industry which imposes ever higher premiums, excludes more and more costs and treatment from coverage, and fails to insure more than about one-third of the poor."[40]

The need for cost controls is imperative under a national health insurance program, since enactment of the program will stimulate demand for health care and thus accelerate the inflation of medical prices, unless some limiting forces are brought to bear.

There is some agreement that a budgetary approach is necessary to control costs and to provide reliable cost estimates. If a prospective budget is used, ceilings will be set on expenditures, based on those of the previous year and broken down by category of service and by locality. The experts now believe that this approach can solve the problem of uncontrollable expenditures. It should be accompanied by abandonment of fee-for-service reimbursement, however, since it is difficult to enforce budgetary ceilings when hospitals and physicians have the privilege of setting fees and calling for services.

Another obstacle to a budgetary approach is its lack of flexibility. For example, what is a hospital to do if its budgeted resources are consumed by an epidemic or some other emergency? Thus, a successful budgetary approach must settle two problems: (1) determining the size of the budget needed for providing optimum services most efficiently, and (2) establishing procedures for enforcing the budget while allowing some needed flexibility.

Former Secretary of Health, Education, and Welfare Elliot Richardson warned that it would take ten years to produce a genuine budgetary system, which would save billions of dollars in national health expenditures. But the proponents of generous programs urge early introduction of national health insurance on the ground that troublesome gaps in benefits prevail now. The less enthusiastic proponents prefer to wait for a genuinely planned program and availability of needed facilities and personnel.

Conflicts of Ideology

President Nixon's views on spending, federal deficits, and intrusion by the federal government in medical markets have contributed greatly to the failure to reorganize medical care in the years since 1968. In a preelection statement in 1968 Nixon said: "I do not favor extension of compulsory health insurance to all persons. The policy would burden our present programs and destroy our highly successful system of health care. Voluntary plans should be extended, but any new federal programs should be geared to the needy."[41]

By 1970, Nixon seemed more disposed to treat the problems: "We face a massive crisis in this area and unless action is taken both administratively and legislatively to meet that crisis within the next two or three years, we will have a breakdown in our medical care system which could have consequences affecting millions of people."[42]

Although the president affirmed that the medical care system bordered on collapse, he sought only modest programs and launched vigorous attacks on proposals for comprehensive group prepayment programs. In his health message of February 18, 1971, Nixon expressed his fear of federal control of a national health program in these terms: "Federal personnel would inevitably be approving the budgets of local hospitals, setting fee schedules for local doctors, and taking other steps which could easily lead to the complete Federal domination of all American medicine. That is an enormous risk."[43]

Secretary of Health, Education, and Welfare Elliot Richardson commented:

Not only are some of the methods of payments untested on a large scale, but there could well be widespread unwillingness on the part of providers to participate, creating serious problems of supply of services. . . . There would have to be created a mechanism for the gathering of cost data to be funneled into a Central Federal Government process with a degree of complexity never envisioned in any Federal proposal to my knowledge.

In Richardson's view, it would require at least a decade to develop a budget system, and gross distortions, inaccessibility, and potentially mass defection of health personnel would prevail.[44] If providers rebelled at federal controls, their cooperation and that of organized medical groups would be lost. The British experience with national health insurance suggests that some such opposition is likely, but that ultimately both doctors and patients are pleased with the national program.

At times Nixon seemed to be supporting the development of health maintenance organizations, but his occasional steps in this direction did not provide substantial sums. Insofar as he supported genuine programs, he tended to minimize the payments to be made by government, especially the federal government.

Granted Nixon faced tough problems. In one year Medicaid ran a $350 million deficit, which had to be paid out of the general budget. Rising demand for Medicaid funds adversely affected other programs, such as those for research and manpower training.

By 1971 Nixon seemed interested in offering a health insurance plan for low-income families, partly financed by government, to largely replace Medicaid; so-called catastrophic medical coverage for middle-income groups; promotion of the health maintenance organizations; and a system of negative tax incentives that would force employers to raise their health insurance benefits to a specified minimum. The financing was to be regressive payroll taxes. Large gaps in benefits were to be left to state and local governments. Poor families were not covered by the catastrophic insurance provisions although higher-income families were. These elements came under criticism when the Secretary of Health, Education, and Welfare was questioned by the Senate Finance Committee:

Senator Ribicoff: Under your bill the employee plans have no limits on hospital care; but there is a 30-day limit for the poor. Is that correct?
Secretary Richardson: Yes.

Senator Ribicoff: Under the employee's plans there are no limits on outpatient physician services; but the poor are limited to seven doctors' visits. Is that correct?

Secretary Richardson: No, eight physician visits.

Senator Ribicoff: The employee gets catastrophic insurance coverage and the poor do not. Is that correct?

Secretary Richardson: Yes.[45]

Nixon's programs did not deal with the problems of lack of control of vast outlays, inflationary medical markets, and major inefficiencies. Expenditures on health have been greatly influenced by Nixon's adverse attitude toward compulsory enrollment, his determination to keep federal spending and deficits in check, and his fear of federal intrusions. By 1973, increasing complaints were heard that the Nixon economy moves were threatening achievement of health goals. Eight private medical schools in the New York area received $120 million from federally supported programs in 1971-72; in 1973-74, they were expected to receive $105 million. When corrected for inflationary price movements, the drop is about $25 million. Dr. John A. Cooper, president of the Association of American Medical Colleges, estimated in May 1973 that 1,400 faculty members would have to be dropped from these colleges unless additional funds could be found. The number of new medical research projects that the schools could support would also be cut by about 40 percent. Total federal funds available to 78 American medical schools amounted to $754 million in 1971-72, but would drop to $671 million in 1972-73. These reductions relate to Nixon's general budgetary policies.[46] Yet the country needs about twice as many doctors as it is now producing each year.

Notes

1. Federal Trade Commission, *Rate of Return for Identical Companies in Selected Manufacturing Industries*, various issues.

2. On these items, see B. Ehrenreich and J. Ehrenreich, *The American Health Empire* (1970), chap. 7.

3. E. Blake and J. Carnoy, "The Vanguard of the Rearguard: Medical Foundations," *Health-PAC* no. 49 (February 1973): 2-14.

4. This average income includes the earnings of interns and residents, ranging from $10,000 to $15,000, as well as the earnings of specialists, with maximums running well over $100,000. A helpful reference point is that physicians who have completed their internship and residency can expect a starting salary of $30,000. Income levels of physicians rise rapidly during their working life and are typically sustained well beyond the normal retirement age of sixty-five, because many physicians continue in practice.

Doctors have the highest earnings of any professional group. The average gross yearly income (of private nonagricultural workers) recently came to about $7,000.

The length of the physician's work day does not appear to influence his earnings. Doctors employed by health maintenance organizations have a regular nine-to-five work day, with night duty limited to a few nights each month, and thus are not on call at all hours of the day and night, but they still receive salaries averaging over $40,000 per year.

5. See A. Gerber, "Our Growing Dependence on Foreign Physicians," *Los Angeles Times*, August 26, 1973; "Flood of Foreign Doctors to U.S.," *U.S. News and World Report*, July 2, 1973, p. 48; and S. Auerbach, "1 in 5 Doctors Got Training outside U.S.," *Los Angeles Times*, June 13, 1973, reviewing an HEW report prepared by R. Stevens and J. Vermeulon of Yale University Medical School.

6. In 1971, 12,000 physicians received licenses, and 4,000 physicians were lost through death and retirement. The 8,000 net gain included 4,300 licensees who were graduates of foreign medical schools.

7. *Your Health Care in Crisis*, Health-PAC Special Report (1972), p. 9.

8. R. Fein, *The Doctor Shortage* (1967), pp. 137-40.

9. It is customary to point to the inferior medical training of many foreign-trained physicians in the United States, implying that substandard care is the result. In 1971, 37 percent of the graduates of foreign medical schools entering the United States failed to pass their tests for American licenses, compared to 9 percent of the graduates of American medical schools. But as the GP-specialist imbalance illustrates, medical knowledge is not one-dimensional, something of which one has simply more or less. The appropriateness of the training, the particular set of skills obtained, and the manner in which these skills complement those of other health care workers are at issue in judging standards of medical care given. For example, some workers might be trained to perform only routine surgical procedures. Dr. Joshua Horn, in *Away With All Pests: An English Surgeon in Peoples China, 1954-1969* (1971), describes just such possibilities. In a system of delivery designed to meet the basic health care needs of all people first, it would be inappropriate to suggest that workers trained to perform only selected surgical procedures have received inferior medical training.

10. A point at issue in the discussion of physicians' incomes is whether the heavy financial and personal toll exacted of medical students looses them on society with an economic vengeance, determined to command high salaries in order to repay debts and recoup income forgone during medical training. It appears that the British system significantly moderates the material appetites of physicians. Medical students live on public subsidies during training and subsequently work for far lower salaries than United States physicians. See D. Blumenthal and J. Fallows, "Health: The Care We Want and Need," *Washington Monthly*, October 1973, p. 16.

11. J. P. Newhouse, "A Model of Physician Pricing," *Southern Economic Journal*, October 1970, pp. 174-83.

12. Calculated from *Compendium of National Health Expenditure Data* and *Economic Report of the President, 1973*.

13. U.S. Senate, Committee on Finance, *Hearings on National Health Insurance*, pp. 124-25.

14. Ibid., p. 122.

15. I. S. Falk, "Financing of Health Care," *Inquiry* (supplement), March 1973, p. 3.

16. The CNHI is an organization composed of supporters of the original Kennedy NHI proposal. Savings in the provision of medical care, as one approach to cutting costs, are discussed in U.S. Senate, Committee on Finance, *Hearings on National Health Insurance*, part 2 (1970), p. 696. See also M. Glasser (of the United Auto Workers) in U.S. Senate, Committee on Finance, *Hearings on National Health Insurance* (April 1971), p. 130.

17. Besides wasting resources, unneeded operations may result in the death of the patient. Estimates of the number of people killed in this manner each year run from 10,000 (*San Francisco Chronicle*, December 17, 1971) to 24,000 (*Washington Post*, July 18, 1972).

18. J. Bunker, "Surgical Manpower: A Comparison of Operations and Surgeons in the United States and in England and Wales," *New England Journal of Medicine*, January 15, 1970. See also H. Denenberg, "A Shopper's Guide to Surgery: 14 Rules on How to Avoid Unnecessary Surgery" (Pennsylvania Insurance Commissioner).

19. Half of the rise in income is due to rising prices. The gains projected for fifty years reflect the accomplishments of 1961-68 and allow for the rise in population in fifty years.

20. L. C. Thurow and R. E. B. Lucas, *The American Distribution of Income: A Structural Problem*, study prepared for the Joint Economic Committee, U.S. Congress (March 17, 1972), p. 7.

21. M. Feldstein, "The Medical Economy," *Scientific American* 229, no. 3 (September 1973): 151. Of course, the terms of credit are frequently unclear, but new legislation requires that the total cost of the item, including finance charges, be clearly noted.

22. Ibid. See also K. J. Arrow, "Uncertainty and the Welfare Economics of Medical Care," *American Economic Review* 51, no. 5 (December 1963): 959-65.

23. See D. Caplovitz, *The Poor Pay More* (1967): "Society now virtually presents the very poor with two options: of forgoing major purchases or being exploited."

24. See L. Mandel, *Credit Card Use in the U.S.*, Institute of Social Research, University of Michigan, Ann Arbor (1973). Collection agencies specializing in medical accounts have blossomed forth.

25. M. S. Feldstein, "A New Approach to National Health Insurance," *Public Interest* 23 (spring 1971): 93-105. For a detailed discussion of postpayment see R. Eilers, "Post-payment Medical Expense Coverage: A Proposed Salvation for Insured and Insurer," *Medical Care*, May/June 1969.

26. For further discussion, see M. V. Pauly, "The Economics of Moral Hazard," *American Economic Review* 58, no. 3 (June 1968): 531-37; R. Zeckhauser, "Medical Insurance: A Case Study of the Tradeoff between Risk Spreading and Appropriate Incentive," *Journal of Economic Theory* 2, no. 1 (March 1970): 10-23; M. S. Feldstein, "The Welfare Loss of Excess Health Insurance," *Journal of Political Economy* 81, no. 2 (March/April 1973): 251-80; P. B. Ginsburg and L. M. Manheim, "Insurance, Copayment and Health Utilization: A Critical Survey," *Journal of Economics and Business* 25, no. 3 (spring/summer 1973): 142-52; M. V. Pauly, "A Measurement of the Welfare Cost of Health Insurance," *Health Services Research* 4, no. 4 (winter 1969): 281-92.

27. R. Zeckhauser, "Coverage for Catastrophic Illness," *Public Policy* 21, no. 2 (spring 1973): 149-72.

28. See A. A. Scitovsky and N. M. Snyder, "Effect of Coinsurance on Use of Physician Services," *Social Security Bulletin*, June 1972, pp. 3-19; C. E. Phelps and J. P. Newhouse, "Effect of Coinsurance: A Multivariate Analysis," *Social Security Bulletin*, June 1972, pp. 20-44.

29. See C. B. Chipman and J. M. Talmadge, "The Evolution of the Right to Health Concept in the U.S.," *Pharos* 34, no. 1 (January 1971): 30-51; J. R. Jeffers, M. F. Bognanno, and J. C. Bartlett, "On the Demand versus Need for Medical Services and the Concept of 'Shortage,'" *American Journal of Public Health* 61, no. 1 (January 1971): 46-63.

30. U.S. Senate, Committee on Finance, *Hearings on National Health Insurance*, pp. 230-32, 240-41.

31. *Los Angeles Times*, November 8, 1970, December 31, 1972, January 25, 1973.

32. J. K. Iglehart, "Regulations Proposed to Enhance HMOs through Phase 4 Cost Control Applications," *National Journal*, December 1, 1973, p. 1880.

33. See H. Klarman, "Major Public Initiatives in Health Care," *Public Interest* 34 (winter 1974): 109. For a description of changes in prices, see L. A. Horowitz, "Medical Care Price Changes in Medicare's First Five Years," *Social Security Bulletin*, March 1972, pp. 16-29.

34. HEW, Social Security Administration, *Medical Care Expenditures, Prices, and Costs: Background Book* (September 1973), p. 41.

35. See Cost of Living Council, "Phase IV Health Care Regulations," *Federal Register*, March 27, 1974, pp. 11376-405.

36. See J. K. Iglehart, "New Federal Health-Care Cost Controls Could Curtail Hospital Services," *National Journal*, September 15, 1973, pp. 1359-66; see also "Stiff Industry Regulations Likely; Congress, HEW Near Agreement," *National Journal*, February 2, 1974, pp. 163-70.

37. For an analysis, see Cost of Living Council, "Control of Hospital Costs under the Economic Stabilization Program," *Federal Register,* January 24, 1974, pp. 2693-700.

38. For discussions of the Nixon policy on medical care, see HEW, Office of Research and Statistics, *National Health Expenditures for Fiscal Year 1972; New York Times,* November 23, 1969, January 12, 1970, January 4, 1971, July 6, 1971, August 6, 1971, August 9, 1971; *Los Angeles Times,* June 25, 1971, November 23, 1972; and *Time,* May 11, 1970.

39. *New York Times,* August 9, 1971.

40. U.S. Senate, Committee on Labor and Public Welfare, *Hearings on National Health Insurance* (1970), p. 723.

41. Ibid., part 2, p. 632.

42. Ibid., p. 746.

43. U.S. Senate, Committee on Finance, *Hearings on National Health Insurance* (April 1971), p. 87.

44. Ibid.

45. Ibid., p. 96.

46. *New York Times,* May 22, 1972, April 25, 1973, May 27, 1973; see also *Los Angeles Times,* August 23, 1970, October 17, 1971; *Business Week,* July 25, 1970; U.S. Senate, Committee on Labor and Public Welfare, *Hearings on National Health Insurance* (1970), pp. 613-15.

2

Costs and
Resource Allocation

In order to place medical care expenditures in perspective, it is necessary to consider the extent of illness-related costs that do not figure in measures of "medical care expenditures." Economists speak of the direct and indirect costs of illness and death. Direct costs of illness, as Dorothy Rice suggests, "comprise the expenditures for prevention, detection, treatment, rehabilitation, research, training, and capital investment in medical facilities. In terms of services or type of medical expenditure, direct costs include amounts spent for hospital and nursing home care, physicians' and other medical professional services, drugs, medical supplies, research, training, and other nonpersonal services."[1] An accounting of the sources and patterns of expenditure of these funds appears in chapter 3.

Indirect costs are the costs of sickness and premature death to the economy in terms of lost labor time and national product. These must be estimated from data on labor force participation rates, changing patterns of earnings at successive ages, and life expectancies for different age and sex groups. Indirect costs raise the total economic costs of illness and death substantially above the costs attributable to direct medical care expenditures alone.

This chapter considers the relative importance of direct and indirect costs of illness and death to individuals and to society. Decisions to provide selected types of medical care carry implications for the direct and indirect costs borne by the citizenry. The allocation of social welfare resources between health care services on the one hand, and education, income maintenance, or other social programs on the other is reviewed, with a focus on alternative uses of resources.

This chapter is primarily descriptive, examining the measures of direct and indirect costs of illness and death and comparing the allocation of resources for different social welfare programs—both domestically and internationally. Statistics on health care expenditures and statistics on morbidity and mortality are juxtaposed for analysis. By way of illustration, several questions are raised: What is the significance of a relatively high infant mortality rate as related to per capita expenditures on health care? Is it important that the United States does not compare favorably with other countries on this score? What are the significant points of comparison on expenditures as they relate to the access to and quality of medical care?

Direct and Indirect Costs

Between 1929 and 1972, the direct costs of morbidity and mortality rose from a few billion dollars to $83.4 billion. It was not until the late 1950s, however, that attention was paid to the indirect costs to the economy of sickness and premature death. This latter category necessarily involves costs to society in excess of direct expenditures, and, viewed in retrospect, they too were escalating over the last half century. The cost-benefit studies of Selma Mushkin, F. D. A. Collings, and Dorothy Rice have contributed significantly to our understanding of the import of indirect costs, as have the research of Rashi Fein, Burton Weisbrod, and Herbert Klarman, among others.[2]

Clarification of Terms

Mushkin and Collings asked: What is the impact of disease on the use, distribution, and availability of economic resources? They defined three types of economic costs: resource-use, resource-transfer, and resource-loss:

The first is actual use of economic resources (manpower and materials) for prevention, diagnosis, treatment, and rehabilitation. This represents the direct price of health programs; it is measured by actual expenditures, both public and private, for health services and their complement of commodities and facilities. In the absence of disease, these expenditures would not be necessary. The second type consists of transfers (of resources or of income) which arise out of mitigating the burdens of sickness. Costs in this category do not, in the first instance, affect the total resources used up by sickness in the economy as a whole, but they do affect the distribution of resources among individuals or families. Many of these transfers are designed to mitigate the impact on family income of losses due to death or disability. The third type, less clearly defined but perhaps more pervasive in effect than either of the other two, is loss of resources occasioned by sickness—human resources lost or impaired as a result of death, disability, and debility caused by sickness.[3]

The direct costs of illness and death were defined above in this chapter, and this cost category is described in detail in chapter 3. The discussion below clarifies the latter two categories of economic cost.

Disease and injury involve the transfer of income between the well and the sick. Mushkin and Collings continue:

The size and importance of these transfers in the American economy have increased rapidly in the last two decades. They take two principal forms. One consists of payments made directly to the sick and disabled (or their survivors) and financed from taxes or contributions levied; social security protection under public and private auspices is the principal example. The other is the hidden re-distribution of the tax burden that comes about through statutory tax provisions designed to assist families and voluntary agencies in meeting problems arising out of sickness. On both these counts, disease takes resources away from those who are well, and who would otherwise have alternative uses for them, and gives them to those who are sick and to survivors.[4]

Finally, the resource-loss due to sickness is described, primarily in terms of the loss to the economy of productive labor time:

The type of sickness cost we have categorized as resource-use relates to the way in which existing economic resources are diverted to the sector of the economy that produces health services. Without sickness and injury, these health services would be unnecessary and the resources would be free for other productive uses. Resource-transfer represents shifts in command over resources between persons or groups, which may be direct costs to one sector of the economy but are of benefit to another. However, sickness and injury also affect the quantity of resources available in the first place. Disease and impairments cause a loss of economic resources, a loss that would cease if disease and injury were to be eliminated. This is also part of the total economic cost of sickness.

The resource lost as a result of sickness is human labor. In order to value the loss in dollars, it is necessary to estimate the output forgone. The question is, if there were no sickness how much would those persons who are now sick have produced?

The effects of sickness upon the amount of human labor available for productive purposes can be summarized under three heads: deaths (loss of workers), disability (loss of working time); and debility (loss of productive capacity while at work).

Essentially, there are two stages in calculating the output forgone: (a) estimating the loss in productive work time, and (b) assigning a money value to the output that this lost work time represents. The result is then a dollar figure which represents the value of the loss in output attributable to deaths, disability, and debility. In other words, it is a rough estimate of the increase in output that would occur if the loss of resources due to sickness were eliminated.[5]

Units of work time lost—whether from short-term disability, debility, or death—are converted to full-time equivalents or man-years as the unit of productive time lost. Estimates developed by the Bureau of Labor Statistics are available on the remaining years of work life for any age group, and these estimates serve as a basis for the calculations.

Estimates of Economic Costs in 1963

Dorothy P. Rice estimated the total economic cost of illness and death to the economy for the year 1963 at $95.9 billion. The breakdown by cost category is shown in table 2.1. Direct expenditures in the amount of $34.3 billion are the costs commonly equated with total health care costs for 1963 (see chapter 3), except that direct expenditures do not normally include the costs of medical training.

TABLE 2.1   Direct and Indirect Costs of Illness, 1963

Category of Costs	Amount (Billions)
Total economic costs	$95.9
Direct expenditures	34.3
By diagnostic category	22.5
Other	11.7
Indirect costs for diagnostic categories	61.6
Mortality	40.6
Morbidity	21.0

Source: D. P. Rice, "Estimating the Cost of Illness," *Health Economics Series* no. 6, May 1966.

Only $22.5 billion of these expenditures, however, could be distributed among the major diagnostic categories. Dorothy Rice explains:

> Distribution by disease of amounts spent for medications and supplies presents problems because many specific drugs and appliances are used for a variety of conditions and illnesses. The function of school health programs included health appraisal, counseling, disease prevention, and control activities in addition to providing emergency service for injury or sudden sickness. Likewise, occupational health emphasizes prevention of illness in addition to emergency care. The proportion of care for emergency services and the types of illnesses treated are not available for the allocation of expenditures for school health and industrial in-plant services.[6]

All indirect costs *are* assigned to diagnostic categories. These estimates of indirect costs include both productive labor lost in the year 1963 by premature death and the present value of lifetime earnings for those who died in 1963, discounted at 6 percent. Approximately 1.8 million persons died in 1963 from all causes. Another 1.5 million were housed in institutions; of these 49 percent were in mental hospitals and 32 percent in nursing homes and homes for the aged. Table 2.2 provides estimates of indirect costs by diagnostic categories. Four diagnostic categories (following the International Classification of Diseases) contributed most significantly to the indirect costs of mortality: diseases of the circulatory system (34.2 percent), neoplasms (17.7 percent), injuries (15.8 percent), and diseases of the nervous system and sense organs (8.2 percent).

If the productivity lost in the year of death (1963) alone were included, indirect costs of mortality would stand at $2.7 billion (in contrast to $40.6 billion for estimated life expectancy), total indirect costs would be $23.8 billion and total economic costs $58.1 billion. As would be expected, under estimation procedures that discount lifetime earnings rather than productivity lost in only a single year, diseases of the circulatory system contribute proportionally less (34.2 percent rather than 44.9 percent), and injuries contribute proportionally more (15.8 percent rather than 8.9 percent). The incidence of injuries resulting in death among the young and middle-aged populations is quite high relative to other disorders, while the present value of lifetime earnings of these age groups exceeds that of the aged. The computation of lifetime earnings is explained by Dorothy Rice:

TABLE 2.2 Direct and Indirect Costs by Diagnosis, 1963

Diagnosis	Amount (Millions)				Percentage			
			Indirect Costs				Indirect Costs	
	Total	Direct Expenditures*	Morbidity	Total Mortality	Total	Direct Expenditures*	Morbidity	Total Mortality
Total	$84,190.1	$22,530.0	$21,042.2	$40,617.9	100.0	100.0	100.0	100.0
Infective and parasitic diseases	1,969.2	501.9	858.0	609.3	2.3	2.2	4.1	1.5
Tuberculosis	916.1	241.4	385.2	289.5	1.1	1.1	1.8	.7
Other	1,053.2	260.6	472.8	319.8	1.3	1.2	2.2	.8
Neoplasms	9,338.5	1,279.0	850.7	7,208.8	11.1	5.7	4.0	17.7
Allergic, endocrine, metabolic, nutritional diseases	2,442.2	902.9	539.5	1,001.8	2.9	4.0	2.6	2.5
Diseases of blood and blood-forming organs	333.5	155.9	41.3	136.3	.4	.7	.2	.3
Mental, psychoneurotic and personality disorders	7,229.8	2,401.7	4,624.0	204.1	8.6	10.7	22.0	.5
Diseases of nervous system and sense organs	6,253.3	1,416.4	1,525.5	3,311.4	7.4	6.3	7.2	8.2
Diseases of circulatory system	19,072.8	2,267.3	2,919.7	13,885.8	22.7	10.1	13.9	34.2
Diseases of respiratory system	6,796.9	1,581.1	3,166.3	2,049.5	8.1	7.0	15.0	5.0
Diseases of digestive system	7,401.6	4,158.7	1,220.1	2,022.8	8.8	18.5	5.8	5.0
Diseases of genitourinary system	2,420.0	1,210.2	497.8	712.0	2.9	5.4	2.4	1.8
Maternity	1,494.5	1,391.1	32.2	71.2	1.8	6.2	.2	.2
Diseases of skin and cellular tissue	436.6	248.1	128.4	60.1	.5	1.1	.6	.1
Diseases of bones and organs of movement	2,757.5	1,430.0	1,225.0	102.5	3.3	6.3	5.8	.3
Congenital malformations	791.6	113.0	41.8	636.8	.9	.5	.2	1.6
Certain diseases of early infancy	1,629.7	30.3	—	1,599.4	1.9	.1	—	3.9
Symptoms, senility and ill-defined conditions	1,491.5	623.7	288.5	579.3	1.8	2.8	1.4	1.4
Injuries	9,940.5	1,702.8	1,810.7	6,427.0	11.8	7.6	8.6	15.8
Special conditions and examinations	977.6	965.8	11.8	—	1.2	4.3	.1	—
Miscellaneous	1,411.1	150.1	1,261.0	—	1.7	.7	6.0	—

Source: D. P. Rice, "Estimating the Cost of Illness," *Health Economics Series* no. 6 (May 1966).

*Direct expenditures for specified health services, including hospital and nursing home care and services of physicians, dentists, nurses, and other health professional personnel; excluded are several types of personal and nonpersonal expenditures, amounting to $11.7 billion, which could not be distributed among the major diagnostic categories.

The estimated cost or value to society of all deaths is the product of the number of deaths and the expected value of an individual's future earnings with sex and age taken into account. This method of derivation must consider life expectancy for different age and sex groups, changing pattern of earnings at successive ages, varying labor force participation rates, imputed value for housewives' services, and the appropriate discount rate to convert a stream of costs or benefits into its present worth.[7]

A third procedure for estimating the indirect costs of mortality aims at estimating the added output in a single year had the cause of death been eliminated. In other words, it considers all the individuals who died prior to 1963 from illness or accident and estimates what their contribution to output in 1963 would have been. No discounting is involved, so the estimates are not sensitive to the discount rate chosen.[8] This method is discussed in the appendix to this chapter. The latter two of the three procedures discussed above appear to have more to recommend them than the single-year earnings method, since they account for a larger portion of estimated losses in output resulting from mortality. Single-year costs seriously underestimate the size of the economic problem.

Similarly, lost output due to disability that continues into future years should be assessed by its present value, since this constitutes the appropriate measure of the indirect costs of the disease. This difficult calculation has not been performed in the estimates of indirect costs of morbidity in this chapter, however.

There are several problems in estimating indirect costs. One of these stems from the way economists prepare national income accounts. The value of the product of women keeping house is excluded from calculations of gross national product (GNP). If it were likewise excluded from calculation of indirect costs in 1963, those costs (estimating output loss for the single year alone) would have been $20.9 billion instead of $23.8 billion. Even when this work product is included, the valuation of the indirect costs of illnesses that are specific to or more common among women is relatively lower because of the wage differentials between men and women.

Multiple diseases and treatment of the side effects of illness also raise problems in estimating indirect costs. Mushkin and Collings explain:

The result of disregarding the presence of multiple diseases is an overestimate of the cost of any single disease. . . . Moreover, the assumption that side effects of other diseases may be disregarded in order to measure the direct effects of the disease in question means that the indirect costs of each disease, taken individually, cannot be added together to make a meaningful total for all diseases.[9]

Theoretically the recurrence of a disease should cause no problem, since indirect costs could be estimated apart from previous costs incurred. But the nature of mental, psychoneurotic, and personality disorders may create problems of estimation in fact, because of the unpredictability of the course of these illnesses.

Economic Costs of Heart Diseases and Cancer

The two leading causes of death by disease in 1962 were cardiovascular diseases, which accounted for 54 percent, and malignant neoplasms (cancer), which caused 16 percent.[10] Analysis of the indirect costs of these diseases illustrates the importance of those costs as a proportion of the total economic costs of illness and death. Between 1900 and 1962, the number of deaths per 100,000 dropped from 1,719 to 945. However, cardiovascular diseases as a cause of death increased both relatively and absolutely (from 264 to 515). Similarly, deaths attributable to cancer rose from 64 to 150. On the other hand, tuberculosis, influenza, and pneumonia declined in absolute and relative terms (tuberculosis from 194 to 5 per 100,000 and influenza and pneumonia from 202 to 32 per 100,000).

According to Dorothy P. Rice, "elimination of cardiovascular-renal disease would add 12 to 14 years of life expectancy at birth depending upon race and sex. Elimination of cancer as a cause of death would add about 2 years of life expectancy."[11] At an earlier period in United States history, the control of tuberculosis and reduction of the severity of influenza and pneumonia significantly increased life expectancy.

Estimates of the total cost of illness for cardiovascular disease and cancer in 1962 are summarized in table 2.3 and described in greater detail in table 2.4. In explaining the computation, Rice says: "Mortality figures (as obtained for 1962 from 'Vital Statistics of the United States') were divided in half on the assumption that the pattern of deaths was approximately symmetrical about midyear. Use of the total number of deaths . . . would have implicitly assumed all deaths occurred on January 1."[12] In other words, to calculate indirect costs of mortality in 1962 it is assumed that half of those who died in 1962 worked the full year and the other half worked none of the

TABLE 2.3   Summary of Costs of Heart Disease and Cancer, 1962

Cost Category	Amount (Billions)
Total economic cost	$43.1
Direct costs	4.3
Indirect costs	38.8
Mortality, 1962	1.7
Mortality, previous years	33.1
Morbidity	4.0

year. The "working" half figure is adjusted downward according to general labor force participation and unemployment rates, and is multiplied by average full-time earnings to estimate this portion of indirect costs.

The appendix to chapter 2 explains the estimation procedures for calculating indirect costs of mortality in previous years. Note particularly that indirect costs in tables 2.3 and 2.4 do not include the present value of *future* losses of output for those who died in 1962. Rather, estimates are prepared for indirect costs of "mortality, 1962" and "mortality, previous years." The intent is to estimate the added output in a single year, 1962, if cardiovascular and cancer death and disability rates had been zero in preceding years.

Note that direct costs are only one-tenth of total costs. The indirect costs of $38.8 billion represent 9.6 million man-years of gainful employment lost. Rice explains:

Approximately 1.2 million persons died in 1962 from heart disease, stroke, and cancer. The losses in output resulting from these deaths are equivalent to approximately 237,000 man-years for those who would have been in the labor force and 205,000 man-years for women who would have kept house. In dollar terms, the losses were $1.7 billion in 1962.

Mortality in previous years comprises the largest share of the indirect costs of these diseases—approximately 85 percent of the total. Of the 33.7 million people who died from heart disease, stroke, and cancer in the period 1900-1961, about 11.5 million would have survived through 1962 and about 8.3 million would have worked or kept house if these major causes of death had been eliminated. In dollar terms, the loss in output amounted to $33.1 billion.[13]

TABLE 2.4   Economic Costs of Cardiovascular Diseases and Cancer by Type of Cost, 1962

Type of Cost	Total Amount (Millions)	Cardiovascular Diseases Amount (Millions)	Percentage	Cancer Amount (Millions)	Percentage
Total	$43,085.9	$31,867.4	74.0	$11,218.5	26.0
Direct costs	4,319.7	3,072.2	71.1	1,247.5	28.9
Personal services and supplies	3,500.4	2,579.7	73.7	920.7	26.3
Hospital care	1,900.8	1,234.8	65.0	666.0	35.0
Nursing home care	322.9	299.8	92.8	23.1	7.2
Physicians' services	873.9	701.4	80.3	172.4	19.7
Drugs	310.1	279.4	90.1	30.8	9.9
Nursing services	92.7	64.3	69.4	28.4	30.6
Nonpersonal services	819.3	492.5	60.1	326.8	39.9
Research	244.5	117.0	47.9	127.5	52.1
Training	37.1	19.8	53.4	17.3	46.6
Other health services	73.3	34.4	46.9	38.9	53.1
Construction	275.4	190.0	69.0	85.4	31.0
Net cost of insurance	189.0	131.3	69.5	57.7	30.5
Indirect costs	38,766.2	28,795.2	74.2	9,971.0	25.7
Mortality	34,781.4	25,824.6	74.3	8,956.8	25.8
1962	1,705.8	1,286.8	75.4	419.1	24.6
Previous years	33,075.5	24,537.8	74.2	8,537.7	25.8
Morbidity	3,984.8	2,970.7	74.6	1,014.2	25.5
Institutionalized	507.9	455.9	89.8	51.9	10.2
Noninstitutionalized	3,476.9	2,514.6	72.3	962.3	27.7

Source: D. P. Rice, "Economic Costs of Cardiovascular Diseases and Cancer, 1962," *Health Economics Series* no. 5, May 1965.

Disease and Death Rates

There has been marked improvement in human longevity over the past several decades. Infant mortality has been reduced by more than half in the last thirty years. Life expectancy, particularly at younger ages, has risen significantly, as childhood diseases have been brought under control. Long-term improvement has been achieved in controlling communicable diseases such as diphtheria, typhoid, measles, pneumonia, influenza, tuberculosis, and gastritis.[14] The development of antibiotics has played an important role.

These improvements have not been matched by gains in the control of degenerative diseases, including major cardiovascular and renal diseases, diseases of the heart, and cancer. The control and cure of medical disorders associated with aging present formidable challenges. The death rate for conditions attributable to old age rises as life expectancy increases. Moreover, diseases of the heart and cancer require longer periods of treatment than did the communicable diseases that were so costly in the early part of the twentieth century. These and other notable changes that have occurred in the health status of the nation influence resource allocation for health services in the future.

The World Health Organization has defined personal health as "a state of complete physical, mental and social well being and not merely the absence of disease or infirmity."[15] Health defined in this way is influenced by a multitude of factors, only one of which is medical care. While only the absence or presence of disease or infirmity conveniently lends itself to direct measurement, nutrition, housing, hereditary traits, safety, and life-style all bear on personal health. Good nutrition and adequate shelter reduce a person's vulnerability to disease and quicken recovery from an illness. These factors correlate with income. Higher incomes are frequently associated with occupations that entail less physical danger on the job. Other stresses associated with competition in businesses and professions take their toll, however, in increased risks of heart disease and stroke.[16] Low-income individuals, on the other hand, face stress due to material insecurity. Those who need to carry more than one job to make ends meet suffer health consequences from their long working hours.

Age-specific death rates for the leading causes of death in 1966 reveal several interesting facets of the sources of poor health.[17] For individuals twenty to twenty-four years of age, motor vehicle accidents, homicide, and suicide are the leading causes of death (excluding war-related deaths). At thirty-five to thirty-nine years, cirrhosis of the liver (a frequent consequence of excessive alcohol consumption) replaces suicide as a leading cause of death. At fifty-five to fifty-nine years, arteriosclerotic heart diseases, lung cancer and other malignant neoplasms of the respiratory system, and cirrhosis of the liver are the leading causes of death.

Differences in the age-specific death rates by race and sex are also found. Between twenty and twenty-four years of age, homicide and motor vehicle accidents cause equal death rates for male and female nonwhites. At ages thirty-five to thirty-nine, the rate of death by homicide is more than double that by motor vehicle accidents.

Females, both white and nonwhite, have a much lower risk of death (on the order of a fourth to a third of the risk for males) at both ages for the three leading causes of death.

Nonwhites and whites at fifty-five to fifty-nine have roughly the same death rates for all three leading causes of death, except that the death rate from arteriosclerotic heart disease for nonwhite females is double that for white females. Again female death rates for all three causes are lower than male rates on the order of a fourth to a third of the risk.

Death rates for the causes cited above have all risen in the 1960s. Deaths due to suicide, homicide, alcohol consumption, and heart disease all reflect stresses of life in our society. Alcohol consumption is a contributing factor in roughly half the fatal motor vehicle accidents, as well as being a cause of cirrhosis of the liver.

Recent research by Dr. M. Harvey Brenner of John Hopkins University has attempted to demonstrate a connection between increases in disease death rates and in mental illness and downswings of the national economy. Some researchers (such as Victor Fuchs and Odin Anderson) have argued that we reach a stage of affluence where further per capita wealth necessarily has a negative effect on health.[18] Work and leisure activities are physically less arduous, dietary strictures are ignored, and individuals become more vulnerable to disease, although cures may also be more readily available. Thus scientific advances have contributed to the increase of some disorders while scientific discoveries have found cures for others. Occasionally science has increased both the incidence and the cure of a single disorder. Heart disease might be a case in point.

Cultural factors also influence prospects for improved health of segments of the population. Nathan Glazer cites evidence that infant mortality rates differ significantly for ethnic and racial groups (even when controlling for income as a proxy for access to health care). Blacks and Puerto Ricans fare substantially worse than Japanese, Chinese, and Jews. Glazer quotes Odin Anderson on this point: "Once the [infant mortality] rate drops below 30, the broad economic and social factors operate with lessening effect and personal behavior factors of the families in the high impact mortality groups involved, particularly the mothers, begin to exercise an increasingly dominant influence."[19]

Indirect Costs of Illness to the Individual Family

In assessing the total cost of illness, estimates were presented for the direct and indirect costs to the economy (or resource-use and resource-loss). The "resource-transfer" cost category was ignored, because it does not affect the total amount of resources used up by sickness in the economy as a whole. Rather it pertains to the distribution of resources among individuals or families. This cost area and the indirect costs of illness and death to the individual family will now be analyzed. In simplest economic terms, the other face of the productive loss to society from ill health is the loss of income and economic security to the individual.[20] The picture is stark indeed for the poorer segments of society.

The calculations made above in this chapter for losses in output associated with illness and death assumed no restrictions on the growth of the national product. In theory, a growing national output or economic pie means that more of the pie is available for everyone to share. However, in an economy that builds on the best technology, hires the most skilled manpower, and pursues the most profitable investment opportunities, certain segments of the society are left behind. Although the total product is increasing at the fastest pace, there is not an equalized distribution of the economic gains. Those in good stead are notably reluctant to empower such a redistribution of wealth. They invoke the vision of increasing the size of the pie once again—maintaining that, in time, there would be more for everybody.

Those who share proportionally less from economic growth, share proportionally more in the indirect costs of illness to the individual through unemployment and limited protection from income loss during short-term sickness or long-term disability. Thus indirect costs of illness and death as measured by the loss of output to the economy must be considered in light of costs to the individual family in terms of economic security. This is especially important because economy-wide perspectives are based on the assumption of full employment (variously defined at 4 or 5 percent unemployment).

Unemployment rates differ considerably by age, race, and sex group. In 1972, 5 percent of whites were unemployed and 10 percent of racial minorities. Among the young (sixteen to nineteen years of age) unemployment ran from 15 to 20 percent. Unemployment and underemployment taken together have been estimated at 25 to 30 percent of the work force of 85 million people.

In the United States, a larger percentage of the work force is unemployed than is employed on farms in agricultural production. This underscores both the productivity of the agricultural sector of the economy and the magnitude of the unemployment problem.

If the economy cannot employ those whose lives would be saved by the elimination of specific diseases, the indirect costs of illness and death are seriously overestimated. As Rice explains, "without the assumption of high employment, losses due to mortality and disability cannot be isolated from losses due to unemployment."

Estimates of the indirect costs of illness described above do not take into account differences in labor market participation and earnings by race. Job discrimination against minorities lowers the estimates of the costs of illnesses that have a higher incidence among minorities than among the population as a whole.

Aggregate measures of indirect costs do not specify how this burden is distributed to individual families. Kathryn H. Allan and Mildred E. Cinsky suggest that the costs to the individual of illness and disability "may be seen as the sum of the factors of unemployment, underemployment, income loss, prevention of normal family life and activities, extraordinary medical expenses and human isolation."[21]

Trends in Costs to the Family

Changes in the burden of personal health care expenditures on the individual can be assessed in two ways—by examining the variation in medical care expenditures as a percentage of disposable individual income (income after taxes), or by comparing the change in disposable individual income to the change in medical care prices. There is only fragmentary evidence from surveys in the late 1950s on how much of a person's income is spent on medical care, and the most recent information is not highly differentiated by race, sex, age, income level, insurance coverage, and so forth, so that it is not very useful for policy purposes. Thus, the best available comparison is between changes in per capita disposable income and changes in medical prices, to determine the shifting capacity of individuals to pay for medical care.

Between 1960 and 1967, medical care prices rose an average of 3.2 percent a year. Physicians' fees increased an average of 3.5 percent annually, and hospital daily service charges rose 7.8 percent annually. For the same period, the consumer price index rose 1.6 percent on the average (1.5 percent, excluding medical care).[22] Per capita disposable income (current dollars) rose an average of 4.9 percent. (In constant dollars it rose 3.4 percent.[23]) Thus, for this period, the ability to pay for medical care was increasing on the average. Still, one large medical bill can easily put a family with low income and savings in the medically indigent class.

The distribution of financial risk for medical care costs, as discussed in chapter 1, is a crucial issue. The distribution has been changed in recent years by the introduction of Medicare and Medicaid in July 1966. In the five years between 1967 and 1971, the medical care price index increased at twice the rate reported in the 1960-67 period—6.6 percent per year as compared with 3.2 percent. Physicians' fees increased at a rate of 6.7 percent and hospital daily service charges, 13.5 percent.[24] For the same period (1967-71) per capita disposable income increased an average of 6.2 percent in current dollars (2.3 percent in constant dollars).[25] Thus the ability to pay for medical expenditures worsened on the average. But again different segments of the population bear different burdens according to their use of services, financial risks, and ability to pay. Patients with heavy utilization of hospital services faced serious financial difficulties. More significantly, since the absolute difference in income between rich and poor in the United States is increasing over time, the capacity of the poor to pay for medical expenses is diminishing. Only full medical insurance coverage (without deductibles and coinsurance provisions) would offer the financial protection most needed by the poor.

Because so much of medical care is financed by third-party arrangements, consumers of medical services have only limited control over medical outlays. They have little to say about the dramatic rise in medical care costs. Those among the poor who cannot receive Medicaid may have to forgo needed medical attention or incur large debts. The rising costs of medical care place the largest burden of personal health expenditures on those least able to bear it—the poor, the aged, and the chronically ill.

Costs to the Disabled

Table 2.5 provides estimates of income from a Social Security Administration survey of noninstitutionalized disabled adults aged eighteen to sixty-four. The disabled population is poorer than the adult population taken as a whole: 28.6 percent of those disabled four to six months had incomes below the poverty level, and 33.2 percent of those disabled seven months or more were below that level. Other findings of the survey show these disabled adults to be older and less educated than the rest of society. The proportion of the population severely disabled was significantly higher among women than among men (40.8 percent as compared to 27.3 percent). Musculoskeletal and cardiovascular disorders account for one-half of all major disabling conditions.[26]

Allan and Cinsky report that men who are occupationally disabled or have secondary work limitations are affected in the type of work and earnings they can get, but the proportion employed is the same

TABLE 2.5   Family Income of Disabled Adults, 1966

Item	Disabled 4-6 Months	Disabled 7 Months or More
Number of families	297,000	15,401,000
Percentage distribution		
Below Social Security Administration poverty level	28.6%	33.2%
Between Social Security Administration poverty and low-income levels	5.7%	8.6%
Above low-income level	65.7%	58.2%
Median unit income	$4,386	$3,923
Percentage with specified source of income		
No income	12.8%	3.4%
Earnings	82.8%	79.4%
Asset income	33.7%	41.3%
Public income maintenance	30.3%	37.6%
Social Security benefit	3.4%	17.8%
Workmen's compensation	14.8%	1.6%
Unemployment compensation	11.4%	2.4%
Public assistance	6.1%	9.3%
Contributions from relatives outside household	10.4%	3.9%

Source: K. H. Allan and M. E. Cinsky, "The General Characteristics of the Disabled Population," *Social Security Bulletin*, August 1972, p. 36.

as for men not disabled. "The family income of the disabled," they explain, "is half that of the general population. Forty percent of the [families] with young children had incomes below the poverty level. . . . Complicating the income problem is the fact that the disabled (in 1965) are less likely than the general population to own health insurance (one-half owned no insurance as compared to one-fifth of the general population in 1965). Yet they need more frequent medical care."[27]

Under certain conditions workers may receive compensation that partially offsets their personal income loss due to disability and illness. Workmen's compensation (medical benefits for *job-related* injuries) and unemployment compensation assist those with short-term disabilities (lasting less than six months). Social Security benefits compensate for loss of income in long-term disabilities (lasting six months or longer).

Jack Schmulowitz has studied disabled workers whose benefits from Social Security were terminated because of recovery and who continued in nonbeneficiary status.[28] The economic security of these individuals was still notably compromised: 11 percent of those surveyed had no earnings in either 1968 or 1969, and 16 percent had an average income of less than $1,800 annually. The occupational distribution of those who were employed showed a lower proportion (26 percent) in white collar employment—professional, managerial, sales, and clerical workers—than for the labor force as a whole (38 percent). The difference was less pronounced for women (51 percent white collar as opposed to 58 percent in the whole population). The median income of the disabled workers surveyed who were employed in professional, managerial, and skilled occupations was only $5,400 in 1970.

Among individuals who suffer short-term disabilities (less than six months) *away from the job*, the low-paid workers, those of minority races, and workers in low-skill occupations had a smaller proportion of their pay replaced (see table 2.6). The statistics in the table, derived from the Health Interview Survey (1968) of the Public Health Service, include only the experience of workers who still had jobs at the time of the survey. Workers who held no job as a result of their short-term illness or disability were excluded. This means that the percentages of income replacement by sickness benefits are lower for the total group of disabled workers. Those least able to compensate

TABLE 2.6   Reimbursements to Disabled Workers by Selected Characteristics, 1968

Characteristic	Percentage of Pay Reimbursed	Percentage of Work-loss Days Not Reimbursed
Type of work		
Professional, technical, and kindred workers	88	14
Managers and officials	89	15
Private household workers	14	58
Operatives	23	50
Laborers (except farm and mine)	17	60
Age		
Seventeen to forty-four	45	42
Sixty-five and over	50	65
Race		
White	48	41
All other	25	50
Family income		
Less than $5,000	26	59
$10,000 or more	65	26

Source: D. N. Price, "Cash Benefits for Short-Term Sickness, 1948-71," *Social Security Bulletin*, January 1973, p. 29.

for income loss are more likely to be required to do so. Excluding states with mandatory temporary disability insurance programs, little more than half the workers in private industry were covered by formal sickness benefit plans in 1971.[29]

The dollar value of protection against income loss because of non-occupational sickness was 36.0 percent of income lost in 1971. Formal paid sick leave plans, which provide for continuation of wages for a specified number of days, and group policies from commercial insurers arranged through the worker's place of employment are the most common forms of protection. Although paid sick leave is received by substantially fewer workers than insurance benefits, it accounts for 62 percent of group benefits paid, largely in the form of full wage-replacement benefits. Again, however, it is the workers at the higher wage and salary levels who are most likely to have paid sick leave plans.

In short, the indirect costs of illness and disability to individuals place a heavier burden on those less able financially to meet such contingencies. Like the indirect costs to the economy in terms of lost output, these costs to the individual could be lessened by elimination of illness and premature death. As illnesses and disabilities are reduced in length, income loss to the family is reduced commensurately. But those families currently unprotected against the costs of illness to the individual cannot wait for medical science and health care delivery systems to reduce morbidity and mortality. To the extent disease and injury can be reduced, problems of both output loss to the economy and income loss to the individual are resolved, but the prospects for remedy in the short term are limited.

Adjustment of Expenditure Data

Health care expenditures in current dollars have risen from 3.5 billion in 1928-29 to $83.4 billion in 1971-72. During that time the population of the United States grew, medical care prices exhibited inflationary increases, utilization of medical care services expanded, the quality of care delivered for a given procedure generally improved, and new and more costly methods of treatment were employed. Each of these factors contributed to the rapid expansion of health care expenditures. Thus, the increase in the quantity of services of standardized quality that were delivered does not equal the increase in expenditures.

Expenditure data can be adjusted to account for these factors. Adjustments for population growth are made by using per capita expenditure data. Price increases in the medical care component of the consumer price index are stated in constant dollars. Changes in the utilization of services per capita and improvements in the quality of care are difficult to measure, however, and adjustments for these factors must be made with an eye to bounding the estimate. Typically these two factors are estimated together as a residual after adjustment for price and population changes. It is estimated, for example, that the growth in expenditures from 1967 to 1971 that is attributable to increased use and improved technology is 26 percent.[30] When international comparisons of expenditure data are being made, an adjustment must be made to account for the exchange rates of the currencies used in the countries under comparison. In comparisons of expenditures for various services within a country (such as health and education), even the statistic for expenditures as percentages of gross national product must be adjusted. For example, price changes in the medical care component of the consumer price index might be different from those for the goods and services used in education. Target populations for expenditures on health differ from those for education, so that refined data on population growth by age group must be considered. And, of course, changes in the utilization of services and the introduction of new methods of producing services require attention in a manner specific to the service.

Double counting of expenditures in two areas of service under comparison may also be a problem when examining expenditures for each service as a percentage of gross national product. Exaggerated claims for the importance of some sector of the economy can be fabricated when the percentage of GNP attributable to that sector subsumes expenditures that could easily be attributed to another sector, were it the focus of the accounting.

Points of comparison for expenditure data must also be selected with care. A dramatic percentage rise in expenditures for some category of service may be cited, but this information is of little value unless the relative importance of the increase is clarified. What is the target group for the expenditure, and how far does the increase go to meet the group's specific medical needs? A 400 percent increase in expenditures for a selected type of care may mean that a long neglected need is now satisfied or that the need is still glaring, since the increase was based on an expenditure that met only a fraction of it. The increase may imply that lavish unnecessary care is being provided or that the suppliers of medical services are reaping sharply increased "profits." These profits may take the form of salary increases for medical professionals, or higher returns to medical supply firms and pharmaceutical manufacturers, or purchases of expensive technology that enhance the reputation of a hospital or doctor while offering only marginal improvement in the quality of care available (since it duplicates technology in use at other medical facilities in the vicinity). A combination of these outcomes could account for a large percentage increase in expenditures. Thus the impact of a percentage increase of an expenditure must be clarified by reference to other data that indicate the significance of change, such as the magnitude of expenditures at the two points being measured.

In assessing the performance of hospitals, cost increases as well as price increases should be examined, since hospitals are typically paid by third-party insurers on a cost-reimbursement basis. Those who pay out of pocket for their hospital expenses constitute a small segment of the population. In past years, hospital costs and prices have risen at similar rates. However, in 1971-72, prices grew at a significantly lower rate than costs.

Noneconomic Costs and Trade-offs

Mushkin and Collings contend:

The accounting of economic gains and losses . . . omits what is perhaps the simplest and most direct economic effect of all. Health is itself an element in the standard of living. Concentration on health as an investment in economic resources—an intermediate product of value in that it helps to increase national output—must not obscure its parallel importance as a final product for human welfare. . . . The value of human life and relief of suffering . . . cannot be disregarded in health programming. Disease prevention and control measures which yield zero or even negative economic returns can be fully justified in terms of human values.[31]

Not only are there considerations other than economic factors that affect health decisions, but also the economic arithmetic itself is sometimes obscured. The extent to which economic calculations figure in the determination of a person's good health is only partially revealed in discussions of health as an investment in economic resources.

In 1970, according to the Bureau of Labor Statistics, 14,200 Americans were killed on the job, while 2.3 million more suffered disabling accidents. Between 1960 and 1970 the number of disabling injuries per million man-hours in manufacturing industries increased 2.7 percent each year on the average. Since 1968, however, the rate of increase has been 4.3 percent each year.[32] Digging a tunnel through a mountain or laying a mile of railroad track in the western states used to involve a predictable toll of disabled and dead laborers. Managers of today's industrial enterprises, too, can assess the cost to the firm of improved on-the-job safety for its workers on the one hand or death and disability benefits on the other. There is considerable evidence to suggest that, particularly for heavy industry, it is often cheaper for the firm to pay benefits after an accident or illness occurs than to protect the worker from disability or death in the first place.[33]

In 1973, the Oil, Chemical, and Atomic Workers' Union struck Shell Oil Company to win the right to participate in making decisions affecting their own health and safety. Workers could not start grievance procedures over health and safety conditions until after an injury had occurred. Shell management maintained that health and safety were concerns of the company, not the workers.

Workers and taxpayers bear part of the cost of disability and death benefits paid out and thus have an interest in protecting the worker from injury and illness. But as consumers they face higher prices for goods and services if workers are successful in gaining their demands for improved working conditions, since the price of these improvements is passed on to the consumer. Job-related injuries are not the random occurrences we associate with the incidence of disease in the population as a whole. The economic trade-offs they involve are sharply in focus.

The economic arithmetic of morbidity and mortality should influence resource allocation decisions. In the absence of disease, the resources now consumed in health care could be used for other purposes, and the people now afflicted would be able to pursue their own material well-being and that of society as a whole.

Social Welfare Resource Allocation

Economic resources are, of course, limited. Money spent on health care has alternative uses in other social welfare programs—education, housing, and so forth. If all people in the United States are to receive adequate essential health care, however, public resources must be used to provide financial access to medical care and to make available high quality medical services. Health care must compete with alternative uses of these resources, most notably for other social welfare programs such as education, nutrition, housing, and income maintenance. Social welfare expenditures have increased over the years, partly from the extension of services to a larger population, partly from higher prices, and partly from a rise in the level and scope of services and programs. The trends in resource allocation for social welfare, both public and private, are examined below, in general terms that suggest the differences in the magnitude of resources committed to different programs.

Public and private social welfare expenditures for income maintenance, health, education, and welfare are shown in table 2.7, and the percentage distribution among federal, state and local, and private expenditures is illustrated in figure 2.8.

TABLE 2.7 Expenditures for Social Welfare, 1950-72

Type of Expenditure	1949-50	1959-60	1964-65	1967-68	1968-69	1969-70	1970-71	1971-72
				Amount (Millions)				
Total	$35,337	$78,704	$117,871	$164,432	$183,796	$209,708	$241,392	$268,433
Public	23,508	52,293	77,175	113,840	127,741	145,965	171,541	192,740
Private	12,160	27,790	42,766	52,679	58,442	66,461	79,370	79,370
Income maintenance	10,723	29,827	42,530	56,153	63,636	72,386	87,376	98,761
Public	9,758	26,292	36,575	47,313	53,466	60,876	74,396	84,251
Private	965	3,535	5,955	8,840	10,170	11,510	12,980	14,510
Health	12,027	25,856	38,892	53,562	59,975	68,058	75,624	83,417
Public	3,065	6,395	9,535	20,039	22,934	25,235	28,576	32,857
Private	8,962	19,461	29,357	33,523	37,041	42,823	47,048	50,560
Education	10,914	21,742	34,228	49,621	54,293	61,991	69,093	75,018
Public	9,366	18,036	28,149	41,055	44,962	51,863	58,114	63,018
Private	1,548	3,706	6,079	8,566	9,331	10,128	10,979	12,000
Welfare and other services	2,004	2,658	4,291	7,183	8,279	9,991	12,555	14,914
Public	1,319	1,570	2,916	5,433	6,379	7,991	10,455	12,614
Private	685	1,088	1,375	1,750	1,900	2,000	2,100	2,300
			Percentage of Expenditures for Specified Purpose					
Public expenditures	65.9	65.3	64.3	68.4	68.6	68.7	70.1	70.8
Income maintenance	91.0	88.1	86.0	84.3	84.0	84.1	85.1	85.3
Health	25.5	24.7	24.5	37.4	38.2	37.1	37.8	39.4
Education	85.8	83.0	82.2	82.7	82.8	83.7	84.1	84.0
Welfare and other services	65.8	59.1	68.0	75.6	77.1	80.0	83.3	84.6
			Percentage of Gross National Product					
Total expenditures	13.4	15.9	18.0	19.9	20.4	22.0	23.9	24.5
Income maintenance	4.1	6.0	6.5	6.8	7.1	7.6	8.6	9.0
Health	4.6	5.2	5.9	6.5	6.7	7.1	7.5	7.6
Education	4.1	4.4	5.2	6.0	6.0	6.5	6.8	6.8
Welfare and other services	.8	.5	.7	.9	.9	1.0	1.2	1.4

Source: A. M. Skolnik and S. R. Dales, "Social Welfare Expenditures, 1971-72," Social Security Bulletin, December 1972, p. 16.

FIGURE 2.8   Percentage Distribution of Social Welfare Expenditures, 1960-72

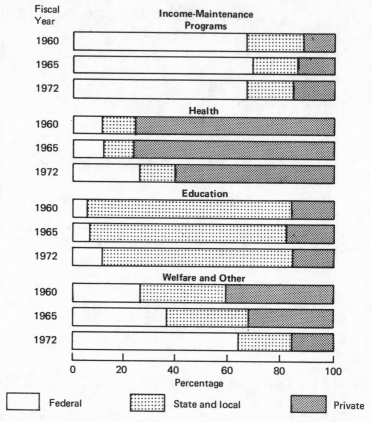

Source: A. M. Skolnik and S. R. Dales, "Social Welfare Expenditures, 1971-72," *Social Security Bulletin,* December 1972, p. 17.

Between 1928-29 and 1971-72, social welfare expenditures rose from 36.3 percent to 52.9 percent of all government expenditures, despite large allocations to military spending. State and local social welfare expenditures exhibited the sharpest rise—from 38.2 percent to 66.1 percent of all state and local expenditures.[34] The federal share of social welfare funding more than doubled from 20.4 percent to 55.0 percent.[35]

The competition of education and public assistance with health for the public dollar is evident. At the state and local levels, education claimed 49.1 percent of non-trust-fund expenditures for social welfare in 1971-72. At the federal level, public assistance claimed the largest share followed by veterans' programs and education. Considering both federal and state and local expenditures, between 1959-60 and 1971-72 social insurance (primarily OASDHI, public employee retirement funds, and unemployment insurance) funded by payroll taxes and employer contributions rose 2.9 times (from $19.3 billion to $75.1 billion); public assistance rose 4.3 times (from $4 billion to $21 billion); education rose 2.5 times (from $17.6 billion to $61.1 billion); while health and medical programs increased 1.8 times (from $4.5 billion to $12.4 billion). (The last three are financed out of general tax revenues.) There is a discrepancy between these statistics and those presented in chapter 3, table 3.5, because of the following: (1) the total for public assistance represents payments under the Social Security Act and (from state and local funds) general assistance; starting in 1968-69 it also includes work-incentive activities; (2) health and medical program expenditures exclude state and local expenditures for domiciliary care in institutions other than mental or tuberculosis and services in connection with OASDHI, state temporary disability insurance, workmen's compensation, public assistance, vocational rehabilitation, and veterans' and antipoverty programs (which *are* included in total expenditures for these programs).[36] It is apparent that public support for education far outpaced expenditures for health and medical programs, and the gap is not narrowing.

The restricted flow of public funds for health and medical programs is indicated by per capita social welfare outlays in 1971-72 (see table 2.9). Per capita expenditures for social insurance were $353.05, education $288.50, and all health and medical programs $155.25. Between 1959-60 and 1971-72, per capita social welfare expenditures (in constant 1971-72 dollars) rose 140 percent from $379.04 to $908.36. For health and medical care alone, the change was 234 percent; for education, there was a 125 percent increase.

How much is spent on medical care depends on the competition among social welfare programs for resources as well as the competition with alternative uses in other sectors of the economy.[37]

Comparison of resource allocations for health care and education is particularly significant. In 1971-72, $83.4 billion was spent on

TABLE 2.9 Per Capita Social Welfare Expenditures, 1929-72

| | Per Capita Expenditures in Current Dollars | | | | | | | | Constant 1971-72 Dollars | | |
| | | | | | | | | | Total Social Welfare Expenditures | | |
Year	Total	Social Insurance	Public Aid	Health and Medical Programs	Veterans' Programs	Education	Other Social Welfare	All Health and Medical Care	Amount (Millions)	Per Capita	Implicit Price Deflators (1971-72=100)
1928-29	$ 31.80	$ 2.78	$ 0.019	$ 2.85	$ 5.31	$ 19.75	$ .62	$ 3.87	$ 9,625.7	$ 78.13	40.7
1949-50	152.56	32.19	16.26	13.44	44.18	43.47	2.92	19.97	39,099.9	254.69	59.9
1954-55	194.66	58.71	17.98	18.58	28.46	66.68	3.71	26.47	47,741.2	285.84	68.1
1959-60	285.42	105.35	22.46	24.45	29.52	96.43	6.24	35.03	69,198.2	379.04	75.3
1964-65	391.28	142.33	31.96	31.77	30.31	142.77	10.51	48.50	96,644.0	491.56	79.6
1967-68	558.44	209.34	54.56	41.61	35.20	199.47	16.16	98.58	132,617.9	652.38	85.6
1968-69	620.62	236.55	65.47	43.87	38.19	215.55	18.47	111.73	143,618.2	699.68	88.7
1969-70	702.04	262.87	79.50	47.02	43.00	245.02	21.27	121.68	156,215.9	753.26	93.2
1970-71	816.47	315.02	101.65	51.91	49.08	269.42	24.41	136.37	176,016.8	839.99	97.2
1971-72	908.36	353.05	120.99	58.41	53.80	288.50	26.77	155.25	192,239.1	908.36	100.0
Percentage change for 1971-72 expenditures (1971-72 prices) from:											
1949-50	+257	+557	+346	+160	−27	+298	+450	+366	+392	+257	
1954-55	+218	+310	+358	+114	+29	+195	+391	+299	+303	+218	
1959-60	+140	+152	+306	+80	+37	+125	+223	+234	+178	+140	
1964-65	+85	+97	+201	+46	+41	+61	+103	+155	+99	+85	
1969-70	+21	+25	+42	+16	+17	+10	+17	+19	+23	+21	
1970-71	+8	+9	+16	+9	+7	+4	+7	+11	+9	+8	

Source: A. M. Skolnik and S. R. Dales, "Social Welfare Expenditures, 1971-72," Social Security Bulletin, December 1972, p. 9.

health and $75.0 billion on education. Total expenditures for health accounted for 7.6 percent of gross national product, while the corresponding figure for education was 6.8 percent. In other words, the total bill for these programs was roughly comparable. But, while 84.0 percent of the expenditures for education came from public funds in 1971-72, only 39.4 percent of outlays for health were public expenditures. Research in health is only 0.3 percent of total expenditures as compared to 4.6 percent for education.[38] Clearly health needs figure lower among public priorities than education. Children are guaranteed eleven to twelve years of schooling at public expense, but no such right to medical care exists. People must by and large fend for themselves to finance essential health care needs, as well as extraordinary medical expenses. Medical care is the single largest cause of personal bankruptcy.

One explanation for this difference in patterns of resource allocation for health and education may lie in our society's view of the individual as the master of his own destiny. Success is seen as the result of hard work, and lack of success is viewed as a sign of personal inadequacy. An individual must have sufficient schooling, however, to avail himself of the opportunity for social mobility. Schools and education lie at the heart of the belief in unbounded frontiers for personal development. As such, public funding and administration of education may be seen as assuring that all people have equal footing in a meritocratic society.

Another explanation for the disparity in public funds for education and health care may lie in the fact that historically the American Medical Association has opposed and forestalled public measures broadening access to health care, whereas professional associations in education encouraged public support of education.

Inequities in the Health of Population Groups

Despite the relatively high levels of aggregate expenditures for health care in the United States, there are vast disparities among groups of Americans in the health care they receive.

The life expectancy of white male Americans at birth is sixty-seven years; that of male Native Americans is more than twenty years less—approximately forty-five years. That is even less than the life expectancy of the population as a whole was at the turn of the century (49.2 years). In 1968, the life expectancy at birth for the white population (both male and female) was 71.1 years but for nonwhites it was only 63.7 years. One health study of Chicago, comparing poor areas to other areas, found that the poor areas had a 60 percent higher infant mortality rate, a 200 percent higher incidence of premature births, 200 percent more new cases of tuberculosis, and a 100 percent higher death rate from cancer of the cervix. In the country as a whole, the maternal death rate for nonwhites is four times that of whites. The incidence of heart disease is three times higher among the poor in inner cities than the national average, and deaths before age thirty-five are four times as high.

Some diseases are unique to certain races (such as sickle-cell anemia among blacks), and some are unique to the poor. A study conducted by the Department of Health, Education, and Welfare in 1973 reported that, among children under the age of six living in deteriorating housing, one out of ten tested had a dangerous level of lead in his bloodstream. The source of this lead poisoning was the old, peeling paint on walls and ceilings in these houses. Diseases caused by rat bites are also restricted to children in poor communities. Protein malnourishment, which leads to irreversible brain damage, strikes at the children of the poor in the rural South. In the United States, middle-aged adults in families with incomes under $2,000 a year are almost three times as likely to suffer chronic conditions that interfere with wage employment or housekeeping as those with higher incomes.

The health of the poor suffers not only from inadequate medical care but also from poor education (resulting, for example, in less awareness of which symptoms require medical attention), poor housing, insufficient heat, and inadequate nutrition (government food stamps and commodity programs attempt to correct this, but reach only a fraction of those in need[39]). Families with incomes less than $3,000 per year are about twice as likely to have diets with inadequate amounts of vitamins A, B, and C as are families with incomes over $7,000 per year.[40]

The necessity to skimp financially means that the poor are less likely to seek preventive health care. Even those who are eligible for Medicare and Medicaid are more likely to be deterred by the deductible and coinsurance provisions from seeking medical attention until an injury or disorder has worsened appreciably. As a result, more extended and expensive medical treatment is required when it is finally sought.

International Comparison of Health Care Expenditures

The United States spends more per capita on medical care than many of the other advanced industrial countries and yet its mortality and morbidity statistics for the population as a whole do not compare favorably. In the early 1960s Brian Abel-Smith conducted the most extensive study to date of international expenditures for health care.[41] When expenditures were matched to indicators of good health, however, the performance of the United States did not stand out among the countries included in the study. The United States was spending more money per capita and as a percentage of GNP than most other countries (see table 2.10), and yet its infant mortality rates were higher and life expectancies lower.[42] Seventeen countries— many with lower per capita expenditures for health care or a lower proportion of their gross national product devoted to health care— have higher life expectancies for males; ten countries have higher life expectancies for females; and infant mortality is lower in twelve countries (see figure 2.11). A ten-year-old boy has a longer life expectancy in thirty-one other countries.[43]

The United States is noted for its refinements of medical science and technology, but these advances do not necessarily reap rewards for the majority of the population. Our comparatively poor performance on major health indicators reveals inadequacies in our patterns of delivering primary health care.

The physician-to-population ratio and the number of hospital beds

TABLE 2.10   Health Expenditures as Percentage of GNP, Seven Countries, 1961-69

Country	Year	Percent of GNP	Year	Percent of GNP
Canada	1961	6.0	1969	7.3
United States	1961-62	5.8	1969	6.8
Sweden	1962	5.4	1969	6.7
Netherlands	1963	4.8	1969	5.9
Federal Republic of Germany	1961	4.5	1969	5.7
France	1963	4.4	1969	5.7
United Kingdom	1961-62	4.2	1969	4.8

Source: J. G. Simanis, "Medical Care Expenditures in Seven Countries," *Social Security Bulletin*, March 1973, p. 39; earlier figures from B. Abel-Smith, *An International Study of Health Expenditure*, World Health Organization Public Health Paper no. 32 (1967).

FIGURE 2.11   International Comparison of Infant Mortality and Life Expectancy

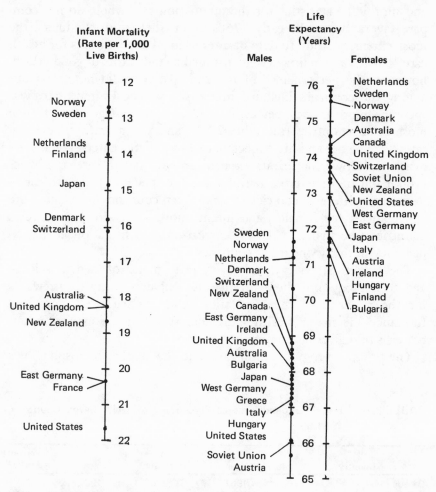

Sources: Adapted from *New York Times*, July 16, 1971; see also *United Nations Demographic Yearbook, 1968* (1969).

Note: The figures on infant mortality are for 1968, while the life expectancy statistics are for different years in the 1960s.

to population are also sometimes taken as indicators of the quality of care afforded the population as a whole. The United States has a high physician-population ratio compared to other countries. Yet our inequitable distribution leads this input, like expenditures, to produce poor output in the health of the nation. A study by economists Victor Fuchs and Marcia Kramer found that variations among states in the quantity of physicians' services available had little or no effect on either infant mortality, or the overall death rate.[44] Apparently, with more and more specialization, increasing the number of physicians does not bring improved primary care. Today, the average physician makes a substantially smaller contribution to the cure of most common disorders than previously, when a larger proportion of doctors were delivering primary care. While the incidence of common maladies is higher, patients are less likely to receive quick medical attention and rapid cure for them.

In the absence of government intervention, priorities for the provision of medical services are set by the market—where individuals bid for the kind of medical care they desire and can afford. Low-income individuals who are excluded from access to quality primary medical care "pull down" national health statistics of morbidity and mortality. Thus, the health of the American populace is a mixed picture: our health care system builds on the best technology and scientific advances, but frequently fails to meet essential medical needs.

A comparison of the health care systems of England, Sweden, and the United States is particularly instructive.[45] England and Sweden provide care at lower cost than the United States, and their populations are healthier and less discontented with their health care delivery systems. In 1965, 85 percent of health care in Britain and Sweden was publicly funded. By 1969, only 38 percent was publicly financed in the United States. The public share of health care expenditures has been rising in this country but it is still far short of that in Britain and Sweden. Nathan Glazer summarizes some of Odin Anderson's observations and indicates trends for various facets of the health care systems in the three countries from 1950 to the late 1960s:

In 1950, Sweden had only 59 doctors per 100,000 population, England 99, the United States a munificent 149. The differences are much smaller in 1967— Sweden is up to 117 and England to 119, while the United States has moved up only slightly to 158. In terms of international comparisons, the United States is still "over-doctored," but not as much.* Similarly, the difference in hospital beds per 1,000 population has declined. In 1950, Sweden was far ahead with 5.7, England had 5.0, the United States only 3.3. We are now all closer—the United States has risen to 4.0, England has dropped to 4.2, Sweden has increased its ratio slightly to 5.9. Also, the differences in the number of nurses have declined. (Some of the earlier differences, however, remain: Sweden still uses considerably less manpower in its hospitals than the United States—1.5 persons per patient-day vs. 2.7 in the United States.)

The variations in the use of hospitals have also diminished. Thus, the United States, whose number of hospital days per 1,000 population was lowest in 1950 (890), shows a rise to 1,132 in 1968. Sweden, whose use of hospitals was greatest in 1950 (1,630) shows a drop to 1,560. England, as in so many of these comparisons, shows the least change. Admissions to general hospitals have risen in all three countries, but the differences are now narrower than they were. Sweden and England have reduced their long average lengths of stay (1950: 15.8 days in Sweden, 15.0 in England; 1968: 11.9 and 11.6) to closer to the short American stay of about eight days in both years. . . .

In all three countries the same proportion of the population sees a physician in a year—just about two thirds—but there are still [fewer] physician visits per capita in Sweden (2.5) than in the United States (4.3) and England (5.9).[46]

---

*It is conceivable that a much higher proportion of American doctors is engaged in research and administration, which would reduce these differences even more. Doctors actually providing medical care in the United States numbered only 130 per 100,000 population in 1967 (Anne R. Somers, *Health Care in Transition: Directions for the Future*, Chicago, Hospital Research and Educational Trust, 1971). I do not have comparable figures for Sweden and England.

These data on health care inputs and medical outcomes reflect the organization and actual operation of the respective health care systems and societal structures of the three countries.[47]

The total costs of illness and death to the individual, the family, and the economy, and the disparities in health among different segments of the population point to the need for clear priorities in allocation of our limited health resources. The function of medical care cannot be defined solely by its impact on the economy or an individual's health. Distinctions must be made between essential, elective, and luxury care, so that differentials in health can be equalized. David Blumenthal and James Fallow explain:

A human medical system must be able to care not only for the majority who are well, but for the minority who are disabled early or sick often. Ill health seems the cruelest of inequalities because we are so powerless to correct it. We all know people denied the span of years, and the vigor during their years of life, that most of us will enjoy. Whenever medicine can compensate for this inequality it has performed its kindest function.[48]

Appendix to Chapter 2

The procedures commonly used to calculate the direct and indirect costs of illness and death are described below for cardiovascular diseases and cancer, to illustrate the difficulties involved in assessing the indirect costs of illness and death for society. The discussion is taken from D. P. Rice, "Economic Costs of Cardiovascular Diseases and Cancer, 1962," *Health Economics Series* no. 5, May 1965.

The direct costs of heart disease, stroke, and cancer . . . represent the dollar value of resources used in connection with these diseases—resources used for prevention, detection, treatment, rehabilitation, research, education, and construction of facilities. In the absence of these diseases, these resources could be utilized for other purposes.

Direct costs alone do not measure the full economic costs imposed upon the Nation by heart disease, stroke, and cancer, since they exclude the loss of output to the economy due to premature death, illness, and disability. The latter are the so-called indirect costs, which are the subject of this discussion.

The direct costs of heart disease, stroke, and cancer are included in the U.S. gross national product (GNP) for 1962. The indirect costs . . . can be employed to indicate how much larger the GNP might have been under certain assumptions (such as full employment), if morbidity and premature mortality had not interfered.

Most calculations of indirect costs are made in terms of the present value of future losses of output that ill or deceased persons would have contributed had they survived and remained healthy. Present value is the sum of the annual losses of output in the future, with each year's loss diminished by a discounting factor.

The aim [here], however, is to develop an estimate of the added output in a single year—1962—had heart disease, stroke, and cancer been eliminated. Cost estimates were, therefore, developed to include: Losses in output due to morbidity in 1962, mortality in 1962, and mortality in previous years. Mortality losses from previous years are calculated because the elimination of heart disease, stroke, and cancer as causes of death and disability in previous years would have led to the survival of many persons through 1962 and to their participation in 1962 production. Discounting does not enter into the calculations in estimating losses of current output for mortality in previous years.

Because of difficulties in measuring the costs of debility or reduced efficiency due to illness and the costs of absenteeism incurred by industry beyond those which can be measured by loss of earnings, these are excluded from the calculations of indirect costs. Information is lacking on which to base estimates of several additional costs attributable to absenteeism among regular workers, such as the costs of administrative time and loss of output due to reduced efficiency.

Transfer payments, such as taxes and relief payments, are not included here among the costs of disease. Transfer payments represent a redistribution of command over resources, rather than their use. It would be double counting to include them in the economic costs of a disease.

Intangible or psychic costs of disease, such as pain and grief, are also omitted. These costs do not directly involve a loss of output and are not readily measurable.

The estimate of losses in output assumes that if it were not for the disease, persons stricken would have had the same employment experience as persons in their age and sex group.[49] Where there is unemployment or substantial underemployment, improved health may result in more unemployment rather than more output. Unless the simplifying assumption of full employment is introduced into the calculation, the effect of disease disability and mortality on output cannot be isolated. If an ill person would be unemployed even if he were in good health, the production losses should be attributed to unemployment, not to the illness.

Population groups (by sex and age) whose potential productive capacity was destroyed or impaired by heart disease, stroke, and cancer were defined in terms of labor force status. Within the labor force, losses in output were computed for both the currently employed and those who would have been employed under conditions of full employment (defined as 4-percent unemployment).

Those not in the labor force who would have contributed to economic output include women keeping house, persons in institutions and those unable to work because of chronic illness and disability. Although the economic contributions of housewives are not included in the national income accounts, omitting the value of their services in calculations of indirect costs would distort comparisons of the costs of illness striking primarily one sex.

Values were placed on the productive time lost by each sex and age class by applying prevailing average (mean) earnings. Implicit is the assumption that average earnings would have remained the same if heart disease, stroke, and cancer had not reduced the size of the labor force.

Average earnings were not adjusted for the value of estimated consumption, contrary to the procedure used by several economists. Consumption is properly viewed as an end in itself and the ultimate goal of economic activity. It then follows that the measure of a person's economic effectiveness should not be influenced by whether or not he consumes what he produces.

Notes

1. D. P. Rice, "Estimating the Cost of Illness," *American Journal of Public Health*, March 1967, p. 424.

2. See especially S. J. Mushkin and F. D. A. Collings, "Economic Costs of Disease and Injury," *Public Health Reports* 74, no. 9 (September 1959); D. P. Rice, "Estimating the Cost of Illness," *American Journal of Public Health*, March 1967, pp. 424-40; D. P. Rice, "Estimating the Cost of Illness," *Health Economics Series* no. 6 (May 1966); D. P. Rice, "Economic Costs of Cardiovascular Diseases and Cancer, 1962," *Health Economics Series* no. 5 (May 1965), and references noted in the first three of these articles.

3. Mushkin and Collings, "Economic Costs."

4. Ibid. See ibid., pp. 799-800 for details on the wide range of cash payments to individuals that mitigate the effects of loss of income due to disability and death.

5. Ibid.

6. D. P. Rice, "Estimating the Cost of Illness," *American Journal of Public Health*, March 1967.

7. D. P. Rice, "Estimating the Cost of Illness," *Health Economic Series* no. 6 (May 1965): 85-86.

8. Discount rates ranging from 2 to 10 percent have been used to estimate the present value of lifetime earnings. A high discount rate greatly reduces the costs of illness and death, particularly those costs associated with illness and death among younger people. In 1963, 10,910 males died between the ages of twenty and twenty-four. A male at age twenty-two had a life expectancy of 47.7 years, so that these deaths resulted in an estimated loss of 520,400 man-years, assuming the working life of an individual extends to the time of death. Ibid., pp. 85-87, 94-95.

In projecting lifetime earnings, allowance should be made for the secular rise of wage rates with increasing productivity (2 to 3 percent per year).

9. Mushkin and Collings, "Economic Costs of Disease and Injury," p. 802.

10. Alcoholism and drug abuse were key factors in reducing the productivity of workers on the job. See the discussion in *Work in America,* Report of a Special Task Force to the Secretary of Health, Education, and Welfare (1973). A high government official estimated that alcoholism cost $2 billion in losses in insurance. U.S. Senate Committee on Labor and Welfare, Subcommittee on Health, *Hearings on Health Services Amendments* (July 1968), pp. 43-46.

11. D. P. Rice, "Economic Costs of Cardiovascular Diseases and Cancer, 1962," *Health Economic Series* no. 5 (May 1965): 599.

12. Ibid.

13. Ibid., p. 612. More than half the man-years lost to gainful employment due to all these diseases occurred among those aged sixty-five and over.

14. See O. W. Anderson and M. Lerner, *Measuring Health Levels in the United States, 1900-1958*, Health Information Foundation Research Series no. 11.

15. "Constitution," in *The First Ten Years of the World Health Organization* (1958), as cited by S. E. Berki and A. W. Heston, "Introduction to the Nations' Health: Some Issues," *Annals*, January 1972, p. ix.

Berki and Heston also reference the social dimension of health. Talcott Parsons, they explain, thought the essence of health was the individual's ability to perform effectively those "roles and tasks for which he had been socialized." (T. Parsons, "Definitions of Health and Illness in the Light of American Values and Social Structures," in E. G. Jaco, ed., *Patients, Physicians and Illness* (1958), p. 176.)

16. C. D. Jenkins, "Psychologic and Social Precursors of Coronary Disease," *New England Journal of Medicine* no. 204 (1971): 244-55, 307-17.

17. *Vital Statistics of the United States*.

18. See N. Glazer, "Perspectives on Health Care," *Public Interest* no. 31 (spring 1973): 113-14.

19. N. Glazer, "Paradoxes of Health Care," *Public Interest* no. 22 (winter 1971): 74-75.

20. Lost output to the economy is not equivalent to forgone earnings. The value of output exceeds the amount of wages paid by the amount of profits—the return to the owners of capital. Wages earned go to consumption, taxes, and savings. Thus it is appropriate to deduct from the total cost of illness and death the additional consumption generated when lives are saved, but only for the period when individuals have not returned to the job.

21. K. H. Allan and M. E. Cinsky, "The General Characteristics of the Disabled Population," *Social Security Bulletin*, August 1972, p. 24.

22. L. A. Horowitz, "Medical Care Price Changes in Medicare's First Five Years," *Social Security Bulletin*, March 1972, p. 17.

23. *Economic Report of the President* (1973), p. 213.

24. Horowitz, "Medical Care Price Changes," p. 17.

25. Inflation associated with the Vietnam War slowed the rise in real income and, in fact, reduced real income for some groups.

26. This survey considered only disability conditions lasting longer than four months, so as to exclude individuals with "short-term impairments resulting from acute illness such as influenza or from injuries such as fractures and lacerations." Ibid., p. 34.

27. Ibid., p. 37.

28. J. Schmulowitz, "Recovery and Benefit Termination: Program Experience of Disabled-Worker Beneficiaries," *Social Security Bulletin*, June 1973, pp. 3-15.

29. Temporary disability programs operate in California, Hawaii, New Jersey, New York, Puerto Rico, and Rhode Island. Railroad workers come under a federally established program.

30. B. S. Cooper and N. L. Worthington, "Medical Care Spending for Three Age Groups," *Social Security Bulletin,* May 1972, p. 3.

31. Mushkin and Collings, "Economic Costs of Disease and Injury," p. 807. For an analysis of the value of good health, see V. Taylor, *How Much Is Good Health Worth?* RAND Publication P-3945 (July 1969).

32. See P. Brodeur, "Annals of Industry: Casualties of the Workplace," *New Yorker* (five-part series), October 29, November 5, 12, 19, 26, 1973. Also see J. A. Page and M. O'Brien, *Bitter Wages: Ralph Nader's Study Group Report on Disease and Injury on the Job* (1972).

33. "In a strange allocation of priorities, while employing only 50 industrial safety inspectors, Ohio employs a force of 103 game wardens." S. Haft, "The Human Costs of Production," *Ripon Forum,* July 1972, p. 39.

34. Excludes federal grants-in-aid (ibid., p. 11). In 1969-70, federal grants to state and local governments included $3.0 billion for education and $1.0 billion for health. This preceded revenue sharing. See S. R. Dales, "Federal Grants to State and Local Governments, 1969-70," *Social Security Bulletin,* September 1971, p. 16.

35. A. M. Skolnik and S. R. Dales, "Social Welfare Expenditures, 1971-72," *Social Security Bulletin,* December 1972, pp. 8, 11.

36. Ibid., p. 5.

37. A more extensive program of income maintenance might well replace many other public programs such as public housing, thereby allowing the individual the opportunity to allocate resources among competing needs and according to personal tastes.

38. See *The Advancement of Knowledge for the Nation's Health, A Report to the President on the Research Programs of the National Institutes of Health* (1967). In 1967, medical research received 36 percent of its funds from the National Institutes of Health, 29 percent from other federal sources, 25 percent from industry, and 10 percent from other sources.

39. See two reports by U.S. Senate, Select Committee on Nutrition and Human Needs, *Hunger—1973* (May 1973), and *Dollars for Food: The Fiscal Year 1974 Budget* (March 1973).

40. T. Davis, N. Gershoff, and D. F. Gamble, "Review of Studies of Vitamin and Mineral Nutrition in the United States (1950-1968)," *Journal of Nutrition Education* (fall 1969), supplement 1, pp. 41-57. Inadequate diets are more common among the poor, but occur even among well-to-do families, apparently because of the increasing consumption of heavily advertised, high-profit, low-nutrition, "junk" foods.

41. B. Abel-Smith, *An International Study of Health Expenditure,* World Health Organization Public Health Paper no. 32 (1967). Abel-Smith anticipated medical outlays would increase 1 percent of GNP every ten years, with an ultimate ceiling of 10 percent of GNP.

42. United States health care expenditures increased to 7.6 percent of GNP in 1971-72, largely as a result of the slowdown in the economy, while medical care costs rose unabated. This illustrates one difficulty in using the share of GNP as a basis of international comparison.

43. *Report of the National Commission on Health Manpower* (1967), vol. 1, pp. 91-92.

44. V. R. Fuchs and M. J. Kramer, *Determinants of the Expenditures for Physician Services in the U.S., 1948-68,* an occasional paper of the National Bureau of Economic Research (1973). J. M. Joyce, "More on Health Care Paradoxes," *Policy Sciences* 3, no. 1 (March 1972): 107-15, similarly examines the relation between health and the number of physicians.

45. The basis for this discussion is the study by O. Anderson, *Health Care: Can There Be Equity? The United States, Sweden and England* (1972).

46. N. Glazer, "Perspectives on Health Care," *Public Interest* no. 31 (spring 1973): 112-13.

47. See ibid.; also L. K. Altman, "Swedish Health Care System," *New York Times* (three-part series), December 23, 24, 25, 1973.

48. D. Blumenthal and J. Fallows, "Health: The Care We Want and Need," *Washington Monthly,* October 1973, p. 19.

49. Not everyone whose death or disability would be prevented would work. Some would be too young, some too old, some unwilling to work, and some unable to find a job. In the normal course of economic activity still others would be looking for work.

3

Sources and Expenditures of Funds

An income-expenditure account of the medical care dollar is necessary for an understanding and analysis of the rising cost of medical care. What are the sources of medical care funds—private individuals, public agencies (federal, state, and local), financial intermediaries (such as private health insurance programs), or philanthropy? How are these funds spent to pay for professional services, hospital care, and drugs? How are expenditures for services distributed in terms of the age, personal income, and geographic location of the recipients of medical care?

Examination of an income-expenditure profile of the medical care dollar and the associated trends in income and expenditures helps clarify who pays for what services and the magnitude of the exchange. This information is necessary to unravel the factors leading to rising medical care costs and the maldistribution of services. It also identifies certain points of leverage bearing on the problems of cost and delivery.

Sources of Medical Care Funds

Public and Private Financing

The amounts spent for medical care and the types of services purchased depend in part on what financial arrangements have been made to pay for the care. Total national health expenditures amounted to $83.4 billion in 1971-72 as compared to $42.1 billion in 1965-66. The distribution of these expenditures between private and governmental sources of funds is portrayed in figure 3.1. The percentage financed by the federal government more than doubled in that time span. This increase was offset by an almost equal percentage reduction in private financing. Still, in current dollars, private expenditures increased from $31.5 billion to $47.0 billion during this period.

Pressures on state and local finances were reflected in the relatively stable percentage of the total financed by state and local governments. The rise in federal expenditures is largely explained by the introduction of Medicare and Medicaid.

Greater detail on the trend from private to public finance of health care from 1928-29 to 1971-72 is provided in table 3.2. While the total outlay for health rose by twenty-three times, public expenditures rose by sixty-nine times. Per capita national health expenditures in current dollars amounted to $29.16 in 1928-29, $141.63 in 1959-60, and $394.16 in 1971-72. Expenditures as a percentage of gross

FIGURE 3.1   Private and Public Shares of National Health Expenditure Funds, 1966 and 1972

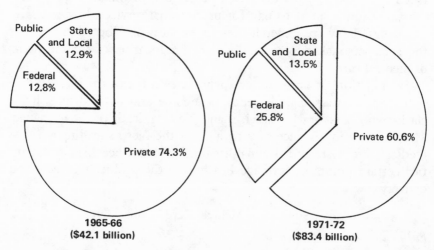

Source: B. S. Cooper and N. L. Worthington, "National Health Expenditures, 1929-72," *Social Security Bulletin,* January 1973, p. 7.

TABLE 3.2 Private and Public Health Expenditures, Total and Per Capita, 1929-72

	Gross National Product (Billions)	Total			Private			Public		
Year		Amount (Millions)	Per Capita	Percent of GNP	Amount (Millions)	Per Capita	Percent of Total	Amount (Millions)	Per Capita	Percent of Total
1928-29	$ 101.0	$ 3,589	$ 29.16	3.6	$ 3,112	$ 25.28	86.7	$ 477	$ 3.88	13.3
1934-35	68.7	2,816	22.04	4.1	2,303	17.84	80.9	543	4.21	19.1
1939-40	95.1	3,863	28.83	4.1	3,081	22.99	79.8	782	5.84	20.2
1949-50	263.4	12,028	78.35	4.6	8,962	58.38	74.5	3,065	19.97	25.5
1954-55	379.7	17,330	103.76	4.6	12,909	77.29	74.5	4,420	26.46	25.5
1959-60	495.6	25,856	141.63	5.2	19,460	106.60	75.3	6,395	35.03	24.7
1964-65	655.6	38,892	197.81	5.9	29,357	149.32	75.5	9,535	48.50	24.5
1965-66	718.5	42,109	211.64	5.9	31,279	157.21	74.3	10,830	54.43	25.7
1966-67	771.4	47,860	237.93	6.2	32,037	159.27	66.9	15,823	78.66	33.1
1967-68	827.0	53,563	263.49	6.5	33,523	164.91	62.6	20,040	98.58	37.4
1968-69	899.0	59,975	292.19	6.7	37,041	180.46	61.8	22,934	111.73	38.2
1969-70	955.1	68,058	328.17	7.1	42,823	206.49	62.9	25,235	121.68	37.1
1970-71	1,010.6	75,624	360.89	7.5	47,048	224.52	62.2	28,576	136.37	37.8
1971-72	1,095.9	83,417	394.16	7.6	50,560	238.90	60.6	32,857	155.25	39.4

Source: B. S. Cooper and N. L. Worthington, "National Health Expenditures, 1929-72," *Social Security Bulletin*, January 1973, p. 5.

national product (GNP) rose from 3.6 percent to 7.6 percent, with
the sharpest rise in the last seven years—up 2.7 percent. Of course,
any rise in expenditures in current dollars must be deflated by the
rise in prices of medical care services and adjusted for population
and utilization changes.[1]

Private expenditures in relation to public outlays for health have
moved steadily downward (see table 3.3).[2] The major increases in
public expenditures in relation to all health expenditures occurred
from 1928-29 to 1949-50 (a yearly average gain of 0.6 percent) and
from 1966-67 to 1967-68 (a gain of 6 percent in the relative share of
public funds). As the last column in table 3.2 shows, there was little
net change in the relative shares from 1949-50 (25.5 percent) to
1965-66 (25.7 percent). But the *federal* share of public expenditures
increased from 15 percent in 1928-29 to 51 percent in 1964-65 and
then to approximately 64 percent in 1971-72.

In current dollars, private expenditures for health grew only 5.7
percent between 1966 and 1969, while public outlays rose 28 percent. But, by 1969-70, the percentage increase in private expenditures
exceeded the percentage increase in public expenditures.

Public funds provided $7.9 billion in 1965-66 and $26.7 billion in
1971-72 for *personal* health care (as distinguished from total health
expenditures, of which it is a part). Medicare contributed $8.8
billion, or 42 percent of the increase, and Medicaid another $5.9
billion for a total of more than $14.7 billion. As might be expected,
expenditures for other major public health programs experienced a
decline in their relative shares of the public dollar.

Note that all Medicare outlays—including premium payments by
individuals for medical insurance under Medicare—are classified as
public expenditures.[3] If these payments were classified as private

TABLE 3.3   Proportions of Private and Public Health Expenditures, 1929-72

	1928-29	1959-60	1971-72
Ratio of private to public expenditures	6½ to 1	3+ to 1	1½ to 1
Percentage of total expenditure from private sources (calendar years)	86.7%	75.4%	60.6%

Source: A. M. Skolnik and S. R. Dales, "Social Welfare Expenditures, 1971-72," *Social Security Bulletin*, December 1972, p. 13.

expenditures, the private share of national health expenditures would rise from 60.6 percent to 62.0 percent for 1971-72 (or $1.17 billion out of the $8.8 billion attributed to public funds for Medicare).[4] The estimated sources of funds for Medicare outlays for both hospital insurance and supplementary medical insurance are given in table 3.4.

Table 3.5 provides a detailed description of the sources and uses of expenditures for health and medical care for selected fiscal years from 1928-29 through 1971-72.[5] Note that the Medicare and Medicaid programs were begun July 1, 1966 (at the start of fiscal year 1967). Table 3.6 distinguishes the federal and the state and local components of public expenditures.[6] The sharp rise in health insurance for the aged (OASDHI) since 1965-66 and the less dramatic but important jump in public assistance (vendor medical payments) from 1959-60 to 1971-72 account for much of the public increase during this period. From 1959-60 to 1965-66 vendor payments rose from 15 percent to 29 percent of all money payments. Vendor payments are a substantially higher proportion of state and local government expenditures than of federal.[7]

TABLE 3.4   Sources of Funds for Medicare, 1970-72

Expenditure and Year	Amount (Millions)	Percentage		
		Payroll Tax	Individual Premiums	General Revenues*
Total Medicare expenditures				
1969-70	$7,149.2	61.2	13.8	24.9
1970-71	7,875.0	60.3	13.0	26.7
1971-72	8,819.2	61.6	14.2	24.2
Hospital insurance expenditures				
1969-70	$4,952.8	88.4	–	11.6
1970-71	5,592.4	84.9	–	15.1
1971-72	6,275.8	90.5	–	9.5
Medical insurance expenditures				
1969-70	$2,196.3	45.0	–	55.0
1970-71	2,282.6	44.9	–	55.1
1971-72	1,543.4	44.4	–	55.6

Source: Adapted from B. S. Cooper and N. L. Worthington, "National Health Expenditures, 1929-72," *Social Security Bulletin*, January 1973, p. 8.

*Includes premium payments by Medicaid.

TABLE 3.5   Sources and Disbursements of Health Expenditures by Program, 1929-72

Type of Expenditure	Amount (Millions)								
	1928-29	1949-50	1959-60	1964-65	1967-68	1968-69	1969-70	1970-71	1971-72*
Total	$3,589.1	$12,027.3	$25,856.2	$38,892.3	$53,562.4	$59,975.1	$68,057.6	$75,624.1	$83,416.8
Private expenditures	3,112.0	8,962.0	19,461.0	29,357.0	33,523.0	37,041.0	42,823.0	47,048.0	50,560.0
Health and medical services	3,010.0	8,710.0	18,816.0	28,023.0	32,017.0	35,294.0	40,464.0	44,571.0	47,665.0
Direct payments	2,900.0	7,107.0	12,576.0	17,577.0	18,899.0	20,316.0	23,253.0	24,674.0	25,070.0
Insurance benefits	–	879.0	4,698.0	8,280.0	10,444.0	12,206.0	14,406.0	16,817.0	19,000.0
Expenses for prepayment	–	274.0	792.0	1,212.0	1,558.0	1,572.0	1,515.0	1,685.0	2,100.0
Industrial in-plant services and philanthropy	110.0	450.0	750.0	954.0	1,116.0	1,200.0	1,290.0	1,395.0	1,495.0
Medical research	–	37.0	121.0	162.0	185.0	190.0	193.0	195.0	195.0
Medical facilities construction	102.0	215.0	524.0	1,172.0	1,321.0	1,557.0	2,166.0	2,282.0	2,700.0
Public expenditures	477.1	3,065.3	6,395.2	9,535.3	20,039.4	22,934.1	25,234.6	28,576.1	32,856.8
Health and medical services	372.5	2,470.2	5,346.3	7,641.2	17,581.1	20,391.5	22,578.9	25,610.9	29,624.8
OASDHI (health insurance for the aged)	–	–	–	–	5,347.2	6,597.7	7,149.2	7,875.0	8,819.2
Temporary disability insurance (medical benefits)	–	2.2	40.2	50.9	54.6	57.7	62.6	68.4	74.2
Workmen's compensation (medical benefits)	75.0	193.0	420.0	580.0	790.0	875.0	985.0	1,100.0	1,200.0
Public assistance (vendor medical payments)	–	51.3	492.7	1,367.1	3,723.2	4,595.6	5,212.8	6,277.5	7,602.7
General hospital and medical care	117.1	886.1	1,973.2	2,515.5	2,927.7	3,009.7	3,382.3	3,737.7	4,235.4
Defense Department hospital and medical care (Armed Forces)	29.2	336.2	820.1	858.5	1,482.9	1,531.1	1,495.9	1,606.1	1,784.8
Military dependents' medical care	–	–	60.1	78.3	165.4	218.4	263.7	350.5	403.0
Maternal and child health programs	6.2	29.8	140.7	223.0	336.8	411.5	431.4	403.3	499.2
School health (educational agencies)	9.4	30.6	101.0	142.2	204.6	225.0	246.6	270.0	295.0
Other public health activities	88.8	350.8	401.2	671.0	1,000.6	1,194.7	1,437.0	1,698.4	2,099.7
Veterans' hospital and medical care	46.7	582.8	879.4	1,114.8	1,342.5	1,430.8	1,651.4	1,873.9	2,255.6
Medical vocational rehabilitation	.1	7.4	17.7	34.2	102.0	118.4	133.8	162.8	179.1
OEO health and medical care	–	–	–	5.6	103.5	126.0	127.3	187.2	176.9

Public expenditures (Continued)									
Medical research	—	72.9	471.2	1,228.8	1,615.5	1,599.7	1,652.8	1,642.6	1,833.8
Medical facilities construction	104.7	522.3	577.7	665.3	842.8	942.9	1,003.0	1,322.6	1,398.2
Defense Department	†	1.1	40.0	31.1	26.8	71.8	52.5	74.1	88.5
Veterans Administration	4.2	161.5	59.6	77.0	49.9	47.9	70.9	85.1	109.9
Other	100.4	359.8	478.1	557.2	766.1	823.2	879.6	1,163.4	1,199.8
Total expenditures as a percentage of gross national product	3.6%	4.6%	5.2%	5.9%	6.5%	6.7%	7.1%	7.5%	7.6%
Public expenditures as a percentage of total expenditures	13.3%	25.5%	24.7%	24.5%	37.4%	38.2%	37.1%	37.8%	39.4%
Personal care expenditures	$3,272.2	$10,400.4	$22,728.7	$33,498.3	$46,323.3	$52,057.3	$59,101.2	$65,669.6	$71,862.4
Private expenditures	2,990.0	8,298.0	17,799.0	26,540.0	30,118.0	33,346.0	38,549.0	42,455.0	45,105.0
Public expenditures	282.2	2,102.4	4,929.7	6,958.3	16,205.3	18,711.3	20,552.2	23,214.6	26,757.4
Percentage from:									
Private expenditures	91.4%	79.8%	78.3%	79.2%	65.0%	64.1%	65.2%	64.6%	62.8%
Direct payments	88.6%	68.3%	55.3%	52.5%	40.8%	39.0%	39.3%	37.6%	34.9%
Insurance benefits	—	8.5%	20.7%	24.7%	22.5%	23.4%	24.4%	25.6%	26.4%
Public expenditures	8.6%	20.2%	21.7%	20.8%	35.0%	35.9%	34.8%	35.4%	37.2%

Source: A. M. Skolnik and S. R. Dales, "Social Welfare Expenditures, 1971-72," *Social Security Bulletin*, December 1972, p. 13.

*Preliminary estimates.
† Data not available.

TABLE 3.6 Federal, State, and Local Health Expenditures by Program, 1929-72

Type of Expenditure	Amount (Millions)								
	1928-29	1949-50	1959-60	1964-65	1967-68	1968-69	1969-70	1970-71	1971-72*
Federal expenditures	$98.3	$1,361.8	$2,917.6	$4,624.7	$13,069.3	$15,227.1	$16,597.7	$18,763.7	$21,559.8
Health and medical services	93.1	1,059.6	2,174.8	3,074.6	11,141.0	13,217.6	14,492.0	16,658.5	19,206.8
OASDHI (health insurance for the aged)	—	—	—	—	5,347.2	6,597.7	7,149.2	7,875.0	8,819.3
Workmen's compensation (medical benefits)	.6	5.2	9.0	11.3	15.3	16.7	20.7	25.9	30.0
Public assistance (vendor medical payments)	—	—	199.8	555.0	1,833.6	2,297.8	2,607.1	3,373.9	4,089.9
General hospital and medical care	8.5	46.4	103.4	137.9	186.6	193.2	283.3	410.8	446.3
Defense Department hospital and medical care (Armed Forces)	29.2	336.2	820.1	858.5	1,482.9	1,531.1	1,495.9	1,606.1	1,784.8
Military dependents' medical care	—	—	60.0	78.3	165.3	218.4	263.7	350.5	403.3
Maternal and child health services	1.2	20.1	34.7	69.1	160.6	192.5	196.0	148.2	234.7
Other public health activities	6.9	63.8	57.3	222.9	426.8	524.7	590.3	677.6	823.2
Veterans' hospital and medical care	46.7	582.8	879.4	1,114.8	1,342.5	1,430.8	1,651.4	1,873.9	2,255.6
Medical vocational rehabilitation	.1	5.1	11.2	21.2	76.5	88.8	107.0	130.2	143.3
OEO health and medical care	—	—	—	5.6	103.5	126.0	127.3	187.2	176.9
Medical research	—	72.9	448.2	1,173.8	1,546.5	1,527.7	1,576.8	1,564.6	1,754.8
Medical facilities construction	5.2	229.3	294.7	376.3	381.8	481.9	529.0	540.6	598.2
Defense Department	†	1.1	40.0	31.1	26.8	71.8	52.5	74.1	88.5
Veterans Administration	4.2	161.5	59.6	77.0	49.9	47.9	70.9	85.1	109.9
Other	.9	66.8	195.1	268.2	305.1	362.2	405.6	381.4	399.8
State and local expenditures	$378.8	$1,703.6	$3,477.5	$4,910.5	$6,970.1	$7,706.9	$8,636.9	$9,812.4	$11,297.0
Health and medical services	279.3	1,410.6	3,171.5	4,566.5	6,440.1	7,173.9	8,086.9	8,952.4	10,418.0
Temporary disability insurance (medical benefits)	—	2.2	40.2	50.9	54.6	57.7	62.6	68.4	74.2
Workmen's compensation (medical benefits)	74.4	187.8	411.0	568.7	774.7	858.3	964.3	1,074.9	1,170.0
Public assistance (vendor medical payments)	—	51.3	292.9	812.1	1,889.6	2,297.8	2,605.6	2,903.6	3,512.9
General hospital and medical care	108.6	839.7	1,869.8	2,377.6	2,741.0	2,816.5	3,099.0	3,326.9	3,789.1
Maternal and child health services	5.0	9.7	106.1	153.9	176.2	219.0	235.3	255.2	264.5
School health (educational agencies)	9.4	30.6	101.0	142.2	204.6	225.0	246.6	270.0	295.0
Other public health activities	81.9	287.0	343.9	448.1	573.8	670.0	846.7	1,020.8	1,276.5
Medical vocational rehabilitation	.1	2.3	6.6	13.0	25.5	29.6	26.8	32.6	35.8
Medical research	—	—	23.0	55.0	69.0	72.0	76.0	78.0	79.0
Medical facilities construction	99.5	293.0	283.0	289.0	461.0	461.0	474.0	782.0	800.0

Source: A. M. Skolnik and S. R. Dales, "Social Welfare Expenditures, 1971-72," Social Security Bulletin, December 1972, p. 14.

*Preliminary estimates.

†Data not available.

In the period following World War II (between 1949-50 and 1971-72), several trends in expenditures for health care appeared. Overall expenditures rose 5.9 times (from $12.0 billion to $83.4 billion). Private expenditures rose 4.6 times (from $9.0 billion to $50.6 billion) and public expenditures 9.5 times (from $3.1 billion to $32.9 billion).

Private direct payments rose 2.5 times (from $7.1 billion to $25.1 billion) while insurance benefits experienced a gain of 20 times (from $0.9 billion to $19.0 billion). Private expenditures for prepayment, while small in magnitude, increased 6 times (from $0.3 billion to $2.1 billion). Industrial in-plant services and private philanthropy increased 2.3 times (from $0.45 billion to $1.5 billion). The percentage of *personal* care expenditures derived from private direct payments dropped to almost half (from 68 percent to 35 percent) while the percentage derived from insurance benefits increased 2.1 times (from 8.5 percent to 26.4 percent).

Public expenditures on medical research increased 23 times (from $0.07 billion to $1.8 billion) during this period, with marked increases between 1959-60 and 1964-65. While public spending for medical facilities construction rose 1.8 times (from $0.5 billion to $1.4 billion), private spending for this construction increased 18 percent in 1972.

Direct and Third-Party Payments

Direct patient outlays for medical care should be distinguished from third-party financing of health expenditures (by private health insurance carriers, government, and philanthropic organizations, among others). For the period from 1949-50 to 1971-72, the percentage of direct payments for *personal* health care was markedly reduced (from 68.3 to 34.9 percent), while the percentage of third-party payments increased (see table 3.7). Incentives for the consumer to control costs were correspondingly muted, and incentives for the providers of services to control costs were also weakened.

The largest rises in third-party payments came (in roughly equal percentages) from private health insurance and government contributions. The largest annual rise of third-party payments occurred from 1966 to 1967 when government payments rose more than nine percentage points and the percentage contribution of private health insurance actually declined. The introduction of Medicare and Medicaid programs (July 1, 1966) was central to these changes.

TABLE 3.7 Direct and Indirect (Private and Public) Payments, 1929-72

		Source of Funds						
		Private				Public		
Year	Total	Total	Direct Payments	Insurance Benefits	Other	Total	Federal	State and Local
		Amount (Millions)						
1928-29	$ 3,165.2	$ 2,883.0	$ 2,800.0	—	$ 83.0	$ 282.2	$ 84.8	$ 197.4
1934-35	2,585.5	2,204.0	2,134.0	—	70.0	381.5	88.7	292.8
1939-40	3,413.7	2,891.0	2,799.0	—	92.0	522.7	133.3	389.4
1949-50	10,400.4	8,298.0	7,107.0	$ 879.0	312.0	2,102.4	978.8	1,123.6
1954-55	15,231.0	11,762.0	8,992.0	2,358.0	412.0	3,469.0	1,582.9	1,886.1
1959-60	22,728.7	17,799.0	12,576.0	4,698.0	525.0	4,929.7	2,102.1	2,827.6
1964-65	33,498.3	26,540.0	17,577.0	8,280.0	683.0	6,958.3	2,839.9	4,118.4
1965-66	36,216.3	28,324.0	18,668.0	8,936.0	720.0	7,892.3	3,349.4	4,542.9
1966-67	41,323.9	28,863.0	18,766.0	9,344.0	753.0	12,460.9	7,470.4	4,990.6
1967-68	46,323.3	30,118.0	18,899.0	10,444.0	775.0	16,205.3	10,407.8	5,797.5
1968-69	52,057.3	33,346.0	20,316.0	12,206.0	824.0	18,711.3	12,290.1	6,421.2
1969-70	59,101.2	38,549.0	23,253.0	14,406.0	890.0	20,552.2	13,410.2	7,141.8
1970-71	65,669.6	42,455.0	24,674.0	16,817.0	964.0	23,214.6	15,411.8	7,803.0
1971-72	71,862.4	45,105.0	25,070.0	19,000.0	1,035.0	26,757.4	17,745.8	9,011.7

Percentage

Year							
1928-29	100.0	91.1	88.5	—	2.6	8.9	2.7	6.2
1934-35	100.0	85.2	82.5	—	2.7	14.8	3.4	11.3
1939-40	100.0	84.7	82.0	—	2.7	15.3	3.9	11.4
1949-50	100.0	79.8	68.3	8.5	3.0	20.2	9.4	10.8
1954-55	100.0	77.2	59.0	15.5	2.7	22.8	10.4	12.4
1959-60	100.0	78.3	55.3	20.7	2.3	21.7	9.2	12.4
1964-65	100.0	79.2	52.5	24.7	2.0	20.8	8.5	12.3
1965-66	100.0	78.2	51.5	24.7	2.0	21.8	9.2	12.5
1966-67	100.0	69.8	45.4	22.6	1.8	30.2	18.1	12.1
1967-68	100.0	65.0	40.8	22.5	1.7	35.0	22.5	12.5
1968-69	100.0	64.1	39.0	23.4	1.6	35.9	23.6	12.3
1969-70	100.0	65.2	39.3	24.4	1.5	34.8	22.7	12.1
1970-71	100.0	64.6	37.6	25.6	1.5	35.4	23.5	11.9
1971-72	100.0	62.8	34.9	26.4	1.4	37.2	24.7	12.5

Source: B. S. Cooper and N. L. Worthington, "National Health Expenditures, 1929-72," *Social Security Bulletin*, January 1973, p. 16.

Total private expenditures for health and medical services have been transformed in much the same way as personal health expenditures. Between 1949-50 and 1971-72, direct payments declined from 79.3 percent to 49.6 percent while insurance benefits increased from 9.8 percent to 37.5 percent (see table 3.8).

The Ultimate Source of Funds

The individual consumer and taxpayer bears the cost of medical care whether the funds derive from direct (out-of-pocket) payments by him as a consumer or from the government, private insurance carriers, philanthropic organizations, or other third parties. Direct payment is now a decreasing proportion of the total medical care bill. Third-party payments (principally government and private health insurance) paid 31.7 percent of the total in 1950 and 65.1 percent in 1972. However, the third parties are presumably less concerned than patients are with keeping quality up and costs down.

The expenditure of public funds means a redistribution of the ability to pay for medical care. The method of taxation, the tax rate schedule, and the tax base that generate the public funds for health expenditures have distributive consequences as important as the pattern of disbursement of these funds. The expenditure of public funds to subsidize research and to develop selected programs for the delivery of services influences the availability of different types of medical care. Again, there are significant distributive consequences,

TABLE 3.8   Total Private Health Expenditures, 1949-50 and 1967-68

	1949-50		1971-72	
Type of Private Expenditure	Amount (Millions)	Percentage	Amount (Millions)	Percentage
Total	$8,962	100.0	$50,560	100.0
Health and medical services	8,710	97.2	47,665	94.3
Direct payments	7,107	79.3	25,070	49.6
Insurance benefits	879	9.8	19,000	37.5
Expenses for prepayment	274	3.1	2,100	4.2
Industrial in-plant services and philanthropy	450	5.0	1,495	3.0
Medical research	37	0.4	195	.4
Medical facilities construction	215	2.4	2,700	5.3

Source: A. M. Skolnik and S. R. Dales, "Social Welfare Expenditures, 1971-72," *Social Security Bulletin,* December 1972, p. 14.

since not all segments of society (differentiated by age, income, sex, race, and residence) have similar problems of access to medical care or the same incidence of various diseases.

The medical care costs that fall to the consumer and taxpayer may be diffused beyond easy recognition, but they are nonetheless a burden that remains with the individual. The amount of this burden on any one person is a function of his or her economic situation and the choices of medical services that situation affords. This set of choices is increasingly influenced by government policy, as government subsidies, tax incentives, and expenditures for health represent a growing proportion of the health care dollar.

Patterns of Expenditure

The purchases made with the medical care dollar relate to or are conditional upon the sources of the funds in several ways. Medical care expenditures, for this discussion, include expenditures for hospital care, nursing homes, professional services (especially physicians' services), drugs, and insurance services. Other items, such as the cost of workmen's compensation and sickness insurance, are included only insofar as they are expenditures for the above services.

The major health expenditures in 1971-72 are listed in table 3.9. In table 3.10 a more detailed list of expenditures is broken into its private and public components. The relative dependence on private funds was especially great for eyeglasses and appliances (96.4 percent), dentists' services (95.0 percent), and drugs and drug sundries (92.5 percent). These are all benefits that are not well covered by health insurance. Public financing was concentrated in hospital care, nursing home care, and research expenditures.

TABLE 3.9   Major Disbursements of Health Care Funds, 1971-72

Type of Service	Amount (Billions)
Hospital care	$32.5
Physicians' services	16.2
Drugs and drug sundries	7.9
Dentists' services	5.0
Medical facilities construction	4.1
Nursing home care	3.5

Source: B. S. Cooper and N. L. Worthington, "National Health Expenditures, 1929-72," *Social Security Bulletin*, January 1973, p. 7.

TABLE 3.10 Private and Public Expenditures by Service, 1971-72

Type of Expenditure	Total	Private			Public		
		Total	Consumers	Other	Total	Federal	State and Local
Total	$83,417	$50,560	$46,170	$4,390	$32,857	$21,560	$11,297
Health services and supplies	77,291	47,665	46,170	1,495	29,625	19,207	10,418
Hospital care	32,460	15,267	14,840	427	17,193	11,220	5,973
Physicians' services	16,150	12,430	12,419	11	3,720	2,803	916
Dentists' services	5,025	4,771	4,771	—	254	165	90
Other professional services	1,655	1,427	1,395	32	228	166	62
Drugs and drug sundries	7,909	7,340	7,340	—	569	303	266
Eyeglasses and appliances	2,037	1,960	1,960	—	77	44	34
Nursing-home care	3,500	1,370	1,345	25	2,130	1,282	848
Expenses for prepayment and administration	2,868	2,100	2,100	—	768	638	130
Government public health activities	2,100	—	—	—	2,100	823	1,276
Other health services	3,587	1,000	—	1,000	2,587	1,763	824
Research and medical facilities construction	6,127	2,895	—	2,895	3,232	2,353	879
Research	2,029	195	—	195	1,834	1,755	79
Construction	4,098	2,700	—	2,700	1,398	598	800
Publicly owned facilities	1,052	—	—	—	1,052	266	786
Privately owned facilities	3,046	2,700	—	2,700	346	332	14

Source: B. S. Cooper and N. L. Worthington, "National Health Expenditures, 1929-72," Social Security Bulletin, January 1973, p. 7.

The distribution of total expenditures for medical services has changed greatly over the years (see figure 3.11). For example, the share spent on hospital care rose from 18 percent to 39 percent from 1929 to 1972. Physicians' and other professionals' services dropped from 48 percent to 27 percent in those years. Drugs and appliances accounted for 20 percent in 1929 and had declined to 12 percent by 1972. Similar changes occurred in *private* medical care expenditures. From 1969-70 to 1971-72, total health expenditures rose 22

FIGURE 3.11   Percentage Distribution of Health Expenditures by Type, 1929 and 1972

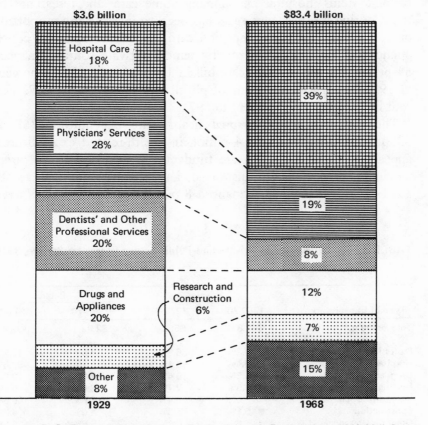

Sources: D. P. Rice and B. S. Cooper, "National Health Expenditures, 1929-68," *Social Security Bulletin*, January 1970, p. 13; B. S. Cooper and N. L. Worthington, "National Health Expenditures, 1929-72," *Social Security Bulletin*, January 1973, p. 7.

percent. Hospital care payments increased 25 percent and drug and appliance payments 22 percent. Physicians' services went up 21 percent and research and construction 21 percent.[8]

The structure of spending for health care varied under private and public auspices. Of the total health care expenditures in 1971-72, $50.6 billion came from private sources and $32.9 billion from public funds. Table 3.12 compares the distribution of private and public funds by type of expenditure for 1969-70 and 1971-72. Clearly expenditures from private funds (direct payments, private health insurance, and philanthropy) are more evenly distributed among professional services, hospital care, and drugs and appliances than public expenditures are. Public funds are directed more toward institutional items—hospital and nursing home care—and research. The trend during the past few years has been to increase the proportion of public funds spent on hospital care, and this is clearly a consequence of the method of reimbursement. Private sources financed 64 percent of the hospital care bill in 1965-66 and only 47 percent in 1971-72. Private payment of physicians' bills went from 93 percent in 1965-66 to 77 percent in 1971-72.

The distribution of *personal* health care expenditures ($71.9 billion out of a total $83.4 billion in health-related expenditures) appears in figure 3.13. Private funds are broken down into direct payment, private health insurance, and philanthropic sources. In 1971-72, direct payments financed 8 percent of hospital care (down

TABLE 3.12   Percentage of Private and Public Expenditures by Service, 1970 and 1972

Type of Expenditure	Private		Public	
	1969-70	1971-72	1969-70	1971-72
Total amount (billions)	$42.8	$50.6	$25.2	$32.9
Professional personnel	36.3%	36.9%	14.0%	13.7%
Hospital care	30.4%	30.1%	51.2%	52.4%
Drugs and appliances	19.5%	18.4%	2.0%	2.0%
Nursing home care	4.5%	2.7%	6.6%	6.5%
Medical research	.5%	.4%	6.6%	5.6%
Construction	5.1%	5.3%	4.0%	4.2%
Other health services	5.6%	6.1%	15.6%	16.6%

Source: B. S. Cooper and N. L. Worthington, "National Health Expenditures, 1929-72," *Social Security Bulletin*, January 1973, p. 7.

from 13 percent in 1970-71), 41 percent of physicians' services (up 2 percent), and 68 percent of other health services, including drugs and sundries (down 2 percent). Government expenditures accounted for 53 percent, 23 percent, and 25 percent of these services, respectively. Private health insurance accounted for 38 percent of hospital care, 36 percent of physicians' services, and 5 percent of other services. Hence third-party payments covered 92 percent of hospital care, 59 percent of physicians' services, and 32 percent of

FIGURE 3.13   Distribution of Expenditures by Source of Funds and Service, 1971-72

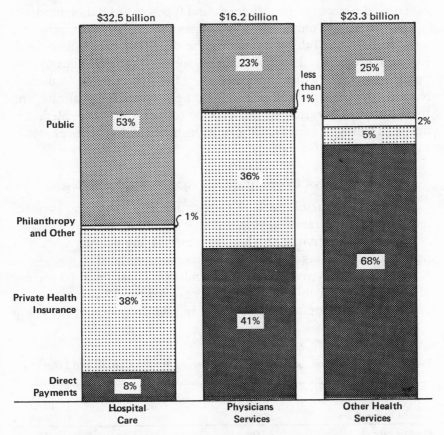

Source: B. S. Cooper and N. L. Worthington, "National Health Expenditures, 1929-72," *Social Security Bulletin,* January 1973, p. 17.

other health services. This means that consumer out-of-pocket payments are low (and decreasing) for hospital care, moderate (and increasing) for physicians' services, and very high for drugs.[9]

The split between the federal government's personal health care contribution and that of state and local governments in 1970-71 is given in table 3.14. In each area of service mentioned above, the split is roughly equal. The breakdown of the public and private sums for personal health care into their specific expenditures for 1970-71 is depicted in figure 3.15. Public funds are spent mostly for hospital care (63 percent) and private funds for professional services (39 percent). Drugs and appliances account for 21 percent of private expenditures and only 3 percent of public spending. Nursing home care used 3 percent of private funds and 9 percent of public funds.

The nature of public spending varies among different programs (see table 3.16). Table 3.17 shows the distribution of public funds for two programs: health insurance for the aged (Medicare) and public assistance (which includes money for Medicaid and Medicare). Note the high proportion of funds that go toward hospital care, and the types of services that are *not* covered (dentists' services—Medicare; drugs and drug sundries—Medicare; eyeglasses and appliances—Medicare and Medicaid).

Distribution of Expenditures by Age, Income, and Region

The distribution of medical care expenditures by age, personal income (and insurance coverage), and region of residence of the recipient of the services provides a picture of the delivery system of health care according to some general measures of need.

Individuals sixty-five years of age and over constituted 10 percent of the population in 1971-72 but accounted for 27 percent of the personal health care outlays of $71.9 billion. In contrast, the group

TABLE 3.14   Federal, State, and Local Personal Health Care Expenditures

Type of Expenditure	Total Public Share	Federal Share	State and Local Share
Hospital care	50%	32%	18%
Physicians' services	25%	18%	7%
Drugs and sundries	7%	3.5%	3.5%

FIGURE 3.15   Shares of Public and Private Funds Spent on Specific Personal
Care Services, 1970-71

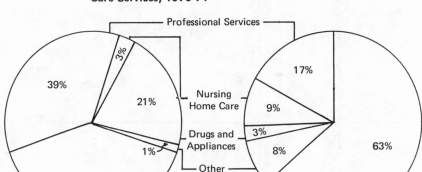

Private Funds
($41.4 billion)

Public Funds
($23.3 billion)

under nineteen years of age comprised 36 percent of the population but consumed only 16 percent of the health outlay, while the intermediate age group (nineteen to sixty-four) spent 57 percent, roughly the proportion suggested by its share of population. These overall proportions have not varied substantially in recent years.

The nature as well as the magnitude of services consumed is markedly different across age groups and is in part conditional on the source of funds. The elderly depend heavily on public resources. Public funds pay two-thirds of the bill for the aged and about one-quarter for the young and intermediate age groups. But the "dependence" of the elderly should be considered in light of their contribution to general tax revenues and Social Security payroll taxes during their working lives. Material security for the elderly against burdensome medical expenses is the aim of Medicare and in part Medicaid.

The extent of insurance coverage by personal income and the type of public assistance by income group are important indicators of the degree to which adequate medical care has been established as a right rather than a privilege determined by the individual's economic circumstances. The regional distribution of expenditures is also a signal in this regard. The Southeast seems to have the greatest shortage of

TABLE 3.16 Public Expenditures by Program and Service, 1971-72

Program and Source of Funds	Amount (Millions)										
	Total	Hospital Care	Physicians' Services	Dentists' Services	Other Professional Services	Drugs and Drug Sundries	Eyeglasses and Appliances	Nursing Home Care	Government Public Health Activities	Other Health Services	Administration
Total	$29,624.8	$17,192.9	$3,719.6	$254.5	$227.5	$569.0	$77.2	$2,129.8	$2,099.7	$2,586.6	$767.7
Health insurance for the aged	8,819.2	6,017.1	2,006.1	—	82.0	—	.8	216.0	—	43.0	455.0
Temporary disability insurance (medical benefits)	74.2	53.7	17.6	—	1.2	.8	—	—	—	—	—
Workmen's compensation (medical benefits)	1,200.0	604.5	510.6	—	36.9	24.0	24.0	—	—	—	—
Public assistance (vendor medical payments)	7,602.7	3,207.0	781.2	185.0	34.3	513.9	—	1,822.8	—	768.2	290.2
General hospital and medical care	4,235.4	4,181.4	7.4	1.7	—	1.3	—	—	—	43.5	—
Defense Department hospital and medical care (including military dependents)	2,187.8	1,393.4	155.2	—	—	—	—	—	—	639.2	—
Maternal and child health services	499.2	74.7	44.7	11.1	36.0	10.7	14.3	—	—	307.7	—
School health	295.0	—	—	—	—	—	—	—	—	295.0	—
Other public health activities	2,099.7	—	—	—	—	—	—	—	2,099.7	—	—
Veterans' hospital and medical care	2,255.6	1,592.1	18.4	47.9	—	4.1	19.7	91.0	—	459.9	22.5
Medical vocational rehabilitation	179.1	69.0	91.7	—	—	—	18.4	—	—	—	—
Office of Economic Opportunity	176.9	86.7	8.8	—	37.1	14.2	—	—	—	30.1	—
Federal	19,206.9	11,220.2	2,803.3	164.8	165.7	302.9	43.5	1,282.1	823.2	1,763.1	637.9
Health insurance for the aged	8,819.2	6,017.1	2,006.1	—	82.0	—	—	216.0	—	43.0	455.0
Workmen's compensation (medical benefits)	30.0	19.5	7.5	—	1.8	.6	.6	—	—	—	—

Federal (continued)

Public assistance (vendor medical payments)	$ 4,089.9	$ 1,715.5	$ 417.9	$ 99.0	$ 18.3	$274.9	—	$ 975.1	—	$ 428.7	160.4
General hospital and medical care	446.3	392.3	7.4	1.7	—	1.3	—	—	—	43.5	—
Defense Department hospital and medical care (including military dependents)	2,187.8	1,393.4	155.2		—	—	—	—	—	639.2	—
Maternal and child health services	234.7	35.1	30.7	7.4	26.5	7.8	8.5	—	—	118.7	—
Other public health activities	823.2	—	—	—	—	—	—	—	823.2	—	—
Veterans' hospital and medical care	2,255.6	1,592.1	18.4	47.9	—	4.1	19.7	91.0	—	459.9	22.5
Medical vocational rehabilitation	143.3	55.2	73.4	—	—	14.2	14.7	—	—	30.1	—
Office of Economic Opportunity	176.9	—	86.7	8.8	37.1	14.2	—	—	—	—	129.8
State and local	10,418.0	5,972.7	916.3	89.7	61.7	266.1	33.7	847.7	1,276.5	823.5	129.8
Temporary disability insurance (medical benefits)	74.2	53.7	17.6	—	1.2	.8	.8	—	—	—	—
Workmen's compensation (medical benefits)	1,170.0	585.0	503.1	—	35.1	23.4	23.4	—	—	—	—
Public assistance (vendor medical payments)	3,512.9	1,491.5	363.3	86.0	15.9	239.0	—	847.7	—	339.5	129.8
General hospital and medical care	3,789.1	3,789.1	—	—	—	—	—	—	—	189.0	—
Maternal and child health services	264.5	39.6	14.0	3.7	9.5	2.9	5.8	—	—	295.0	—
School health	295.0	—	—	—	—	—	—	—	—	—	—
Other public health activities	1,276.5	—	—	—	—	—	—	1,276.5	—	—	—
Medical vocational rehabilitation	35.8	13.8	18.3	—	—	—	3.7	—	—	—	—

Source: B. S. Cooper and N. L. Worthington, "National Health Expenditures, 1929-72," *Social Security Bulletin*, January 1973, p. 9.

TABLE 3.17   Percentage Distribution of Expenditures on Selected Public Programs, 1971-72

Type of Service	Health Insurance for the Aged (Federal)	Public Assistance (Vendor Medical Payments)		
		Total	Federal	State and Local
Total expenditures (millions)	$8,819.2	$7,602.7	$4,089.9	$3,512.9
Hospital care	68.3%	42.1%	42.0%	42.5%
Physicians' services	22.8	10.3	10.2	10.3
Dentists' services	–	2.4	2.4	2.4
Other professional services	0.9	0.4	0.4	0.5
Drugs and drug sundries	–	6.8	6.7	6.8
Eyeglasses and appliances	–	–	–	–
Nursing home care	2.4	24.0	23.8	24.1
Government public health activities	–	–	–	–
Other health services	0.5	10.1	10.5	9.6
Administration	5.2	3.8	3.9	3.7

Source: B. S. Cooper and N. L. Worthington, "National Health Expenditures, 1929-72," *Social Security Bulletin*, January 1973, p. 9.

physicians (and the highest physician income) of any region, a deficiency that is compounded by the low per capita income of its population.

Age Distribution of Expenditures

Expenditures for medical care vary greatly among age groups. The average medical care bill for an aged person reached nearly $1,000 in 1971-72, compared with $358 for a person between nineteen and sixty-four years of age and $147 for an individual under nineteen. Despite the increase in third-party payments, the average out-of-pocket payments for aged persons ($276) were $10 higher in 1972 than the 1971 amount in current dollars, but slightly less in real terms. In 1971-72, expenditures per capita on personal health care for those sixty-five and over were about three times as large as the outlays for those under sixty-five years of age ($441 as compared to $155).

The aged person used out-of-pocket expenditures of $225 to pay a little more than one-quarter of his bill in 1971; in 1966—the year before Medicare became operational—he paid about $234 or half his medical expenses from his own funds. After adjustment for population and price increases, the 1967 to 1971 growth in expenditures attributable to increased use and improved technology was 26 percent.[10] If the proportion of income spent out-of-pocket for medical care were known, we could then assess whether the financial burden for the aged at each income level had been reduced by Medicare. It is clear, however, that the Medicare program did increase utilization of medical services.[11]

Whatever the category of care, bills were higher for the aged than for the rest of the population. Expenditures per capita on hospitals for those sixty-five and over in 1971-72 were ten times those of the young; physicians' services were four times higher for the aged; and all other health services were six times higher (see table 3.18). More detailed estimates are provided in table 3.19 for 1968-69 and 1971-72. These figures point to the heavy burden of hospital care, nursing home care, and outlays for drugs and sundries for the old.

From 1965-66 to 1971-72, the contribution of public funds to personal health care for the aged increased $10.5 billion or from 30 percent to 66 percent of the total expenditure. For the nonaged, the public funds increased $8.3 billion or 7 percent. (While there has been a sharp decline in the relative contribution of private funds, the amount of private funds spent on personal health care for the aged was close in magnitude in 1971-72 to that in 1965-66. Expenditures from private funds varied from $5.8 billion in 1965-66 to $6.8 billion in 1971-72. In constant dollars, the magnitude of private expenditures would be smaller. It appears, however, that public dollars did not significantly substitute for private dollars when

TABLE 3.18   Per Capita Personal Health Care Expenditures by Age Group, 1971-72

Type of Expenditure	Age Group			
	All Ages	Under 19	19-64	65 and Over
Total	$340	$145	$358	$981
Hospital care	153	46	169	484
Physicians' services	76	46	80	177
Other health services	111	53	109	320

Source: B. S. Cooper and N. L. Worthington, "Age Differences in Medical Care Spending, Fiscal Year 1972," *Social Security Bulletin*, May 1973, p. 10.

TABLE 3.19 Specific Per Capita Expenditures by Source of Funds and Age Group, 1969-72

Type of Expenditure	All Ages			Under 19			19-64			65 and Over		
	Total	Private	Public	Total	Private	Public	Total	Private	Public	Total	Private	Public
1968-69, total	$253.61	$162.46	$ 91.16	$111.03	$ 83.13	$27.90	$270.76	$205.90	$64.86	$710.22	$224.80	$485.42
Hospital care	108.91	51.15	57.77	27.04	15.03	12.01	124.93	78.95	45.97	336.17	34.13	302.04
Physicians' services	57.69	44.63	13.07	37.50	33.94	3.56	59.18	52.13	7.05	127.64	43.68	83.97
Dentists' services	18.62	17.48	1.13	11.68	10.45	1.23	24.00	22.97	1.03	15.14	13.81	1.33
Other professional services	6.29	5.32	.97	4.08	3.46	.62	6.46	5.96	.51	13.91	8.98	4.93
Drugs and drug sundries	31.57	29.88	1.69	16.85	16.10	.74	33.45	32.14	1.32	78.06	70.57	7.49
Eyeglasses and appliances	8.49	8.24	.25	3.85	3.69	.16	9.79	9.45	.34	19.25	19.09	.15
Nursing home care	12.01	3.71	8.30	.82	.45	.37	2.80	.65	2.14	107.52	33.67	73.86
Other health services	10.03	2.05	7.98	9.22	—	9.22	10.15	3.66	6.49	12.52	.87	11.65
1971-72, total	$339.56	$213.13	$126.43	$146.86	$105.55	$41.28	$358.25	$265.10	$93.15	$981.42	$337.21	$644.21
Hospital care	153.38	72.14	81.24	45.54	24.40	21.13	168.92	104.60	64.33	483.83	74.18	409.65
Physicians' services	76.31	58.73	17.58	45.64	40.65	4.98	79.63	69.38	10.25	176.53	68.81	107.72
Dentists' services	23.74	22.54	1.20	14.23	13.15	1.08	31.35	30.15	1.21	17.79	16.10	1.69
Other professional services	7.82	6.74	1.08	4.67	4.02	.64	8.17	7.46	.71	18.09	13.37	4.72
Drugs and drug sundries	37.37	34.68	2.69	19.97	18.90	1.06	40.02	37.76	2.26	89.98	78.50	11.48
Eyeglasses and appliances	9.62	9.26	.36	4.31	4.14	.17	11.15	10.62	.53	21.66	21.41	.25
Nursing home care	16.54	6.47	10.06	1.13	.28	.85	3.86	.56	3.30	147.81	63.84	83.97
Other health services	14.77	2.55	12.22	11.39	—	11.39	15.15	4.58	10.57	25.74	.99	24.74

Source: B. S. Cooper and N. L. Worthington, "Age Differences in Medical Care Spending, Fiscal Year 1972," Social Security Bulletin, May 1973, p. 6.

Medicare and Medicaid were introduced.) Table 3.20 provides estimates of the personal health expenditures for three age groups by type of expenditure and source of funds for 1968-69 and 1971-72.

The aged received 11 percent of private and 52 percent of public funds in 1967-68. In 1971-72, public expenditures were 49 percent of the total, while private funds spent for health care of the aged had increased to 15 percent (see table 3.21). The percentage distribution of personal health care expenditures by source of funds for each age group in 1971-72 is displayed in table 3.22.

The group sixty-five and over depended largely on public sources of finance. Its public funds in 1970-71 were twice its private funds. While there was a slight decline in this dependence (from 67.6 percent in 1967-68 to 65.6 percent in 1971-72) the aged still depended almost three times as much on public funds as the under-sixty-five group in 1971-72. The ratio of public to private funds varies greatly according to the service, as table 3.23 indicates. Federal funds yielded 81 percent of government money for personal health care for the aged in 1971-72 (the remainder coming from state and local governments) and only 52.8 percent for the other age groups (see table 3.24).

Medicare explains a good part of the rise of public funds for the aged. This program financed 45 percent of the medical bill for the aged in 1967-68 (see table 3.25). Medicare's contribution to public funds for the aged rose by 11 percent between 1966-67 and 1967-68.

The effect of Medicare and Medicaid programs is suggested by the changes in the percentages of public funds spent on personal health care for the aged in various categories of services from 1966-67 to 1967-68 (table 3.23). The largest movement occurred in the category of physicians' services—the relative contribution of public funds rose by almost two-thirds. The new legislation built on a system that had provided rather limited insurance coverage of physicians' services. Hence there was room for a relatively large gain in this category. The increase of about two-fifths in the public contribution for nursing home care also reflects large additional resources for this service made available under the new legislation.

However, the proportion of personal health expenditures for the aged met by Medicare dropped from 46 percent in 1968-69 to 42 percent in 1971-72. Three factors contributed to this significant drop.[12] Controls on the use of extended care facilities, which are

TABLE 3.20 Personal Health Expenditures by Source of Funds and Age Group, 1969-72

| | Amount (Millions) | | | | | | | | | | | |
| Type of Expenditure | All Ages | | | Under 19 | | | 19-64 | | | 65 and Over | | |
	Total	Private	Public	Total	Private	Public	Total	Private	Public	Total	Private	Public
1969, total	$52,057	$33,346	$18,711	$ 8,397	$6,287	$2,110	$29,825	$22,681	$ 7,144	$13,838	$4,380	$ 9,457
Hospital care	22,356	10,499	11,857	2,045	1,137	908	13,761	8,697	5,064	6,550	665	5,885
Physicians' services	11,842	9,160	2,682	2,836	2,567	269	6,519	5,742	777	2,487	851	1,636
Dentists' services	3,821	3,589	232	883	790	93	2,644	2,530	114	295	269	26
Other professional services	1,292	1,092	200	309	262	47	712	656	56	271	175	96
Drugs and drug sundries	6,480	6,133	347	1,274	1,218	56	3,685	3,540	145	1,521	1,375	146
Eyeglasses and appliances	1,743	1,692	51	291	279	12	1,078	1,041	37	375	372	3
Nursing home care	2,465	762	1,703	62	34	28	308	72	236	2,095	656	1,439
Other health services	2,058	420	1,638	697	—	697	1,118	403	715	244	17	227
1972, total	$71,862	$45,105	$26,757	$11,459	$8,236	$3,221	$40,654	$30,084	$10,571	$19,753	$6,787	$12,966
Hospital care	32,460	15,267	17,193	3,553	1,904	1,649	19,169	11,870	7,300	9,738	1,493	8,245
Physicians' services	16,150	12,430	3,720	3,561	3,172	389	9,036	7,873	1,163	3,553	1,385	2,168
Dentists' services	5,025	4,771	254	1,110	1,026	84	3,558	3,421	137	358	324	34
Other professional services	1,655	1,427	228	364	314	50	927	846	81	364	269	95
Drugs and drug sundries	7,909	7,340	569	1,558	1,475	83	4,542	4,285	257	1,811	1,580	231
Eyeglasses and appliances	2,037	1,960	77	336	323	13	1,265	1,205	60	436	431	5
Nursing home care	3,500	1,370	2,130	88	22	66	438	64	374	2,975	1,285	1,690
Other health services	3,126	540	2,587	889	—	889	1,719	520	1,199	518	20	498

Source: B. S. Cooper and N. L. Worthington, "Age Differences in Medical Care Spending, Fiscal Year 1972," *Social Security Bulletin*, May 1973, p. 4.

TABLE 3.21   Age Distribution of Public and Private Personal Health Expenditures, 1971-72

	Public		Private		Total	
Age Group	Amount (Billions)	Percent	Amount (Billions)	Percent	Amount (Billions)	Percent
Total	$26.6	100	$45.1	100	$71.9	100
Under 19	3.2	12	8.2	18	11.5	16
19-64	10.6	39	30.1	67	40.7	57
65 and over	13.0	49	6.8	15	19.8	27

Source: B. S. Cooper and N. L. Worthington, "Age Differences in Medical Care Spending, Fiscal Year 1972," *Social Security Bulletin*, May 1973, p. 4.

included in the nursing home category, were tightened in 1969-70, and, as a result, payments to these facilities declined in both 1970-71 and 1971-72. Extended care facilities received 18 percent of the nursing home bill for the aged in 1968-69 but only 7 percent in 1971-72. In current dollars the drop was from $367 million to $216 million.

Additionally, physicians declined to accept assignment of Medicare claims in an increasing number of cases. If a physician accepts assignment, he accepts Medicare's determination of a reasonable charge, and the patient is billed for the unmet part of his annual $50 deductible plus 20 percent of the remaining amount. (A $5.30 monthly premium is also paid as a condition of participation in the supplementary medical insurance program.) However, if the physician does not accept assignment he can charge more than the "reasonable charge" and the patient pays the difference. In 1968-69, the assignment rate (exclusive of hospital-based physicians) was 61 percent; in 1970-71, 60.0 percent; and in 1971-72, 56.4 percent. This, in part, accounted for the decline of Medicare's contribution to physicians' services for the aged—from 61 percent in 1968-69 to 56 percent in 1971-72. An additional factor has been tighter regulation of reimbursement of charges for physicians' services.

Finally, Medicare's share of the hospital bill for the aged has also decreased. The decrease in the average length of stay for the elderly is one factor. Since the aged individual is responsible for a hospital deductible roughly equivalent to one day of care, the proportion of the medical bill paid out-of-pocket goes up as the average length of

TABLE 3.22   Source of Funds for Personal Health Expenditures by Age, 1966 and 1972

Source of Funds	All Ages Amount (Millions) 1966	1972	All Ages Percentage 1966	1972	Under 65 Amount (Millions) 1966	1972	Under 65 Percentage 1966	1972	65 and Over Amount (Millions) 1966	1972	65 and Over Percentage 1966	1972
Total	$36,216	$71,862	100.0	100.0	$27,974	$52,113	100.0	100.0	$8,242	$19,753	100.0	100.0
Direct payments	18,668	25,070	51.5	34.9	14,286	19,520	51.1	37.5	4,382	5,553	53.2	28.1
Third-party payments	17,548	46,792	48.5	65.1	13,688	32,593	48.9	62.5	3,860	14,200	46.8	71.9
Private health insurance	8,936	19,000	24.7	26.4	7,627	17,860	27.3	34.3	1,309	1,140	15.9	5.8
Government	7,892	26,757	21.8	37.2	5,432	13,792	19.4	26.4	2,460	12,966	29.8	65.6
Philanthropy and industry	720	1,035	2.0	1.4	629	941	2.2	1.8	91	94	1.1	0.5

Source: B. S. Cooper and N. L. Worthington, "Age Differences in Medical Care Spending, Fiscal Year 1972," *Social Security Bulletin*, May 1973, p. 14.

TABLE 3.23   Public Funding of Specific Health Services for the Aged, 1967-68

Type of Expenditure	Percentage from Public Funds	
	1966-67	1967-68
Total	59.5	70.2
Hospital care	91.7	89.9
Physicians' services	45.6	74.0
Drugs and drug sundries	9.3	11.2
Nursing home care	53.9	77.3

Source: D. P. Rice and B. S. Cooper, HEW, *Outlays for Medical Care of Aged and Nonaged Persons, Fiscal Years 1966-68,* Research and Statistics Note no. 12, July 16, 1969, table 3.

stay goes down. Medicare's proportion of the hospital bill of the aged dropped from 66 percent in 1968-69 to 62 percent in 1971-72 as a result of this and because some outlays for care are not covered or only partially covered by Medicare. Thus, a greater financial burden is placed on the aged.

The distribution of Medicare benefits and the use of its services have been uneven. Medicare includes seven types of benefits. The largest share of expenditures in 1971-72—72 percent—went for in-patient hospital stays; physicians' services took the next largest portion, 24 percent, and extended care facilities took 2.5 percent.

Per capita expenditures under Medicare have more than doubled since 1965-66. In 1967, 20 percent of the population insured under Medicare used no covered services and another 20 percent were hospitalized.

Costs are incurred by a small percentage of the covered group. Thus 7.5 percent of the persons served were reimbursed for costs of $2,000 or more, and this constituted around 40 percent of total reimbursements; 25 percent of the persons served were reimbursed less than $50, accounting for 6 percent of total reimbursements.[13]

The distribution of medical services by age can be further described in terms of the claims different age groups make on various public programs. In 1971-72, Medicare and Medicaid together accounted for over 85 percent of public expenditures for the aged.[14] In 1971-72, the aged received 100 percent of the funds allocated to health insurance for the aged and one-third of public assistance (vendor payments). The under-nineteen group received 40 percent

TABLE 3.24 Personal Health Expenditures by Program and Age Group, 1971-72

Program	Total				Federal				State and Local			
	All Ages	Under 19	19-64	65 and Over	All Ages	Under 19	19-64	65 and Over	All Ages	Under 19	19-64	65 and Over
Total	$26,757	$3,221	$10,571	$12,966	$17,746	$1,861	$5,408	$10,475	$9,012	$1,357	$5,163	$2,491
Health insurance for the aged	8,364	—	—	8,364	8,364	—	—	8,364	—	—	—	—
Temporary disability insurance	74	—	74	—	—	—	—	—	74	—	74	—
Workmen's compensation (medical benefits)	1,200	—	1,157	43	30	—	30	—	1,170	—	1,127	43
Public assistance (vendor medical payments)	7,312	1,280	3,320	2,713	3,930	688	1,784	1,458	3,383	592	1,536	1,255
General hospital and medical care	4,235	423	2,578	1,234	446	140	264	42	3,789	283	2,314	1,192
Defense Department hospital and medical care (including military dependents)	2,188	766	1,357	66	2,188	766	1,357	66	—	—	—	—
Maternal and child health services	499	340	159	—	235	160	75	—	264	180	84	—
School health	295	295	—	—	—	—	—	—	295	295	—	—
Veterans' hospital and medical care	2,233	—	1,703	530	2,233	—	1,703	530	—	—	—	—
Medical vocational rehabilitation	179	36	140	3	143	29	112	2	36	7	28	1
Office of Economic Opportunity	177	81	83	13	177	81	83	13	—	—	—	—

Source: B. S. Cooper and N. L. Worthington, "Age Differences in Medical Care Spending, Fiscal Year 1972," Social Security Bulletin, May 1973, p. 8.

TABLE 3.25   Trend in Public and Private Funding of Health Care for the Aged,
1966-68

Source of Funds	1965-66	1966-67	1967-68
Total expenditure (billions)	$ 7.9	$ 9.4	$11.4
Public	31%	60%	70%
Medicare	—	34%	45%
Other public	—	26%	25%
Private	69%	40%	30%

Source: Adapted from D. P. Rice and B. S. Cooper, HEW, *Outlays for Medical Care of Aged and Nonaged Persons, Fiscal Years 1966-68,* Research and Statistics Note no. 12, July 16, 1969, chart 3.

from public assistance (Medicaid), 13 percent from general hospital and medical care, and 24 percent from Defense Department hospital and medical care. The intermediate age group received 31 percent of its share of public funds from Medicaid; general hospital and medical care programs (primarily state and local mental hospitals) yielded 24 percent; Veterans Administration 16 percent; and the Department of Defense 13 percent.

Health Insurance Coverage and Distribution of Services by Income

Coverage by health insurance is related to age, retirement status, family income, and health status. Logically then, health care expenditures vary with income, health status, and age.

From 1950 to 1970 benefits from private insurance for hospitals rose three times as much as gross enrollment for hospital care. The increase in benefit expenditures for physicians' services over the same period was 2-1/3 times the rate of increase in gross enrollment for the type of care. The higher rate of increase in benefit expenditures is due to rising costs of medical care, some expansion of benefits, and higher utilization.[15] The portion of consumer expenditures met by private insurance likewise increased from 1950 to 1970 (see table 3.26).[16]

There are three main categories of private health insurance providers: the Blue Cross and Blue Shield associations, commercial insurers (offering group and individual policies), and independent plans (including community, employee-employer-union, and private group clinic arrangements).

TABLE 3.26   Percentage of Consumer Expenditures Met by Private Insurance

Year	Total	Hospital Care	Physicians' Services
1950	12.2%	37.1%	12.0%
1955	21.7	56.0	25.0
1960	27.8	64.5	30.0
1965	31.8	71.2	32.8
1970	40.3	73.2	48.1

Source: HEW, Office of Research and Statistics, *Background: Medical Care, Costs and Prices* (1972), p. 101.

The commercial insurance companies carry the lowest proportion of high-risk persons, and the independent plans the highest proportion. Correspondingly, the commercial plans have the lowest average premiums, because they enroll the low-risk population and provide for substantial cost-sharing.[17] Independent plans have the highest premiums because of their higher risk subscribers, more comprehensive medical benefits, and less extensive cost-sharing features.

The amount of cost-sharing by each type of plan is mirrored by the percentage of persons covered who had *no* doctor visits: 49.6 percent of those covered by commercial insurers did not see a doctor once, 36.1 percent of Blue Cross-Blue Shield members saw no doctor, and 33.4 percent of those covered by independent plans saw none. Benefit restrictions discourage the demand for care, since part of the medical care costs must be paid out-of-pocket.[18] Benefit payments for hospital care per insurance enrollee in 1970 ranged from $18 for individual policies from commercial insurers to $66.01 (3-2/3 times as much) for Blue Cross.

Table 3.27 portrays the split of consumer health expenditures between premium payments and out-of-pocket expenditures. Out-of-pocket expenditures were highest for Blue Cross-Blue Shield, but the percentage of consumer expenditures paid out-of-pocket was about equal (43 percent) for Blue Cross-Blue Shield and commercial insurers. This reflects differences in the populations served and variations in the scope of coverage.

Table 3.28 provides estimates of the percentage of persons covered under private insurance plans by type of care and age for 1971. These estimates of coverage of health services are adjusted so as to eliminate

TABLE 3.27   Distribution of Consumer Expenditures by Type of Insurer

Type of Insurer	Average Premium	Out-of-Pocket Expenditures	Consumer Expenditures on Health Care
Commercial insurers	$208	$156	$364
Blue Cross-Blue Shield	257	190	447
Independent plans	271	52	323

Source: Dr. Milton Roemer, testimony before the Senate Subcommittee on Anti-Trust and Monopoly, June 7, 1972.

duplication or multiple coverage. The actual financial protection offered by private health insurance is far less than that suggested by these percentages. The proportion of consumer expenditures for health care that are met by these plans varies widely among individuals. As a result of deductibles and coinsurance provisions, the full cost of health care services is rarely met. This is especially true for physicians' office and home visits, dental care, and drugs. Only 6.2 percent of consumer expenditures for health services, other than hospital care and physicians' services, were paid by health insurance.

There are significant variations among age groups in health insurance coverage. Table 3.29 shows the percentage of persons aged sixty-five and over covered by health care insurance.[19] As a result of Medicare, only a small fraction of the aged have no financial protection against the cost of medical care. However, close to one-half of this age group feels it necessary to supplement the protection offered by the Medicare program.

Over one-fifth of the population under age sixty-five has no private health insurance. A portion of this group receives medical care services under public assistance. Again, financial protection even for those with some insurance can be quite limited.

At incomes under $3,000, 36 percent were covered by hospital insurance and 35 percent under surgical insurance. At incomes of $10,000 or more, 92 and 91 percent were covered under these two categories. The tremendous financial burden that some families face despite health insurance is illustrated by the fact that the percentage of family income spent on health care can vary from less than 5 percent to well over 20 percent.

TABLE 3.28 Persons Covered by Private Health Insurance by Service and Age Group, 1971

	All Ages		Under 65		65 and Over	
Type of Service	Number (Thousands)	Percent of Civilian Population	Number (Thousands)	Percent of Civilian Population	Number (Thousands)	Percent of Civilian Population
Hospital care	157,996	76.9	147,345	79.8	10,651	51.2
Physicians' services:						
Surgical services	152,562	74.2	142,753	77.3	9,809	47.2
In-hospital visits	148,514	72.3	140,685	76.2	7,829	37.7
X-ray and laboratory						
examinations	145,207	70.7	137,463	74.4	7,744	37.3
Office and home visits	95,825	46.6	91,493	49.5	4,332	20.8
Dental care	15,348	7.5	15,155	8.2	193	0.9
Prescribed drugs (out-of-hospital)	106,985	52.1	103,672	56.1	3,313	15.9
Private-duty nursing	104,730	51.0	101,450	54.9	3,280	15.8
Visiting nurse service	110,215	53.6	106,190	57.5	4,025	19.4
Nursing home care	38,636	18.8	33,434	18.1	5,202	25.0
HIAA* estimates						
Hospital care	179,900	87.5	168,513	91.2	11,387	54.8
Surgical services	165,449	80.5	155,841	84.4	9,608	46.2

Source: M. S. Mueller, "Private Health Insurance in 1971," *Social Security Bulletin*, February 1973, p. 4.

*HIAA is the Health Insurance Association of America, an association of insurance companies.

TABLE 3.29   Percent of Persons Sixty-five and Over Covered by Health
Insurance, 1971

Coverage	Hospital Insurance	Medical Insurance
No insurance	3%	4%
Medicare	94%	92%
Supplemental private insurance	48%	43%
Private insurance alone	3%	4%

Source: M. S. Mueller, "Private Health Insurance in 1971: Health Care Services, Enrollment
and Finances," Social Security Bulletin, February 1973, p. 3.

Regional Distribution of Expenditures

Per capita expenditures for health care vary greatly by region.
This, like other aspects of the distribution of expenditures, is significant if it reflects a discrepancy between health care needs and the
ability to pay for services. It also indicates the efficiency of utilization of health care resources.

Health care needs vary across income groups as ability to pay
varies. Moreover, ability to pay is also determined by the prices of
services. The Southeast region of the United States appears to have
the greatest shortage of physicians as well as the highest physician
income. The pairing of a shortage of health personnel and low per
capita income places an unusually heavy burden of medical care
expenses on low-income groups.

Regional variations for five different categories of services are
shown in table 3.30. The region with the highest per capita expenditures has an index almost two times that of the lowest for nonfederal
hospital care, while the highest region is four times the lowest for
psychiatric hospital care. The lowest per capita expenditures occur
typically in the southern regions and the highest in the Northeast or
Pacific region. These differentials in per capita expenditures are
generally much larger than per capita income differentials among
regions. Income differentials thus explain only a part of the health
care expenditure differentials.

In 1966, the per capita expenditures for hospital care services of
physicians and dentists were 4.1 percent of per capita income for the
United States as a whole. Regional variations ranged from 3.8 percent for the South Atlantic region to 4.7 percent for the Pacific

TABLE 3.30   Index of Expenditures by Region and Type of Service

	Index of Per Capita Expenditures						
Region	Non-federal Hospital Care	General Hospital Care	Psychiatric Hospital Care	Physicians' Services	Dentists' Services	Private Health Insurance	Index of Per Capita Personal Income
United States	100	100	100	100	100	100	100
Northeast	135	129	173	91	99	111	110
Middle Atlantic	122	121	137	103	116	114	112
South Atlantic	81	81	76	84	85	80	87
East North Central	105	103	112	99	91	121	109
East South Central	71	73	58	77	71	71	71
West North Central	99	101	87	84	86	98	96
West South Central	73	76	43	90	71	74	82
Mountain	85	88	69	106	124	87	89
Pacific	107	108	105	148	149	104	112

Source: HEW, *Per Capita Expenditures for Hospital Care,* Research and Statistics Note (August 1969), p. 6.

states, or a differential of less than one-quarter. Here expenditure differentials are small compared to per capita income differences, but this should not be the only point of comparison.[20]

Both the prices of services and the quantity of services consumed figure in the total expenditure for health services. Prices are influenced by the availability of health manpower, the efficiency of its utilization, and the demand for services. The quantity of services consumed depends on the type of service and the income of the recipient of medical care.

As described in chapters 5 and 6 on health manpower, there are large variations in health manpower among regions, among states, and among urban and rural areas of a state. This has an impact on the price of medical services. The number of physicians per 100,000 population in 1966 ranged between 69 (Mississippi and Alaska) and 199 (New York). Similarly, the ratio of dentists varied between 25 (Mississippi) and 69 (Oregon).[21]

The large number of medical specialists in urban areas accentuates the disparity in physician-population ratios. In California, for example, the physician-population ratio varies from 243 (in greater metropolitan areas) to 149 (in adjacent-to-metropolitan areas) to 112 (in isolated rural areas).[22]

Regional differentials in hospital care are significant as measured by both admission rates and days of care per capita. The regional distribution of expenditures may reflect disparities in the availability of services, in the need for services, and in the ability to pay for services. Further, these differences may result from inefficiencies in the supply of services. Expenditure data by region do not clarify these points, and further examination is required.

This chapter has surveyed the sources of medical care funds and their patterns of expenditure to offer an income-expenditure accounting of the medical care dollar. Beyond its descriptive value, such a profile forms a statistical basis for inquiring into the cost and distribution of medical care services.

Notes

1. For example, 47.2 percent of the $54.7 billion increase from 1949-50 to 1970-71 in personal health care expenditures reflected the rise in prices, 16.8 percent was the result of population growth, and 36 percent was attributable to greater utilization of services and the introduction of new medical techniques. D. P. Rice and B. S. Cooper, "National Health Expenditures, 1929-71," *Social Security Bulletin*, January 1972, p. 9.

2. A. M. Skolnik and S. R. Dales, "Social Welfare Expenditures, 1971-72," *Social Security Bulletin*, December 1972, p. 13.

3. This is in accordance with the convention employed for social insurance in the Social Security Administration social welfare expenditure series, where all outlays under various government programs, including those financed through employee contributions are treated as public outlays. See A. M. Skolnik and S. R. Dales, "Social Welfare Expenditures, 1971-72," *Social Security Bulletin*, December 1972.

4. Since tax-supported expenditures have distributive consequences and offer incentives to individuals to behave in particular ways, they may best be considered "public" expenditures. Premium payments are tied to "public" expenditures under Medicare, and in only this sense are public outlays.

5. There are several explanatory notes that should be given about how these figures are derived. (For specific details on definitions, methodology, and sources of data, see B. S. Cooper and N. L. Worthington, "National Health Expenditures, 1929-72," *Social Security Bulletin*, January 1973, pp. 14-19, 40.)

Health expenditures (public and private) for medical training and education are excluded from estimates of total health expenditures. Exceptions include sums from the Department of Defense and the Veterans Administration, and expenditures in hospitals where such expenditures are not separable from the costs of hospital operation. Federal expenditures on medical training and education were $1.3 billion in 1971-72.

The cost of physicians' services appears under the cost of hospital care in several instances: expenditures by the Veterans Administration and the Department of Defense for physicians' services; services of staff physicians of hospitals; etc. Self-employed physicians' services in hospitals are not counted as hospital expenditures.

The cost of drugs used in hospitals is included in hospital care, while anesthesia and X-ray services are sometimes hospital care expenditures and sometimes expenditures for physicians' services.

Research expenditures of drug and medical supply companies are excluded from "expenditures for medical research," since they are included in the cost of the product.

It could be argued that estimates of consumer expenditures are biased downward, since they are typically calculated as a residual—total expenditures less public expenditures and receipts from philanthropy. Admittedly this bias on estimates would be difficult to measure. There are instances, however, where consumer expenditures are included as public expenditures. One example is premium payments under Medicare (see table 3.3); another is workmen's compensation payments.

6. There is some duplication in the amounts designated for Medicare and Medicaid. Medical vendor expenditures under the public assistance programs include the premiums paid into Medicare's supplementary medical insurance trust fund for medical insurance coverage for old-age assistance. Disbursements from the supplementary medical insurance trust fund also include these payments and are thereby counted twice. The amount of premiums paid by states to "buy in" to Medicare for those elderly unable to meet supplementary medical insurance premiums but eligible for old-age assistance under Medicaid rose from $32.1 million in 1966-67 to $137.9 million in 1971-72.

7. HEW, *Social Welfare Expenditures under Public Programs in the United States, 1929-66*, Report no. 25, tables 2-3, p. 210.

8. B. S. Cooper and N. L. Worthington, "National Health Expenditures, 1929-72," *Social Security Bulletin*, January 1973, p. 7.

9. Note that "expenses for prepayment" of health insurance (operating expenses, additions to reserves, and profits) are excluded from personal health care expenditures. This difference between insurance premiums and insurance benefits are counted as consumer expenditures. They are "out-of-pocket" expenditures but they do represent personal health care outlays per se.

10. In all these calculations of personal health costs, the net cost of insurance—the difference between health insurance premiums and benefits paid plus operating expenses—is excluded.

11. This figure was 17 percent for individuals under nineteen years of age and 10 percent for individuals nineteen to sixty-four years of age. B. S. Cooper and N. L. Worthington, "Medical Care Spending for Three Age Groups," *Social Security Bulletin*, May 1972, p. 3.

12. This discussion is based on B. S. Cooper and N. L. Worthington, "Age Differences in Medical Care Spending, Fiscal Year 1972," *Social Security Bulletin*, May 1973, pp. 10-12.

13. *Social Security Bulletin*, December 1971, p. 27.

14. In 1971-72, expenditures for services in intermediate care facilities were added to the Medicaid program (and are classified under "other health services" in the tables). This program affected mainly the aged.

15. HEW, Research and Statistics, *Background: Medical Care, Costs and Prices* (1972), pp. 94-95.

16. Note that consumer expenditures (premiums plus out-of-pocket expenditures) are not necessarily equal to health care costs.

17. Commercial insurance companies have the highest operating costs per enrollee, however—more than three times the Blue Cross rate in 1971. In other words, operating expenses, additions to reserves, and profits consume a large proportion of the insurance premium relative to benefits paid out.

18. Since persons insured by commercial plans are typically healthier, fewer people in this category seek medical care. Also the cost of physicians' visits, if paid out-of-pocket, would be less prohibitive for this group.

19. Prior to Medicare, the aged depended on individual insurance with limited coverage obtained at high rates. According to a 1959 study in Michigan (cited in *Hospital and Medical Economics*, chap. 14), those sixty-five and over were the only age group for which premium payments and out-of-pocket expenditures exceeded the cost of services received. For all other age groups, direct outlays were less than benefits received, the difference being the consequence of access to medical clinics, welfare, insurance paid by an employer, etc.

20. HEW, *Per Capita Expenditures for Hospital Care*, Research and Statistics Note (August 1969), p. 8.

21. HEW, *Health Manpower, United States, 1965-67*, pp. 17-18.

22. HEW, *Health Manpower Source Book*, section 19 (1965), p. 15.

PART II

Productivity and Medical Personnel

4

Labor Productivity

Over the last twenty years (1952-72), labor productivity for the work force in the private economy has been rising at an average rate of 3 percent a year.[1] But the rise in productivity in the medical care sector has generally been substantially less. Some sources explain the difference as the result of inadequate use of capital and lack of planning in the finance and delivery of medical services.

Increasing labor productivity contributes to both increased output and price stability. If the wages of workers increase more than their productivity increases, the price of medical services will rise over time.[2] On the other hand, if wage increases are matched by gains in labor productivity, unit labor costs will be stable; and if labor's share of national income remains unchanged, prices would remain relatively stable. "In fact, the price level generally moves very closely with the ratio of compensation per hour to productivity per hour except for cyclical or other short-term interruptions."[3] Then, only if demand for services increased beyond the supply capacity would prices be pushed higher.

The productivity of physicians, dentists, and allied health workers is examined in this chapter, with a view toward weighing the relative emphasis to be placed on increasing labor productivity as opposed to increasing medical manpower in order to increase output. A 1 percent increase in the productivity of our 200,000 practicing physicians would be roughly equivalent to increasing the supply of physicians by 2,000 (although the "increased supply" would be immobile). If this increased productivity is achieved by greater reliance on auxiliary personnel, the cost of this reliance should be measured against the cost of increasing the supply of physicians. However, the picture is complicated by the fact that physicians have closely guarded professional prerogatives that hamper placing new responsibilities in the hands of auxiliary personnel, while the supply of physicians has not increased substantially despite an excess of qualified candidates for medical schools.

For various reasons, the supply of physicians has been unresponsive to the growing demand for their services. The increased demand was in part stimulated by federal programs that improved financial access to medical services by the poor and the aged. In theory additions to the supply of physicians could be placed where they are most needed, and productivity gains could release physicians to practice in the areas of most pressing medical need. But, if past experience is any gauge, physicians will locate their medical practices to suit their own purposes, not the needs of the community at large. Financial inducements to physicians (in the form of a home, automobile, and guaranteed income) to locate in a specific community do alter physician preferences, but at the price of increasing the cost of medical services.

The medical care industry is similar in many respects to other segments of the expanding service sector of the economy.[4] The production of services is necessarily labor-intensive, so that capital investment in new technology can contribute only to a limited extent to expanding output. Shortages of medical personnel, especially physicians, and growing wage demands from historically underpaid hospital workers have focused attention on the need to increase labor productivity as a short-term solution and as a contributory factor in the long-term solutions.[5]

Definition and Measurement

Most simply, labor productivity is the ratio between the real or physical volume of output and the number of man-hours worked to produce the service.[6] It refers not to an activity but to the results of an activity (the final product or service) and its relationship to labor input. Increased labor productivity means more efficient organization of production or more efficient use of labor.[7] To the consumer, the manner in which the service is rendered may be as important as the number of services provided, but for measuring labor productivity as defined this fact must be ignored.

It is difficult to define the output of medical services in real or physical terms. There is no concept of output unique to the industry, such as tons of steel or kilowatt-hours of electricity. No single measure adequately describes the impact of services on the patient's health. The number of physicians' visits, for example, is only a crude measure of services rendered. When more refined measures of output are specified, they often rely on data for measurement that are not readily available.

As a result, the price or dollar value of the output (the cost of the services) is sometimes taken as a proxy for the physical volume of output. Prices are tied closely to wage rates, since labor is the principal input to health services. Hence the ratio of total sales (deflated for price increases) to man-hours paid (which, unlike hours worked, includes paid holidays, vacations, sick leave, etc.) may show no change, giving a picture of no change in labor productivity.[8]

Not only is output measured in value terms but labor input is as well. Man-hours expended in the delivery of services is a composite of man-hours contributed by workers from different occupational categories (physicians, nurses, allied health professionals, cooks, maintenance employees, etc.). Their contributions are weighted according to the wages and fees they are paid.

There are significant problems in substituting market values for physical measures of output and input to calculate labor productivity. Problems in the delivery of medical services influence the relative pay scales of different workers, and third-party reimbursement systems influence medical care prices in ways that distort productivity. The dilemma is even more acute in measuring total factor productivity, which can *only* be measured in value terms, since the factor input is an aggregation of inputs (such as capital and labor) that are combined according to market prices.[9]

Labor and Total Factor Productivity

Labor is one input—the most important one—in the production of medical services. Each of the other factors of production, including capital, also has a measure of productivity. Thus labor productivity taken by itself is an incomplete measure of productivity. A complete measure includes the contribution of materials and other purchased "intermediate products," land, and capital goods (structures, equipment, and inventory stocks), as well as labor.[10] By taking advantage of economies of scale in providing care, and by coordinating the delivery of medical services that might otherwise be fragmented, the health industry can improve total factor productivity, reducing costs per unit of output.

Use and Misuse of the Concept of Productivity

Labor productivity indexes are used for analyzing the productive capacity of labor and projecting manpower needs under the existing methods of delivering services. Productivity measures relate to technical change, the accumulation of human and physical capital, and the organization of production.

In the face of sharply rising prices for medical care, public officials look to increased labor productivity to reduce costs. Services in the medical sector are necessarily labor-intensive; capital cannot be substituted for labor on a broad scale to increase the productivity of those workers who are not displaced by the capital. Greater potential for boosting labor productivity lies in reorganization of delivery, which may or may not depend on the introduction of new technology. When new technology is introduced (substituting capital for labor), the productivity of labor that remains on the job is increased. Total output of the economy is raised, too, if the displaced workers are reemployed at other tasks. However, introducing new technology may create new jobs only for highly skilled labor while lower skilled labor is displaced.[11]

The usual unit of labor input in labor productivity indexes is man-hours worked by all employees. All classes of employees are counted equally, regardless of their varying contributions to the service provided. One alternative to this approach is to weight man-hours worked by compensation per occupational class. This assumes that wage differentials reflect true productivity differentials because of differences in education, experience, or skill. This may not be the case in fact.

Wage differentials tend to reflect more than productivity differentials. Our economic system builds on the best and most skilled individuals and rewards them accordingly. The contribution of the employee with fewer skills is undervalued, because pay differentials reflect both productivity differentials and incentives to motivate advancement up the organization's ladder. In a large hierarchical organization with many levels of responsibility and authority, there must be corresponding levels of compensation. Sufficient pay differentials must exist from one level to the next to make promotion attractive, or to give a financial incentive for undertaking the additional education required to become a physician, for example.[12] Just as profits are commonly seen as a guide to investment and a means to encourage innovation, so pay differentials in excess of productivity differentials are maintained to attract the most skilled personnel (those who can command the highest fees). The larger and more complex the organization, the larger the pay differential from top to bottom (reducing economies of scale in this respect).

Physicians' fees are not tied to gains in productivity as much as to their economic power in the market. Physicians hold the corresponding power to influence reorganization of delivery to increase output. But if this entails reducing their personal income, they may be expected to resist it.

Technology and Labor Productivity

As defined, labor productivity is a relationship between output (a final product or service) and labor input. However, factor productivity depends somewhat on the degree of technological development. New technology contributes to labor productivity, but it also influences jobs so that some skill categories, mainly the lower-skill occupations, become less productive.

New technology has varying effects on employees of a hospital. It alters the demand for labor, since there is a new mix of tasks to be accomplished. Some workers are displaced from their jobs, while others from the same skill category are retained to operate the new equipment. Workers with specialized training are needed to maintain the equipment and to direct others in its use. The skills of physicians and nurses may be upgraded to enable them to use the technological development in their treatment or diagnostic tasks.

The productivity of all employees whose jobs are affected by the new technology is increased, although this is done in part at the expense of workers who are displaced from their jobs.

The full gain of productivity from new technology may not be realized because of inherent factors in its introduction. The lower-skilled workers who are not displaced now must operate the new equipment. Their new jobs generally are more specialized and standardized. As a result, these workers tend to have a reduced work incentive, since they have even less opportunity to demonstrate individual initiative on the job or to assume responsibility for the quality of their work.

Thus, technology restructures jobs and often diminishes the worker's identification with the tasks he performs. Labor productivity, it has been shown, is related to a worker's understanding of the importance of his job—feeling responsibility for the results of his work and seeing the relationship between his task and the service rendered to people needing it.

In industries where unions are strong, they may engage in productivity bargaining, demanding that pay raises and other benefits be tied to any gains in labor productivity.[13] These demands are warranted if the productivity gains are not attributable mainly to capital investment and technological advance. In service industries, this is the case, since production is labor-intensive. But productivity bargaining in the medical care industry is not likely to be successful, because of the difficulty of measuring real increases in labor productivity. Unions may also be reluctant to enter into agreements that eliminate jobs when unemployment is high. They tend to push instead for restrictive work practices—rules designed to protect the employment of union members. Ironically, important instances of restrictive practices or job redundancy in the medical care industry result from physicians' protection of their own roles by preventing allied health personnel from performing tasks for which they are trained.

Economic criteria, such as cost reduction, and administrative criteria, such as control over the delivery of services, influence the nature of technology employed. Still, a comparative study of health services in Sweden, England, and the United States indicated that substantial differences in the mix of personnel and facilities appear even when fairly similar medical technology is used.[14]

Measurement of Medical Productivity

Difficulties in defining the output and assessing the quality of medical services pose formidable barriers to the measurement of productivity in the medical care industry. Physicians' visits and patients' days in the hospital are frequently taken as general indexes of performance or productivity for physicians and hospital staff. Since the early 1900s, the average length of stay at hospitals has been reduced from forty to eight days. In a generation, doctors have doubled their output of visits. But these are clearly not precise measures of output or improvement in the patient's condition.

The increase in the number of physicians' visits over time may indicate an increase in physician productivity, but it also reflects an increase in the number of paramedical personnel. A drop in the average length of hospital stay over a period of several years can indicate better prevention and treatment of disease as well as increased utilization of ancillary services. Hospitals tend to charge less than cost for daily service and more than cost for ancillary services, which are needed in the first days of the patient's stay. Thus, there is a clear economic incentive to shorten the length of the hospital stay, quite apart from improvement in the patient's condition. There is also an economic incentive to get the patient into the hospital where services such as X-ray treatment or diagnosis will be reimbursed by medical insurance.

Just as the quality of schooling is frequently measured in terms of inputs, such as expenditures per pupil, rather than outputs, such as the student achievement, so doctors often define the quality of medical services by inputs, such as physicians' formal degrees or hospital accreditation, rather than by outputs, such as morbidity, disability, and mortality rates.

Another problem in measuring productivity arises when a patient has multiple disorders. The treatment prescribed affects the whole patient, making it difficult to isolate the impact on each disorder and to assign costs of treatment to each disorder.[15]

When meaningful physical measures are unavailable, productivity is measured by determining the value of the input and output. As the prices of medical services rise, however, it is hard to separate the increase into quality and cost changes.[16]

Delivery and Productivity

The organization of delivery of medical services and of financial reimbursement is a significant factor affecting labor productivity. R. S. Daniels explains:

Physician productivity is a complicated concept which involves a variety of factors. Included among them are the characteristics of the health delivery system, particularly the organization and funding; the social and geographic characteristics of the population served; the negotiations between the provider and the recipient about the quality of the health service; the relative emphasis on crisis, the episodes of illness, prevention of illness, and continuity of health care; the relationship between physician, hospital and patient; and the use of human and physical resources. . . .

The health delivery system and physician productivity are influenced by a complicated mix of economic, social and personal forces which must be better evaluated and understood. Deficiencies in our current data include inadequate methodology to assess the quality of health care, the shortcomings of simple production figures to describe a complicated transactional process, and insufficient information about the social and personal factors which determine physician attitudes and activities.[17]

Over the years, the emphasis has been placed in the health care industry on finding increasing sums of money as the means of solving health problems. But the emphasis now is shifting to more equitable financing of medical care. Techniques for increasing productivity thus stimulate the response of personnel and facilities to the escalating funds being made available. Plans for national health insurance and the development of more health maintenance organizations are part of this trend.

Physician Productivity

The shortage of medical personnel and rising medical care costs brought about concern for improving physicians' productivity. Their productivity may be measured in various ways. One team of researchers has discovered 200 different measures of performance for physicians.[18] The number of visits provided by physicians in private practice is one common measure of productivity.

From 1947 to 1964, the median gross income of physicians in private practice rose at an annual rate of over 6.7 percent, with physicians' fees increasing an average of 3 percent. The *Report of the National Advisory Commission on Health Manpower* (1967) concluded that, since hours of work did not change greatly, the excess of 6.7 over 3.0 (3.7 percent) measured a rise of productivity. Undoubtedly, most of the advances in physicians' productivity over the long run have taken the form of seeing more patients in the same amount of time. Note, however, that an increase in the number of visits handled could signal a decline in productivity, if the quality of service has deteriorated.

House calls over a generation have dropped from 40 percent to 8 percent of physicians' contacts. This shift from house to office and clinic visits has saved doctors a great deal of transportation time. Improvements in medical science, more capital equipment, and more auxiliary personnel at both the hospital and the office have contributed to higher physician productivity. Advances in chemotherapy and the easy and quick prevention of infectious diseases have shortened the course of treatment now required for many conditions, thereby freeing the physician's time. The formation of group practices among specialists has permitted individual physicians to use their time more intensively. Physicians practicing alone devote about the same time to professional activities as physicians in partnerships and groups, but they see one-fifth fewer patients and receive one-fifth less income.

Information technology has entered the medical care field especially in laboratory data systems, patient monitoring systems, and business systems. The productivity of auxiliary medical personnel has been enhanced in particular.[19] Training programs for physicians' assistants, pediatric public health nurse practitioners, and other paramedical personnel have been established in the United States.[20] Paramedical personnel could release physicians from many of the routine tasks they now perform.

The structure of medical practice (solo or group practice) and the method of reimbursement (fee-for-service, salary, or capitation plan) may have a significant impact on physician productivity. Group practice potentially can offer economies of scale, improved technology, review of practice by peers, and other advantages of size, such as greater specialization and accessibility to capital markets.[21] Although group practice may operate with any of the three reimbursement schemes, it is most often coupled with prepayment or capitation plans, while solo practice is generally based on fee-for-service. Some analysts argue that this is what provides more incentives to groups to reduce medical care costs.[22] But this is still an open question.

Hospital Productivity

Since hospitals offer a wide variety of services, it is all but impossible to assemble an overall index of hospital performance (i.e., total factor productivity). Neither the number of services offered nor the number of hospital days is an adequate measure. One approach to the problem is to study the number of employees necessary to staff a general hospital adequately for acute diseases. It may be argued that the lower the number of employee-hours per patient per day the higher the productivity. One study revealed that Swedish nonteaching hospitals average 6.0 employee-hours per patient-day, while Israeli hospitals average 7.6. Israeli teaching hospitals averaged 9.1 hours. Three group-practice hospitals in the United States ranged from 11.7 to 12.6 employee-hours per patient-day, and the median among nine United States community hospitals was 12.6 hours. The differences may relate in part to varying products—for example, fewer frills are provided abroad.[23] A large rise in the number of hospital personnel per patient may point to either a reduction of productivity or an improvement in quality. Hospital personnel averaged 73 per 100 patients in 1945 and 114 per 100 in 1960.

The 1965 Medicare legislation provided that the program was to be neutral about the method of delivery of services: it would not include incentives for altering the delivery system to provide greater efficiency and economy. This feature was won by the professional medical associations. However, utilization review committees were established to check on hospital admissions, lengths of stays, and integration of outpatient and emergency services with hospital care.[24] In Philadelphia, a physician review board checked on excessive admissions to hospitals and lengths of stays. It estimated the average length of stay for sixteen classifications of hospitals. The hospitals were divided into ten categories on the basis of length of stay, with differential payments ranging from 200 percent of the basic rate for the first day to 75 percent for days in excess of the average for the appropriate category.

Coordinating hospital services within a community and better planning within each hospital could contribute significantly to productivity. Duplication in services could be avoided where demand warranted sharing services. Medical care is largely a personal service, and the normal occurrence of emergencies excludes the use of many administrative techniques for raising productivity.

Increased output achieved through economies of scale or higher occupancy rates should be distinguished from productivity gains from more efficient use of factor inputs. With economies of scale, costs per unit of service drop. Larger hospitals also seem to have higher occupancy rates, more lengthy stays, higher expenses per patient-day, and smaller relative financing by patient income. More costly procedures and services help explain the higher cost. Frequently there is also redundancy of expensive equipment among nearby hospitals, so that none of the technology is used to capacity.

Some economists have suggested guidelines to determine whether a hospital should continue in operation: if occupancy falls below 75 percent, the hospital should be closed. Of course, consideration should be given to the overall medical requirements of the community and the nature of the services provided by each hospital. A hospital bed unoccupied costs about 75 percent of its costs when occupied. Excess capacity is a troublesome problem, since it leads to increased use and waste.

Reimbursement formulas for services rendered by hospitals, extended care facilities, and professional personnel are important in determining the productivity of the health care industry. Over the years, hospitals have been reimbursed on the basis of costs or customary and reasonable charges, so that providers are guaranteed recovery of costs, regardless of the quality of their performances. When reimbursement is based on costs, the incentives to keep costs down are admittedly weakened, and hence productivity is affected adversely.[25] In the late 1960s, almost two-thirds of the Blue Cross plans reimbursed hospitals on a cost basis. A 1968 study by the Social Security Administration discussed the history of hospital cost reimbursement, giving attention to the cost items that some argue should be applied to the hospital patient's bill. These include educational and research costs, funds required for replacement, modernization, and growth, and amortization of the principal of capital indebtedness.[26]

There are various ways third parties could try to hold costs down. For example, insurance companies could set ceilings on daily costs or limit the rise of daily costs from year to year. Recognition could be given to justifiable variations in costs incurred by different hospitals providing the same services, but efficiency in plant operation must be encouraged. When a hospital's costs depart substantially from those of other hospitals of similar size, scope of service, and utilization in the same geographic area, maximum reimbursement should be negotiated between third parties and hospitals. A target for costs can be defined and the efficient hospital given part of the difference between the target and its lower costs, while high-cost hospitals are penalized.[27]

Various studies have been made of the savings in admissions and hospital days according to the type of insurance program used. Estimates of savings in admissions range from one-fifth to two-fifths (see table 4.1). Insurance coverage of hospital benefits alone results in excessive use of hospitals and low use of less expensive alternatives. To economize on hospital admissions, insurance should cover both hospital and out-of-hospital care (including extended care facilities' services, home services, etc.), so as to encourage the most appropriate care and minimize the total cost of illness. This, by itself, would provide no particular incentive to physicians to eliminate unnecessary care. However, prepayment of physicians on a capitation basis would provide this incentive and discourage unnecessary recourse to surgery. The reimbursement formula must also take into account the objective of maintaining or improving quality; otherwise, economizing may be accomplished by deterioration in the quality of care.

Increasing Medical Output

According to Jerome Mark, "productivity measures for service-type industries are not reliable measures for identifying either the magnitude or the direction of change in productivity."[28] Nonetheless, analysis of labor and total factor productivity in the provision of

TABLE 4.1   Number of Hospital Admissions by Type of Coverage

Coverage	Admissions per 1,000 Enrollees
Steelworker experience	
Standard Blue Cross contract	135
Private insurance contract	146
Kaiser Foundation Health Plan	113
All United States Blue Cross plans	136
Group practice plans	
Kaiser Foundation Health Plan, California	97
Group Health Cooperative, Seattle	93
Group Health Association, Washington, D.C.	79
Health Insurance Plan of Greater New York	78

Source: W. J. McNerney, *Hospital and Medical Economics* (1962), vol. 1, p. 515.

medical services is useful for discussing proposed measures to increase output. Just as the quality of medical care cannot be defined precisely but steps can still be taken to improve quality, so even if changes in productivity cannot be measured accurately, delivery systems can be designed to improve output. The National Commission on Productivity undertook a study in 1973 at the request of the Cost of Living Council to examine productivity improvement opportunities in the health services industry.

The study will explore the incidence of inflation by sector (nursing home, hospital, physicians), the anatomy of recent large increases in health care expenditures by sector and the structural arrangements that may impede productivity improvements, such as the bias of government and private health insurance toward hospitalization, the most expensive mode of service, and away from outpatient care.[29]

Factors that contribute to the growth in output of medical services include (1) increased inputs (labor, equipment, etc.), (2) improved quality of labor through education, (3) achievement of economies of scale and higher utilization, and (4) technical change or advances in knowledge. Various measures have been proposed to increase the output of medical services by increasing manpower inputs, and increasing the productivity of labor.[30] Each proposal must be analyzed in the context of the need for reform of the finance of medical services (to reward efficiency) and the need for reorganization of delivery of medical care (to increase total factor productivity). Increased productivity raises output, contributing to economic growth, if the hours worked are not reduced. However, some gains in productivity are translated into a reduced work schedule (for physicians as well as hourly workers) permitting more leisure time.

Without proper financial control, increasing inputs to medical care would prove wasteful and would lead to further inflation in medical care prices. Overutilization and waste of medical resources would be equivalent to a decline in productivity. Productivity analysis serves as a guide to organization of production in the way that cost-effectiveness analysis aids in decisions about what services to provide. Both productivity analysis and cost-effectiveness analysis are guides to resource allocation.

Proposals to increase medical manpower (or free medical manpower from present tasks) urge greater attention to preventive medicine and breaking down occupational rigidities. Reducing the incidence or severity of disease by early diagnosis is an alternative in the first instance to increasing the number of physicians to cure diseases that might have been avoided or treated less expensively before they became far advanced. One salutory effect of rising food prices is that families may be paying greater attention to the importance of a balanced diet to protect their pocketbooks as well as their health.

Another alternative to increasing the number of physicians is to alter the task allocation between physicians and paramedical personnel. The division of labor now is bound by tradition, assigned by status, and reinforced by legal restrictions. New categories of health personnel offer a potential for breaking the rigidity of the present system.[31] Sylvester Berki and Alan Heston note:

> Entry of new manpower is limited both by training capacities and by the licensing system, which not only requires legal legitimization prior to practice but which countenances fifty licensing standards in fifty states, as well as a variety of certification procedures administered within medical specialties that will determine, for example, whether a heart surgeon can make his own examination of the lungs of his patient.[32]

Proposals to upgrade the place of preventive medicine and physician assistants offer significant potential to lessen the physician shortage if professional, legal, and political difficulties can be overcome.

Notes

1. National Commission on Productivity, *Second Annual Report* (March 1973), p. 62.

2. Wages of workers, as used here, include wages paid to low-skilled hospital workers as well as the fees collected by highly trained physicians. This aggregation is misleading since it does not suggest the differences in ability to command higher incomes and to shape the organization of delivery to enhance productivity.

3. H. Stein, "The Meaning of Productivity," in *The Meaning and Measurement of Productivity*, Bureau of Labor Statistics Bulletin no. 1714 (September 1971), p. 1.

4. V. Fuchs, *The Service Economy* (1968). Over one-half of GNP is attributable to service industries, and two-thirds of the labor force is employed in these industries, but the productivity of service sector employees is 30 percent to 50 percent lower than the productivity of factory workers. The comparison may be inappropriate, however, because of differences in the nature and valuation of the output.

5. For a review of the need to improve productivity throughout the economy,

see "Productivity: Our Biggest Undeveloped Resource," *Business Week* (special issue), September 9, 1972, p. 79.

6. See J. W. Kendrick, "The Productivity Factor in Phase 2," *National Industrial Conference Board Record,* March 1972, pp. 28-29. For further discussion of the measurement of productivity, see J. W. Kendrick and D. Creamer, *Measuring Company Productivity: Handbook with Case Studies,* National Industrial Conference Board Studies in Business Economics no. 89 (1965). On an introductory level, see S. Fabricant, *A Primer on Productivity* (1969); also *International Encyclopedia of the Social Sciences* (1968), s.v. "productivity."

7. Irving Siegel argues, "conventional productivity measures 'do not so much reveal the changing intrinsic efficiency of labor as the changing effectiveness with which labor is used in conjunction with other factors of production.' " See "Measurement of Productivity," in National Commission on Productivity, *Conference on an Agenda for Economic Research on Productivity* (April 1973), p. 18.

8. The price indexes used to deflate the value of output are conceptually equivalent to indexes that use physical quantities combined with price weights. See J. W. Kendrick, "The Productivity Factor in Phase 2," *National Industrial Conference Board Record,* March 1972, pp. 32-33.

9. Labor and capital are aggregated using their unit costs as weights. These weights can also be viewed as the proportion of current dollar output earned by each input (factor share).

10. See M. I. Nadiri, "Some Approaches to the Theory of Measurement of Total Factor Productivity: A Survey," *Journal of Economic Literature,* December 1970, pp. 1137-1177. Economic depreciation plays a crucial role in measurement of capital input productivity and total factor productivity. Depreciation depends on the decline in the efficiency of capital goods. See an exchange of views between D. W. Jorgenson and Z. Griliches, and Edward F. Denison, *The Measurement of Productivity,* Brookings Institution Reprint no. 244 (1972).

11. See J. A. Mark, "Concepts and Measures of Productivity," in *The Meaning and Measurement of Productivity,* Bureau of Labor Statistics Bulletin no. 1714 (September 1971), p. 11, for estimates of productivity gains from the shift of workers between sectors in the private economy, and the shift from production to nonproduction work in manufacturing.

12. See S. Marglin, "What Do Bosses Do? The Origins and Functions of Hierarchy in Capitalist Production," Harvard Institute of Economic Research, Discussion Paper no. 222 (November 1971), for an analysis of the relation between hierarchy, technology, and the organization of production.

13. See National Commission on Productivity, *Productivity Bargaining: The British and American Experience* (1972).

14. O. W. Anderson, "Styles of Planning Health Services: The United States, Sweden, and England," *International Journal of Health Services* 1, no. 2 (May

1972): 106-20. See also E. A. Krause, "Health and the Politics of Technology," *Inquiry*, September 1971, pp. 51-59.

15. On the relationship between costs, product mix, and level of output in the hospital, see R. E. Berry, Jr., "Product Heterogeneity and Hospital Cost Analysis," *Inquiry*, March 1970, pp. 70-75.

16. See M. W. Reder, "Some Problems in the Measurement of Productivity in the Medical Care Industry," in V. R. Fuchs, ed., *Production and Productivity in the Service Industries* (1969), pp. 95-131. See also A. Scitovsky, "Cost of Medical Treatment: Reply," *American Economic Review*, September 1968, pp. 938-40.

17. R. S. Daniels, "Physician Productivity and the Hospital," *Inquiry*, September 1969, pp. 57-78.

18. P. B. Price et al., "Measurement of Physician Performance," *Journal of Medical Education*, February 1964, pp. 203-11.

19. G. O. Barnett and A. Robbins, "Information Technology and Manpower Productivity," *Journal of the American Medical Association*, July 28, 1969, pp. 546-48.

20. C. U. Letourneau, "The Assistant Physician," *Hospital Management* 105 (April 1968): 55. See also E. H. Estes, "The Critical Shortage—Physicians and Supporting Personnel," *Annals of Internal Medicine*, November 1968, pp. 957-62.

21. F. E. Graham II, "Group vs. Solo Practice: Arguments and Evidence," *Inquiry*, June 1972, pp. 49-60; also M. W. Reder, "Some Problems in the Measurement of Productivity in the Medical Care Industry," in V. R. Fuchs, ed., *Production and Productivity in the Service Industries* (1969), pp. 115-21.

22. J. P. Newhouse, "The Economics of Group Practice," *Journal of Human Resources*, winter 1973, pp. 37-56.

23. "Staffing the General Hospital for Acute Diseases," *Medical Care*, January-March 1965, pp. 11-13.

24. See H. M. Somers and A. R. Somers, *Medicare and the Hospitals* (1967), pp. 62-70.

25. See M. W. Reder, "Some Problems in the Measurement of Productivity in the Medical Care Industry," in V. R. Fuchs, ed., *Production and Productivity in the Service Industries* (1969), pp. 107-13; W. J. McNerney, *Hospital and Medical Economics* (1962), vol. 2, pp. 970-71; U.S. Senate, *Hearings on Health Care in America* (1968), pp. 517-20.

26. HEW, Social Security Administration, *Reimbursement Incentives for Hospital and Medical Care, Objectives, and Alternatives* (1968), pp. 1-25.

27. See M. V. Pauly, "Efficiency, Incentives and Reimbursement for Health Care," *Inquiry*, March 1970, pp. 114-31.

28. J. A. Mark, "Concepts and Measures of Productivity," in *The Meaning and Measurement of Productivity*, Bureau of Labor Statistics Bulletin no. 1714 (September 1971), p. 14.

29. National Commission on Productivity, *Second Annual Report* (March 1973), p. xix.

30. Useful references on the analysis of manpower projections include H. E. Klarman, "Economic Aspects of Projecting Requirements for Health Manpower," *Journal of Human Resources* 4, no. 3 (fall 1969): 360-76; I. Butler, "Health Manpower Research: A Survey," *Inquiry*, December 1967, pp. 5-41; W. L. Hansen, "An Appraisal of Physician Manpower Projections," *Inquiry*, March 1970, pp. 102-13.

31. S. E. Berki, "The Economics of New Types of Health Personnel," *Macy Conference on Intermediate Level Health Personnel in the Delivery of Direct Health Services*, Williamsburg, Va., November 12-14, 1972; E. Forgotson and J. Forgotson, "Innovations and Experiments in Uses of Health Manpower—A Study of Selected Programs and Problems in the United Kingdom and Soviet Union," RAND Corporation Publication P-4074 (April 1969).

32. S. E. Berki and A. W. Heston, "The Nation's Health: Some Issues," *Annals*, January 1972, p. xii. For a discussion of medical licensure laws, see E. H. Forgotson and J. L. Cook, "Innovations and Experiments in the Uses of Health Manpower—The Effect of Licensure Laws," *Law and Contemporary Problems* 35, no. 4 (winter 1967): 731-50; M. Friedman, "Occupational Licensure," *Capitalism and Freedom* (1962), chap. 9, pp. 137-60.

5

Professional Manpower

Medical personnel are increasingly in demand. In 1930 Americans saw a physician an average of two to three times a year; by 1964 the figure had risen to more than five times. The annual admissions to general hospitals in those years increased from 56 per thousand population to 145. Average hospital stays were 0.9 days per year per person in 1930 and 1.3 days in 1964. Moreover, increasingly complex and intense medical care is being given to patients.[1]

Additional health manpower is clearly needed. Rising income and higher educational achievement encourage the public demand for more and more medical care, and there is a deficit of personnel currently. The large rise in the number of older people in the population also contributes to the deficit. Thus from 1930 to 1980, the population aged sixty-five and over will increase 2½ times, as compared to 2 times for all ages. Older people require more medical attention than the population as a whole (see table 5.1). From 1950 to 1965, the demand for health care rose 25 percent for all ages but 50 percent for those sixty-five and over.[2]

One factor contributing to the personnel shortage is the strenuous competition among fields for highly skilled manpower. Professional, technical, and kindred workers rose from about 5 million in 1950 to

TABLE 5.1   Health Care of Older Population Compared to Total Population

Health Care or Need	All Ages	65 and Over
Bed disability, days per year	8	16
Physicians' visits, per person, per year	5.3	6.8
Annual hospital days, per 100 persons	85.1	177.8

Source: HEW, *Physicians for a Growing America: Report of the Surgeon General's Consultant Group on Medical Education* (1959), p. 5.

more than 8 million in 1963. The proportion of white collar workers rose from 35 to 45 percent, while service workers rose only from 10 to 13 percent, from 1947 to 1965.[3]

The Increase in Medical Personnel

The number of medical personnel of all types rose from 1955 to 1965, ranging from an 8 percent increase in pharmacists to a 70 percent increase in clinical laboratory personnel. The rise in physicians (20 percent) was somewhat greater than the population growth and the rise in dentists less (15 percent).

Within each professional category, the rate of growth varied among types of employment (see table 5.2).[4] While estimates of personnel vary to some extent, as assumptions and definitions vary, the general trend is clear in all sources. From 1900 to 1967, for example, the rise in the number of physicians has been relatively small, while the increase in nurses has been tremendous.[5]

Much has been said in recent years about the need to combine increases in professional manpower with the larger influx of semi-professional and technical help. This mix of personnel has been proceeding at a great rate since at least 1900. In that year, health occupations employed 350,000 workers, 35 percent of them physicians and 9 percent dentists. By 1967, employment was up to 3,362,000. Physicians had dropped to 9 percent and dentists to 3 percent. The outstanding rise during that period was from 4 percent to 20 percent for registered nurses (see table 5.3). From 1950 to 1967, the rise in nurses was about five times the rise in physicians and dentists.

In that same period, health personnel rose 100 percent but

TABLE 5.2 Trends in the Supply of Health Manpower

Profession and Employment	Manpower (Thousands)				Percentage Increase, 1955-65
	1950	1955	1960	1965	
Physicians (M.D. and D.O.)	233	255	275	305	20
Active physicians (M.D.)	209	228	247	278	22
Private practice (M.D. and D.O.)	168.1	169.9	179.2	190.7	12
Training (M.D.)	21.4	31.0	37.6	43.5	40
Other nonfederal (M.D.)	16.8	25.2	27.3	34.4	37
Other federal (M.D.)	12.6	13.0	14.2	18.9	45
Nursing and related personnel	734	886	1,085	1,366	54
Professional nurses in practice	375	416*	504	600*	44
Practical nurses in practice	138	172*	206	266*	55
Aides, orderlies, and attendants employed	221	298*	375	500	68
Radiologic technologists[†]	31	45*	60	70	56
Clinical laboratory personnel[†‡]	30	50	68	85	70
Dentists and allied personnel[§]	170	197	221	241	22
Total dentists	87.2	94.9	101.9	109.3	15
Active nonfederal dentists	75.3	76.1	82.6	86.3	13
Dental hygienists (active)	7.0	9.8*	12.5	15.1	54
Dental assistants (employed)	55.2	68.9*	82.5	91.0	32
Dental laboratory technicians (employed)	21.0	23.0*	25.0	25.5	11
Pharmacists (active)	101	109*	117	118	8

Source: HEW, *Health Resources Statistics,* Public Health Service Publication no. 1509 (1965).

*Based on a straight-line interpolation between the closest available data points.
[†]All figures are rough estimates.
[‡]Excludes physicians.
[§]Includes all dentists, whether active or inactive.

TABLE 5.3 Estimated Employment in Health Occupations, 1900 and 1967

Health Occupation	Number of Workers		Percentage of Workers	
	1900	1967	1900	1967
Total	350,000	3,362,000	100	100
Physicians (M.D. and D.O.)	123,000	305,500	35	9
Medical-related personnel	60,000	651,300	17	19
Dentists	30,000	98,700	9	3
Dental-related personnel	5,000	137,000	1	4
Registered nurses	12,000	659,000	4	20
Other nursing personnel	109,000	1,095,000	31	33
Environmental personnel	} 11,000	65,000	} 3	2
All other health personnel		350,500		10

Source: HEW, *Report to the President and the Congress: The Allied Health Professions Personnel Training Act of 1966, as Amended* (1969), p. 21.

physicians rose only about 40 percent. But for the period from 1967 to 1980 the anticipated rise for all health personnel is 50 percent and for physicians it is 33 percent, indicating a change in the trend. [6] Another indication is the fact that the ratio of physicians to total health personnel has declined rather modestly in later years as compared to the earlier years of the 1900-67 period (see table 5.4). But

TABLE 5.4   Ratio of Physicians to Total Number of Health Personnel

Year	Proportion of Physicians	Average Drop in Percentage per Year
1900	35%	—
1950	13%	0.44
1967	9%	0.23
1980*	8%	0.08

*Estimate.

the small improvement of the ratios for 1967-80 comes in the face of strong measures by the federal government to increase the number of physicians.

Estimates of the supply and requirements for health personnel are subject to reservations.

Any discussion of requirements for allied health manpower must recognize that the assumptions underlying an analysis of supply versus demand are not agreed upon, and that much essential data are not available. The most important lack is an objective against which our present ability to provide health services can be measured. These difficulties are especially apparent in attempting to determine or forecast requirements for medical and dental allied manpower, since requirements are related more to rising standards and demands for health care than to simple growth in population.

There are, however, a number of estimates of national needs for allied health manpower which, while not based on uniform assumptions or definition of requirements, are in sufficient agreement to allow some general conclusions to be drawn. Among these concepts or approaches to the determination of present requirements for allied health manpower are: budgeted vacancies, ratios to total population, professional judgments of need, ratios to patient populations, requirements per unit of service, and staffing patterns.

Since the production and employment of trained allied health manpower over the next decade are of immediate interest and importance, "requirements" is given the special meaning of the number of workers who could find employment without major changes in the health system, in manpower utilization patterns, or in the economics of health care. The term is not used here to represent the number of health workers that would be necessary in order to have a fully effective or adequate health system, or to achieve some improved level of national health.[7]

Thus, estimates of health personnel calculated by different sources differ to some extent (see table 5.5).

TABLE 5.5   Estimates of Health Workers and Physicians

Source or Basis of Estimate	For Year	Total Number of Health Workers	Number of Physicians
Department of Health, Education,	1967	3,362,000	305,000
and Welfare	1975	4,421,000	361,000
	1980	5,038,000	407,000
Public Health Service	1966	2,786,000	297,000
Professional judgment	1975	3,735,000	400,000
Estimates by personnel in	1975	3,798,000	425,000
the most populous regions			
Bureau of Labor Statistics	1975	3,978,000	390,000

Sources: HEW, *Report to the President and the Congress: The Allied Health Professions Personnel Training Act of 1966, as Amended* (1969), p. 34; HEW, *Health Manpower Perspective: 1967,* p. 15.

Health Personnel and the Labor Force

The number of health personnel has been rising proportionally much more than the labor force as a whole, largely because of rising incomes for health workers, rising expenditures for health care, and the growth of health facilities, especially hospitals. In 1900, health occupations accounted for 342,700 workers, 1.2 percent of the civilian labor force. In 1940, there were 1,059,000 workers, 2.1 percent; in 1960, 2.9 percent; in 1966, 3.7 percent; and in 1975, these occupations are projected to reach 4.3 percent. The rise is especially large in the latest period. From 1900 to 1975 the growth rate was .04 percent per year, while from 1960 to 1975 it will be .10 percent.

The growth in employment in health occupations reflects major changes in the composition of the labor force, with white collar workers now outnumbering blue collar workers, and service workers outnumbering farm workers. From 1940 to 1965, growth in employment in health occupations as a proportion of the total labor force mirrored growth in employment in the service sector of the economy.[8] And of seventy-one industries, only seven grew more rapidly than health in the 1950s.[9]

The importance of the expansion of health facilities for increased employment in health services is suggested by the following: in the decade 1950-60, the number of persons employed in all health services rose 54 percent, but the number employed in hospitals rose 70 percent while all other employment in health services rose only 32 percent.[10]

Trends in the growth of health personnel reflect current social developments and concerns to some extent. Thus the number of medical personnel rose 34 percent from 1950 to 1960, but environmental personnel increased 92 percent and research personnel 300 percent. Still, these fast-growing fields accounted for only 1.0 and 1.3 percent of all health manpower in 1960.[11]

The Need for Additional Health Manpower

A comparison of allied health requirements and supplies of manpower available for the years 1967, 1975, and 1980 reveals the current and anticipated deficits. The requirements for dental allied manpower in those years are 165,700, 202,000, and 246,000, respectively, and the deficits will be 28,700, 63,000, and 95,000. In 1966, professional and technical personnel in hospitals were estimated at 1,332,100. To give optimum care, the country needed 257,200 or 19 percent more. By 1975, 2,000,000 more will be needed.

A broader picture of health occupations shows personnel of 2,417,000 in 1965 and a rise to 3,735,000 (about a 50 percent increase) by 1975, in estimates based on professional judgments. A somewhat smaller rise is estimated by personnel in the region with the largest number of personnel. The 1965-75 growth estimates (professional judgment) vary by categories. For example, physicians are expected to increase by almost 40 percent, but professional and technical personnel exclusive of physicians, dentists, and nurses will rise more than 80 percent. Auxiliary personnel continue to increase more than professionals, but not as much more as in earlier years, and the rate of advance is uneven.

A more detailed study covering twenty-nine occupations in hospitals found that hospital personnel numbered 1,380,800 in 1966 and that 108,000 more were urgently needed. The researchers estimated that 275,000 additional workers would be required to provide optimum care.[12]

The Shortage of Physicians

A shortage of physicians is evident from various guides: those now practicing can earn spectacularly high incomes; the public has difficulty obtaining appointments; there are long queues for physicians' services; manpower has been diverted away from practice and into teaching, research, and administration; rising demands are being made on interns and residents; and long hours are kept by many physicians. This last indicator, moreover, leads to understatement of the deficits: at normal working hours per day, the shortage of physicians would be much greater than it is generally estimated by simple count.

It was recently estimated that only 85 percent of the openings for interns and residents were being filled.[13] From 1931 to 1959, the number of physicians enrolled in training programs rose from 7,200 to 37,110, a rise about eight times as great as the rise in the number of physicians as a whole.[14]

Authorities generally stress more doctors as the major solution to the problem of supply deficiencies. But it is clear that merely increasing the number may fail to solve a key issue—optimum distribution. The simple solution of more doctors may be merely therapy imposed on a malfunctioning system. Health professionals and facilities must be used more efficiently, services must be distributed more fairly to all sectors of the population, and medical care must be offered at costs within reasonable bounds.[15]

In discussions of the doctor shortage, much attention has been devoted to the physician-population ratio (PPR). This crude ratio may be very misleading, since it is affected by such factors as the mix of capital and physicians, the substitution of drugs for physicians, and the type of medical practice. Greater use of capital and drugs may bring a reduced PPR; psychiatric practice, which is costly in manpower, increases the PPR. The changing age structure of the society and movements of population to denser areas tend to increase the PPR without alleviating the shortage of physicians.

From 1870 to 1929, the number of physicians rose from 60,000 to 152,503, but the population rose substantially more, so that the PPR declined from 150 to 125.[16] From 1931 to 1959, the PPR for active physicians rose from 121 to 128. But the ratio of active *nonfederal* physicians to the *civilian* population was roughly unchanged; and the PPR for physicians in private practice dropped from 108 to 92.[17]

Although a falling PPR concerned many by the 1950s, it was possible to improve the ratio by what Dr. Louis Lasagna called "statistical legerdemain":

In 1964, after a conference called by the Health Resources Advisory Committee, all interns and residents, the June medical graduates, physicians with temporary foreign addresses, and others whose addresses were temporarily not known were included in the calculation of the physician-population ratio. As a result, the ratio "rose" but there were no more doctors than before.[18]

From 1959 to 1967, the number of physicians rose from 241,000 to 294,000. During this period the proportion of physicians who graduated from United States schools declined from 92 to 82 percent. The estimated supply of active physicians was 311,000 in 1968, and it is expected to be 361,500 in 1975. The PPR for this period is expected to rise from 151 to 160.[19] The sources of medical graduates for these years are given in table 5.6. The large rise of

TABLE 5.6   United States and Foreign Medical Graduates

	1968	1975
Graduates of United States schools	7,973	9,770
Graduates of foreign schools	5,000	3,000
Deaths of physicians	4,360	4,970

Source: HEW, *Health Manpower Source Book,* section 20 (1969), p. 76.

United States graduates (about one-fourth) is offset by a decline of foreign graduates by 2,000 and loss through death of 610 more doctors than in the earlier year.

Table 5.7 shows the movement of the PPR from 1870 to 1975. The ratio has risen in recent years, especially since 1963.

It must be clear by now that the significance of the PPR is limited. The supply of physicians available depends on the type of physician and the population segment being measured. Table 5.8, for example, shows three kinds of PPRs. The number of federal physicians accounts for a substantial difference in these ratios.

TABLE 5.7   Periodic Changes in Physician-Population Ratio

Period	Average Annual Change in PPR
1870-1920	minus 0.40%
1931-1959	plus 0.25%
1959-1967	plus 0.60%
1963-1967	plus 1.75%
1968-1975	plus 1.30%

Many aspects of medical practice have an impact on the PPR. Especially important is the productivity of the doctors. The National Advisory Commission on Health Manpower notes that although the supply of doctors in relation to population is rising, there are substantial shortages, because less-than-effective use is made of physicians. The commission estimates that there is a real shortage of primary doctors and that from 1965 to 1975, there will be a 50 percent increase in the services *directed* by physicians. Inefficiencies arise in part from the failure of doctors to use the referral process adequately and to use the information available to primary physicians effectively. Inadequate initial access to the primary physician is also subject to criticism.

The economy as a whole increases man-hour output by 3 percent a year on the average. If medicine performed as well, the increase in available doctors' services would more than equal the services available from the annual output of United States medical school graduates.[20]

TABLE 5.8   Physician-Population Ratios, 1963 and 1967

Physician and Population Segment	Physicians per 100,000 Population	
	1963	1967
All physicians, active and nonactive, to total population	149	158
Nonfederal physicians providing patient care to civilian population	124	130
Nonfederal physicians in office-based practice providing patient care to civilian population	99	100

Source: HEW, *Health Manpower, United States, 1965-1967,* p. 16.

The view of many is that the portion of the health care sector devoted to delivery of medical services has not shared the great advances of the rest of the economy in technology. The National Advisory Committee on Health Manpower reported in 1967:

While medicine has participated in the scientific revolution, the provision of care has been little affected by the technological changes. Computers are now a major aid to management in almost every industry, but not in the health care sector. Increasing substitution of capital for labor and advances in communication and transportation have taken place in many service industries, but not in medical care. Yet, it is only by exploiting the innovations and technologies of other sectors and by developing new techniques appropriate to its own problems that the health care system can adequately respond to social change and scientific advance.[21]

Any rise in the number of physicians depends most on an increased output of medical school graduates. From 1930 to 1960, the number of graduates rose steadily. Expansion of existing schools and development of new schools helped. If the expansion rate of these years were to continue until 1975, there would then be 9,000 new graduates each year. Assuming an annual influx of 750 graduates from foreign institutions, the number of physicians would rise to 318,400 by 1975. But to maintain a PPR of 141, 330,000 physicians would be required, and an annual graduate rate of 11,000 would be needed.[22]

The number of students who enter medical schools depends on the number of qualified applicants, when there are fewer applicants than openings. However, at present the number of openings appears to be the constraint. The number of medical school applicants is far outpacing the positions open to first-year medical and osteopathic students.[23]

Growth of the Specialties

The number of active physicians in specialties has been increasing in recent years more rapidly than the number in general practice or in training (see figure 5.9). Almost every specialty increased in number of practitioners. Only pulmonary diseases, colon and rectal surgery, and occupational medicine declined slightly.

General practitioners are declining both absolutely and relatively. In recent years only a small percentage of medical students have chosen general practice. Increased specialization involves large risks

FIGURE 5.9   Active Physicians by Type of Practice

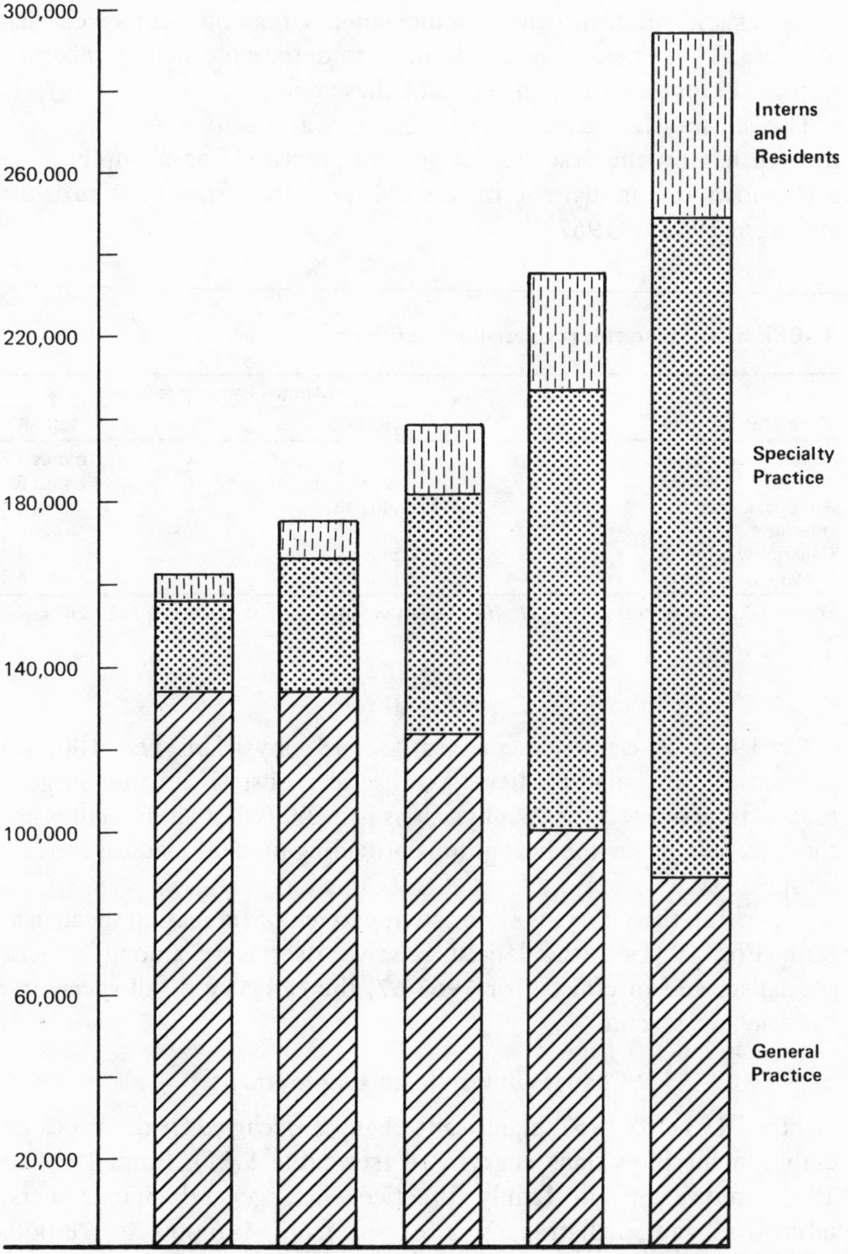

Source: HEW, *Health Manpower Source Book,* section 20 (1969), p. 43.

to doctors, as medical practice changes in response to technical advances and other institutional movements, making some specialties obsolete. These risks suggest the need to deflate physicians' incomes to some extent to offset the costs of these risks.

The substantial increases in specialty practice to some extent fill the gap left by the desertion of general practice. For example, table 5.10 shows the annual rise in selected specialties from 1931 to 1960 and from 1963 to 1967.

TABLE 5.10   Increases in Specialty Practitioners

	Annual Percentage Change	
Type of Practitioner	1931-60	1963-67
General practitioners	minus 0.7	minus 1.5
All active physicians	plus 2.0	plus 3
All specialists	plus 13	plus 6
Internists	plus 15	plus 5
General surgeons	plus 10	plus 4
Surgery specialists	plus 67	plus 4

Source: Calculated from HEW, *Health Manpower Source Book*, section 20 (1969), tables 41, 42.

By 1965, internists accounted for 45 physicians per 100,000 population; internal medicine, pediatrics, obstetrics, and surgery together accounted for 79 physicians per 100,000. (These figures are the "average in six medical groups providing prepaid medical service, by specialty."[24])

In general, then, there is a consistent pattern of increasing specialization. For 1931-60 the largest relative rises were among surgery specialists and internists; for 1963-67, the category of all specialists had the largest gain.

Changes in Physician Employment

From 1931 to 1957, significant changes occurred in the types of employment physicians engaged in (see table 5.11). From 1950 to 1965, physicians in family practice, i.e., general practitioners, internists, and pediatricians, dropped from 116,000 to 98,000. Physicians not in private practice experienced the largest proportional increase in numbers—from 17 percent to 34 percent. This group

TABLE 5.11   Increase in Physicians by Type of Employment, 1931-57

Type of Employment	Percentage Rise
All employment situations	46%
Private practice	16%
Hospital service	274%
Teaching, research, and other	268%
Retired	79%

includes doctors in teaching, research, public health, and industry. Those in training programs rose from 21,000 to 43,000—roughly double, like those in nonprivate practice.[25]

In 1966, general practitioners depended almost wholly on office-based practice, while substantial numbers of specialists engaged in hospital and other practice (see table 5.12). From 1950 to 1965, the proportion of medical and osteopathic doctors in private practice dropped from 72 to 63 percent. Offsetting this were gains in nonfederal practice (from 7 to 11 percent) and in training (from 9 to 15 percent).[26] The type of employment varied among the major specialties in 1963, as shown in table 5.13.

Comments on the Shortage

Experts estimated in 1968 that we would need 16,000 medical graduates each year to maintain present standards and that a genuine shortage of 50,000 doctors existed. About 5,000 communities had no doctor. The ratio of physicians devoting themselves to family medicine fell from 76 per 100,000 population in 1950 to 50 per 100,000 in 1968.[27]

TABLE 5.12   Percentages of Physicians in Different Employment Situations

Employment Situation	All Specialties	General Practice	Medical Specialties
Office-based practice	65%	91%	59%
Hospital training	16%	1%	18%
Hospital-based practice	12%	7%	13%
Other professional activities	7%	1%	10%

Source: Calculated from HEW, *Health Manpower, United States, 1965-1967*, p. 19.

TABLE 5.13   Types of Employment Among Major Specialties, 1963

Type of Employment	Number of Active Physicians	Percentages by Major Specialty				
		General	Medical	Surgical	Psych. and Neurol.	Other
Total	261,730	32	21	30	7	10
Private practice	174,974	39	20	32	5	4
Training						
Intern	9,517	89	6	4	*	1
Resident	29,002	2	29	44	13	12
Federal service	18,551	21	25	25	9	20
Other nonfederal	29,686	12	24	15	14	35

Source: HEW, *Health Manpower Source Book,* section 18 (1964), table 18, p. 31.

*Less than 0.5 percent.

Shortages are common in most specialties. For example, the ratio of pediatricians to children under fifteen was 1:6,135 in 1961. One expert estimated that the average pediatrician cares for approximately 1,000 children. Using this guideline, we would need over 69,000 pediatricians, more than six times the number in full-time practice in 1961. However, if the role of the pediatrician excludes general care of children, the 1961 ratio is "not far from adequate."[28]

The shortage of doctors relates to the narrow sources from which they are drawn. A study by W. J. McNerney and his associates throws some light on these problems. For thirty years, according to that study, the physician-population ratio has been constant at 141 (per 100,000). Increased productivity has helped to solve the problem of deficits but it also contributes to increased demands for medical personnel.

There are many reasons to be pessimistic about the ability of further increases in productivity to close the gap between demand and supply. These are:

1. The supply of physicians currently being graduated, and the supply to be expected through presently planned medical school expansion, will fall far short of maintaining the present physician-population ratio.

2. Demand per unit of population is growing for many reasons. . .; this should necessitate an *increased* physician-population ratio.

3. Effective demand apparently will increase with every increase in the adequacy of health insurance coverage.

4. The improvements due to centralization of care in the hospital and in the

office may have reached their limit. Less than 10 percent of doctors' visits are now in the home; and, in fact, increasing concern with hospital effectiveness may have the effect of *increasing* home calls.

5. A fuller exploration of another type of centralization of care—group practice— may increase the physician's productivity. Aside from developments such as this (i.e., social organization as a technique to increase productivity), however, the contribution *specialization* may make to *productivity* may have already reached its limit. For example, the greater the number of cases transferred from the general practitioner to the internist and the psychiatrist, the greater is the number of physicians needed, for the internist and psychiatrist can see fewer patients per unit of time than can the general practitioner.

6. Some developments of medical science may render diagnosis and treatment more effective, but also require more medical manpower for their exploitation. The personnel requirements for open heart surgery, for the repair of congenital anomalies, and for the use of radioisotopes and high voltage radiation therapy illustrate this point. Many of these developments are the result of specialization, and produce further specialization; in any event specialization and scientific advance can reinforce demand, rather than damp it.

7. Research and teaching will themselves require a greater and greater supply of physicians, thus reducing the numbers available for direct patient services.

8. The other health professions and skills, which have absorbed much of the increased demand for physician's services, are themselves in short supply.[29]

The total PPR must be used carefully, as noted earlier, because it includes physicians who do not render direct patient care. It is still a better indicator of the supply of doctors than the ratio of active physicians in private practice to civilian population, however. The latter excludes interns and residents, who contribute substantially to patient care.

The pool from which physicians are drawn should be broadened. Whereas in the first sixty years of the nineteenth century, 28 percent to 35 percent of college graduates entered the practice of medicine, only 2 percent entered in the 1950s.

It is apparent that a simple increase in number of applicants is not enough, but that it is also of prime importance to increase the quality of applicants. If it is granted that competition with other learned disciplines has practical limits, and that it is not desirable to deplete any other productive profession, then new pools of talent must be sought. Are there such pools? It would seem that there are, judging, for example, by the extremely small number of women and Negroes among practitioners and students of medicine.

Another pool of potential talent exists among low-income families. The failure of the young man or woman from such a family to become a serious candidate for medical school admission may stem from his inability to go to college, or even to finish high school. It is evident that the enormous expense and the long duration of a medical education has adversely influenced the selection of students from among low-income groups in the population.

Counts and Stalnaker surveyed medical students for the 1952-53 school year regarding the occupations and incomes of their fathers.* The fathers of about one-half of the students were in the professional, executive, or managerial groups—10 percent were physicians, 16 percent belonged to other professions, 25 percent were executives or managers. The average income of the fathers was about $7,000 in 1952. The distribution was as follows:

Under $5,000 income	29%
$5,000-$7,499	24%
$7,500-$10,000	15%
Over $10,000	23%
Did not answer	6%

The Bane report cities unpublished figures indicating that for senior students in 1959, six out of ten fathers were in the professional or managerial group. With regard to income, 20 percent of the families of the students had incomes under $5,000; 40 percent had incomes between $5,000 and $9,999; and 40 percent had incomes of $10,000 a year or over.[†]

Among other measures, the tapping of whatever pools of talent there are among women, Negroes, and low-income families would seem to require two broad kinds of financial measures—strong government aid to medical schools to prevent drastic rises in tuition, and generous scholarship aid to talented applicants.[30]

---

*S. Counts and J. M. Stalnaker. "The Cost of Attending Medical School." *The Journal of Medical Education,* Vol. 29, No. 2, February 1954.

†U.S. Public Health Service. *Physicians for a Growing America.* Report of the Surgeon General's consultant group on medical education, Frank Bane, Chairman, Washington, D.C.: U.S. Government Printing Office, 1959.

Shortages are revealed also by the great dependence on foreign-trained doctors.[31] By 1967, graduates of foreign medical schools accounted for 2,281 licentiates, 24 percent of the total.

The role of the foreign medical graduate seems conclusive evidence of an actually existing shortage of medical manpower. Moreover, there are many negative aspects in this solution of the problem.

The countries from which these physicians come need physicians more than we do; we are draining their supply, and in some cases depriving them of future leaders and teachers. In the interests of our long-range national goals we ought rather to be in a position to *export* physicians, as does the Soviet Union.

Furthermore, doubts have been repeatedly expressed as to the adequacy of the medical education of some of these foreign medical graduates. These doubts were confirmed quite dramatically by the results of the examinations given by the Educational Council for Foreign Medical Graduates, composed of representatives of the American Medical Association, the American Hospital Association, and the Federation of State Medical Boards.

Of the 8,713 foreign physicians who took the September 1960 examination, 2,481 failed; 2,456 achieved grades between 70 and 74 and were given a two-year extension with the opportunity eventually to take a make-up examination; and 3,776 passed with an average grade of 75 percent or better. In other words, 44 percent passed, 28 percent received an extension, and 28 percent failed.

The hospitals employing those who failed face loss of accreditation if they keep the doctors, or severe physician shortages if they do not; the physicians involved face loss of professional standing and loss of visas, necessitating return to their home countries. The organizations concerned face problems of foreign relations, medical education, and health manpower.[32]

Geographic Distribution of Medical Manpower

The availability of health personnel varies among cities, among concentrations of population in Standard Metropolitan Statistical Areas (SMSAs), among states, and among regions. In California, for example, the PPR ranges from a minimum of 119 for Bakersfield to a maximum of 296 for San Francisco (see table 5.14). The less populous the area, the lower its PPR (see table 5.15).

TABLE 5.14 Physician-Population Ratios in California Standard Metropolitan Statistical Areas

SMSA Identification	Number of Counties	Number of Persons	PPR
009 Anaheim	1	800,500	176.0
016 Bakersfield	1	303,500	119.3
066 Fresno	1	381,700	138.1
105 Los Angeles	1	6,337,400	230.2
155 Sacramento	3	672,900	146.3
162 San Bernardino	2	880,100	153.7
163 San Diego	1	1,125,400	189.7
164 San Francisco	5	2,740,000	296.2
165 San Jose	1	715,400	239.6
166 Santa Barbara	1	189,400	225.4
180 Stockton	1	258,900	148.4
194 Vallejo	2	209,100	186.0

Source: HEW, *Health Manpower Source Book,* section 19 (1965), p. 11.

TABLE 5.15   Physician-Population Ratios in Metropolitan and Rural Areas of California

Type of Area	PPR
Greater metropolitan	243
Adjacent to metropolitan	149
Isolated rural	112

Source: HEW, *Health Manpower Source Book,* section 19 (1965), p. 15.

For general practitioners there were only small variations in the PPRs in 1963, ranging from 38 for lesser metropolitan areas to 30 for isolated areas. But in the specialties the picture is entirely different: the PPRs range from 80 for greater metropolitan areas to 27 for isolated areas.

The ratio of all health personnel is highest in the greater metropolitan areas and then declines in lesser metropolitan, adjacent-to-metropolitan, isolated semirural, and isolated rural areas respectively. The ratios vary from one category of personnel to another (see table 5.16).[33] Comparing greater metropolitan areas to isolated rural

TABLE 5.16   Ratios of Health Personnel to Population by Area, 1962

Type of Personnel	Number per 100,000 Population				
	Greater Metro-politan	Lesser Metro-politan	Adjacent to Metro-politan	Isolated Semi-rural	Isolated Rural
Dentists	71.0	52.0	38.7	40.6	27.4
Nurses					
Total	492.7	509.3	388.3	350.6	195.7
Active	327.5	339.6	254.2	242.8	125.9
Pharmacists	81.2	65.2	51.3	56.0	45.3
Physicians					
Total	205.3	153.0	91.5	100.4	59.1
M.D.	195.4	145.3	85.6	94.2	53.0
D.O.	9.9	7.7	5.9	6.2	6.1
Sanitarians	4.6	6.9	5.8	6.3	3.9
Sanitary engineers	4.1	3.5	1.5	1.5	0.3
Veterinarians	7.5	10.6	17.3	16.5	15.6
General hospital beds per 1,000 population	4.0	3.9	3.2	4.1	2.0
Effective buying income per capita	$2,526	$2,070	$1,654	$1,551	$1,207

Source: HEW, *Health Manpower Source Book,* section 19 (1965), p. 13.

ones, the ratios were 2½ to 1 for dentists, 3 to 1 for active nurses, 3½ to 1 for physicians, and 2 to 1 for hospital beds.

For counties of less than 50,000 and those from 50,000 to 1 million, the ratio of active nonfederal physicians to population changed little from 1959 to 1967. But for counties of 1 million or more, the ratio rose from 158 to 185 per 100,000. Thus, the large communities continued to improve their position in these years, although the general practitioner ratio dropped from 47 to 32, and this reflected an especially large drop for large communities. Specialty practice rose from 45 to 64 doctors per 100,000.[34]

Fifteen SMSAs with populations from 1 million to 2 million had PPRs ranging from 130 (Patterson) to a maximum of 218 (Seattle). For SMSAs with populations of 2 million to 5 million, the minimum was 131 (Pittsburgh) and the maximum 296 (Washington, D.C.).[35]

Large variations in PPRs among states are evident (see figure 5.17). These appear, to a significant extent, to reflect differences in the sizes of the communities they include. From 1931 to 1957 the ratio of nonfederal physicians to civilian population for the country as a whole scarcely changed, but it varied greatly among regions (see table 5.18). The advantage held by rich areas clearly increased in these years.

In the next decade, northern superiority was expected to decline greatly.[36] In fact, by 1965, of the fifteen states that exceeded the national average of 147, eight were in the Northeast, three in the Pacific, three in the Middle West, and one in the Rocky Mountain region. The bottom fifteen states included eight in the South and seven in the Mountain and Western regions. New York was the *state* with the highest PPR, 217, although the District of Columbia PPR was even higher—375. Alaska was lowest at 71, followed by Mississippi at 74.[37] Still, on the whole, practicing physicians were more numerous in the Northeast than in the South, as the lists of the top and bottom five states show (see table 5.19).

In 1957, Mississippi had the lowest ratio, 73, while New York had the highest, 219. By regions, the East South Central area had the lowest, 92, and the Middle Atlantic the highest, 183.[38] These are indeed large differences.

A comparison of professional activity in SMSAs and non-SMSAs is interesting because it shows that large communities have a greater concentration of physicians in the specialties and a smaller

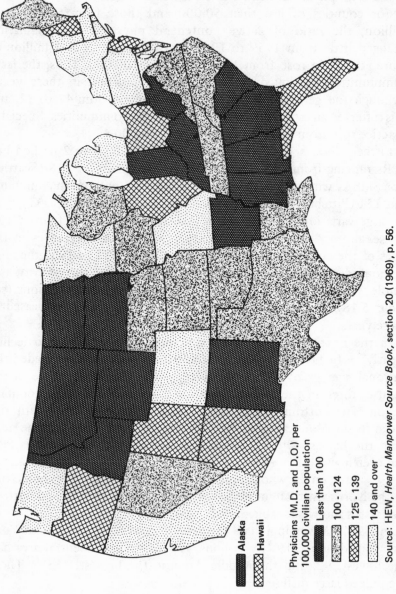

FIGURE 5.17   Active Nonfederal Physician-Population Ratios by State, 1967.

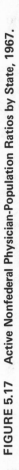

Alaska

Hawaii

Physicians (M.D. and D.O.) per
100,000 civilian population

Less than 100

100 - 124

125 - 139

140 and over

Source: HEW, *Health Manpower Source Book*, section 20 (1969), p. 56.

TABLE 5.18   Movement in Regional PPRs, 1931 and 1957

Region	1931	1957
New England	140	164
East South Central	95	85

Source: HEW, *Physicians for a Growing America: Report of the Surgeon General's Consultant Group on Medical Education* (1959), p. 82.

concentration in general practice. The SMSAs show heavy concentration in medical specialties (90 percent) and hospital-based practice (93 percent), although they have only 85 percent of total physicians and only 75 percent of hospital beds (see table 5.20).

Mobilizing Students

In the 1960s, much federal legislation was enacted to improve the medical manpower situation. The government provided grants, loans, and "forgiving" loans to medical students, to help stimulate increases in enrollment. It was clear that additional funds were needed; but funds without increased manpower and facilities would not be enough. It was necessary to provide new programs, acquire additional faculty members with higher levels of educational achievement, and construct new facilities. The government stressed the need for creating new medical schools and increasing the enrollment capacity of existing schools. The resulting leap forward is documented in table 5.21. The American Medical Association supported the building program, but expressed little enthusiasm for increased enrollments, perhaps in fear of excessive competition.[39]

The increase in students was 1.26 percent per year from 1930-31 to 1960-61, while from 1960-61 to 1967-68 it was 2.0 percent per

TABLE 5.19   States with Highest and Lowest PPRs

Top Five		Bottom Five	
State	PPR	State	PPR
New York	199	Alaska	69
Massachusetts	181	Mississippi	69
Colorado	168	Alabama	75
Connecticut	164	South Carolina	76
Maryland	152	Arkansas	78

Source: HEW, *Health Manpower, United States, 1965-1967*, pp. 17-18.

TABLE 5.20 Distribution of Nonfederal Physicians by SMSA and Non-SMSA

	Total	SMSA		Non-SMSA	
		Number	Percentage	Number	Percentage
Total physicians	272,891	230,518	84.5	42,373	15.5
Total patient care	243,333	204,941	84.2	38,392	15.8
Solo, partnership, group, or other practice					
General practice	64,063	43,821	68.4	20,242	31.6
Medical specialties	38,921	35,022	90.0	3,899	10.0
Surgical specialties	55,170	47,765	86.6	7,405	13.4
Other specialties	28,946	25,917	89.5	3,029	10.5
Hospital-based practice	56,233	52,416	93.2	3,817	6.8
Other professional activity*	16,346	15,022	91.9	1,324	8.1
Inactive	13,212	10,555	79.9	2,657	20.1
Number of hospitals	5,583	2,718	48.7	2,865	51.3
Number of hospital beds	743,275	556,331	74.8	186,944	25.2
Resident population	195,195,000	141,379,000	72.4	53,816,000	27.6
Income					
Per capita	$2,367	$2,598		$1,762	
Per household	7,990	8,675		6,122	

Source: American Medical Association, *Distribution of Physicians, Hospitals and Hospital Beds in the U.S.* (1966), vol. 2, p. 10.

* Includes medical school faculty, administration, and research.

TABLE 5.21   Medical Schools and Enrollments, 1900-68

Period	Number of Schools	Number of Students	First-Year Students	Graduates
1900	160	25,171	–	5,214
1930-31	76	21,982	6,456	4,735
1960-61	86	30,288	8,298	6,994
1967-68	95	34,538	9,979	7,573

year. For graduates during these periods, however, the increases were 1.6 and 1.14 percent per year, respectively. Thus, while the expansion of enrollments was greater in the later period than in the earlier period, the rate of increase of the number graduating was declining.

From 1947-48 to 1967-68, the number of medical school applicants increased only moderately, although from 1960-61 to 1967-68 a rise from 14,397 to 18,724 occurred. Strenuous competition for entry was reflected in a rise in the number of applications filed by each applicant—from 3.0 in 1947-48 to 5.0 by 1967-68.[40]

The quality of students, of course, helps determine the quality of physicians. In the late 1950s average grades of entering students on the Medical College Admission Test ranged from a high level of over 600 for some schools to under 450, a low level, for others. The percentage of students withdrawing because of poor academic standards rose sharply in this period.

One of the problems facing medical students was financial need. Whereas the average scholarship or fellowship for medical students was $512, for graduate students in five other fields scholarships averaged $1,365 to $1,675. Thus there was severe competition from other fields for students who might otherwise have gone into medicine.

The Shortage of Dentists

The supply of and national requirements for dentists present problems similar to those relating to physicians. The shortage of dentists may well be even more serious than the shortage of doctors. The rise of the supply of dentists since 1900 and especially since

TABLE 5.22   Increases in the Supply of Dentists, 1850 to 1968

Period	Percentage Increase in Supply
1850-1900	200
1900-1950	126
1950-1968	0 (no change)

1950 (see table 5.22) has been inadequate to meet the need, especially when allowance is made for the rising income level of the population and the understatement of needs because of the elective nature of dental treatments.

Regional variations in the dentist-population ratio are large, indicating poor distribution of dental manpower (see table 5.23 and figure 5.24).

From 1930-31 to 1968-69 the number of dental students both entering and graduating roughly doubled. Projections to 1974-75 indicate a further rise, varying from a high estimate of 24 percent to a low estimate of 15 percent. The number of graduates is expected to increase 23 percent. The number of dental school applicants has been rising to some extent (see table 5.25).

The forecasted dentist-population ratio for 1975 is 49 per 100,000. With income steadily rising and growing public knowledge of the need for dental care, this clearly is not enough.[41]

TABLE 5.23   Highest and Lowest Dentist-Population Ratios by Region and State, 1968

	Dentists per 100,000 Population	Region or State
Maximum region	59	Middle Atlantic
Minimum region	32	East South Central
Maximum state*	69	Oregon
Minimum state	25	Mississippi

Source: HEW, Health Manpower Source Book, section 20, 1969, p. 81.

*The District of Columbia had a ratio of 92, exceeding the highest state.

FIGURE 5.24　Active Nonfederal Dentist-Population Ratio by State, 1968

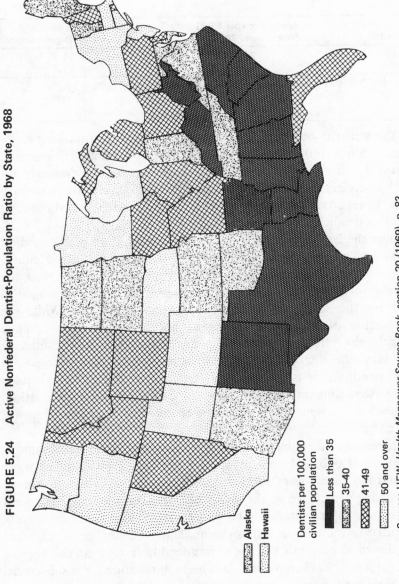

Alaska

Hawaii

Dentists per 100,000
civilian population

Less than 35

35-40

41-49

50 and over

Source: HEW, *Health Manpower Source Book*, section 20 (1969), p. 83.

TABLE 5.25   Dental School Applicants in Relation to Eligible Population Segments

Period	Applications per 1,000 Persons Aged 20	Applications per 100 Bachelors' Degrees Granted
1960-61	2.7	1.6
1967-68	2.7	1.8

Source: HEW, *Health Manpower Source Book,* section 20 (1969), p. 78.

Trends in Manpower

The statistics outlined in this chapter indicate the following major trends. Since 1900, the number of medical personnel has increased markedly, in part because of the large increase in demands for health services, which is related to increased income, rising population, educational advancement of the public, and increased numbers of older people in the population.

Over the last seventy years or so, the contribution of the medical team has grown greatly, while that of the physician has declined. The number of auxiliary personnel increased much more than the number of physicians, and vigorous campaigns have been waged to increase the supply of auxiliary personnel even more. While the proportion of physicians among all health professionals dropped sharply, the ratio of professional nurses to physicians skyrocketed.

Today the demand for more personnel throughout the health field continues. It is not easy to determine the standards of adequate manpower, but budgeted vacancies, ratios to total population, professional judgments of need, and requirements per unit of service are all helpful.

In response to rising incomes and rising interest in health among the general public, health manpower has been growing much more than total manpower, so that health occupations account for an increasing percentage of the civilian labor force, especially in recent years (and in projections). The growth of physical facilities has contributed to increases in employment. Thus, the number of personnel employed in hospitals has risen considerably faster than the number of health personnel employed elsewhere. But despite these substantial absolute and relative improvements in available manpower, large deficits are anticipated for 1975 and 1980.

Severe competition among fields for top quality personnel

accounts for some of the deficits in the medical field. The number of professional, technical, and kindred workers in all areas has increased substantially since 1950.

Although estimates of the deficits in health occupations vary, all sources agree that they exist at serious levels.

Merely turning out more doctors and spending more money will not solve the doctor shortage, however. The problem of getting doctors into the impoverished areas still remains. The present lack of optimum distribution is suggested by the varying rates of growth in different regions. Although the number of physicians enrolled in training programs rose about eight times as fast as the total number of physicians from 1931 to 1959, there was still an urgent need to improve the delivery system, exploit technological advances, and make more effective use of the referral system and of the primary physician. According to one estimate, a 3 percent rise in productivity (the national average) would add as much health care as the annual output of American medical school graduates.

In a 1962 study, however, W. J. McNerney, president of Blue Cross, expressed doubts that rising productivity would solve the shortage of doctors. The current and prospective increases in medical school enrollments and graduates are inadequate to maintain the present inadequate physician-population ratio. Demand is rising per person; effective demand will rise with every increase of health insurance coverage; and gains from centralization of practice and group practice are declining, McNerney felt. Improvements in treatment add to rather than diminish the need for manpower, while nonpractice needs for physicians are on the rise.

One way to attack the shortage is to broaden the applicant base. If rising productivity is not a solution, perhaps an increase in the reserves from which medical manpower is drawn will help. Future doctors are now drawn disproportionately from families with high economic status.

Much has been made of the physician-population ratio (PPR), which fell from 1880 to the 1950s but since has been rising (especially since 1960 and in projections for the 1970s). This index should be used with caution, however. The value of the PPR is dependent on the categories of population and doctors studied. The mix of factors such as capital, technology, and drugs used and types of practices or specialties that predominate may raise or lower the PPR without a commensurate effect on the level of health care available. In a 1965-67 study, for example, the ratios of physicians providing patient care in office-based practice, those providing patient care to the civilian population, and all physicians to the total population were 100, 130, and 158, respectively, a considerable range.

Another trend is the greater dependence on foreign-trained doctors. The percentage of all physicians graduated from United States medical schools has been declining, although it is still the bulk of the total. Some studies show, however, that foreign-trained physicians tend to be less competent than those trained in the United States. A smaller percentage of the foreign-trained applicants passed the licensing examination, for example.

As medicine has become more complex, the shift to specialization has accelerated. Growing numbers of specialists in pediatrics, obstetrics, internal medicine, and general surgery have not been adequate to offset losses in direct patient care from the decline of general practice. Moreover shifts to training, education, research, government, and military service further reduced the number of available general practitioners.

Specialists are concentrated largely in office-based practice, hospital training programs, and hospital-based practice, in declining order. In the early 1960s there were widespread shortages even in the specialties.

The available personnel are badly distributed. There are wide variations in physician-population ratios among Standard Metropolitan Statistical Areas. Concentrated-population areas had higher general practice PPRs and much higher specialty PPRs than isolated areas. In general the ratios continue to drop from the most populated greater metropolitan areas to the most isolated rural areas. Moreover, from 1959 to 1967, the larger communities continued to improve their relative position.

Notes

1. U.S. Department of Health, Education, and Welfare (HEW), *Health Manpower Perspective: 1967*, p. 5.

2. Ibid., passim.

3. U.S. Department of Labor, Bureau of Labor Statistics, *Some Facts Relating to Health Manpower Outlook*, by H. Bienstock (1967), pp. 1, 5.

4. Also see HEW, *Report to the President and the Congress: The Allied Health Professions Personnel Training Act of 1966, as Amended* (1969).

5. Estimates of health personnel for 1900, 1950, 1967, 1975, and 1980 are given in ibid., pp. 22, 34.

6. Ibid.

7. U.S. Senate, Committee on Labor, Subcommittee on Health and Public Welfare, *Hearings on Allied Health Professions Training* (1970), p. 216. The details of the estimates for 1950-60, 1950-67, 1967-75, and 1980 may be found in several sources: HEW, *Health Manpower Source Book,* section 18 (1964), table 5; HEW, *Report to the President and the Congress* (1969), p. 22; and HEW, *Health Manpower Source Book,* section 21 (1970), table 14.

8. Ibid., p. 4.

9. HEW, *Health Manpower Source Book,* section 18 (1964), pp. 2-3.

10. Ibid., p. 7.

11. Ibid., p. 15.

12. HEW, *Indicators,* January 1967, pp. 5, 7.

13. See U.S. Senate, Committee on Government Operations, Subcommittee on Executive Reorganization, *Hearings on Health Care in America* (1968), vol. 1, p. 158.

14. HEW, *Health Manpower Source Book,* section 20 (1968), p. 33.

15. *Report of the National Advisory Commission on Health Manpower* (November 1967), vol. 1, p. 2.

16. HEW, *Health Manpower Source Book,* section 20 (1968), p. 31.

17. Ibid., p. 32.

18. L. Lasagna, *Life, Death, and the Doctor* (1968), p. 27.

19. HEW, *Health Manpower Source Book,* section 20 (1968), p. 70

20. Ibid., pp. 1-5, 13-14, 81.

21. *Report of the National Advisory Commission on Health Manpower* (November 1967), vol. 1, pp. 74-75.

22. HEW, *Physicians for a Growing America: Report of the Surgeon General's Consultant Group on Medical Education* (1959), p. 2.

23. HEW, *Health Manpower Source Book,* section 18 (1964), p. 36.

24. HEW, *Health Manpower Perspective: 1967,* p. 75.

25. Ibid.

26. HEW, *Health Resources Statistics, Health Manpower* (1965), p. 102.

27. Senate Subcommittee on Executive Reorganization, *Hearings on Health Care in America,* vol. 1, pp. 119-21.

28. HEW, *Health Manpower Perspective: 1967,* Appendix C, pp. 69-71.

29. W. J. McNerney, *Hospital and Medical Economics* (1962), vol. 1, pp. 631-32.

30. Ibid., pp. 673-74.

31. See especially ibid., pp. 630-32, 643, 663-64, 673-75, and HEW, *Health Manpower Source Book,* section 20 (1968), p. 69.

32. McNerney, *Hospital and Medical Economics,* p. 630.

33. HEW, *Health Manpower Source Book,* section 18 (1964), p. 25; section 19 (1965), p. 13.

34. HEW, *Health Manpower Source Book,* section 20 (1968), table 52.

35. HEW, *Health Manpower Source Book,* section 19 (1965), p. 9.

36. HEW, *Health Manpower Source Book,* section 20 (1968), p. 77.

37. HEW, "State Data and State Rankings," part 2 of *HEW Welfare Trends,* pp. 5-10.

38. HEW, *Health Manpower Source Book,* section 20 (1968), pp. 51-53.

39. Important sources of materials are: U.S. Senate, Committee on Labor, Subcommittee on Health and Public Welfare, *Hearings on the Health Manpower Act of 1968* (March 1968); Senate Report no. 1307, *Health Manpower Act of 1968;* U.S. Senate, Committee on Aging, Subcommittee on Health of the Elderly, *Hearings on Costs and Delivery of Health Services to Older Americans,* part 1 (June 1967), part 3 (October 1968); U.S. Senate, Committee on Government Operations, Subcommittee on Executive Reorganization, *Hearings on Health Care in America* (1968), vol. 1; HEW, *Report to the President and the Congress: The Allied Health Professions Personnel Training Act of 1966, as Amended* (1969).

40. See HEW, *Health Manpower Source Book,* section 20 (1968), pp. 2-7, 15.

41. Ibid., pp. 72-83.

6

Allied Health Personnel

More than 100 specialties are considered allied health occupations. Bringing those offering these medical services together with the population in need of the services is an important and difficult task. Emphasis is now being placed on allied health occupations because of their neglect in the past and the rising needs for these personnel, now and in the future.

An excellent summary of the issues involved in building up allied health personnel is given in the U.S. Department of Health, Education, and Welfare's *Report to the President and the Congress: The Allied Health Professions Personnel Training Act of 1966, as Amended:*

The great advances in prevention, diagnosis, therapy, and rehabilitation developed through research in the past two decades; improvements in education and understanding by the public of health care; increasing awareness of the availability of health services; shifts in the size, age composition, and distribution of the population; and a growing conviction that adequate health care is a right have heightened the disparity between the demand for health services and their timely availability to individuals and the community.

Recent legislation designed to improve health services . . . has had a major influence on the demand for health personnel. In response to recognized needs, legislation has also been passed within the last decade which has been directed specifically toward increasing the supply and the quality of health personnel. . . .

The increasing complexity of social problems and the necessity for confronting such technological problems as the contamination of our environment, together with the potential benefits to be derived from the application of advances in science and technology to such problems, have greatly increased the demand for individuals skilled in the health professions and technologies to provide the array of services which are now possible. Demands and expectations for health services that must be provided by professional and technical workers in the field of personal and environmental health services exceed the supply and the present capacities of the educational and other institutions which prepare them.

The many types of skills required to provide the potential range of services essential to the maintenance of health, the prevention of illness, and the care and therapy required by those who have become ill must be brought together in such a way that they are effective and efficient. However, effectiveness and efficiency in the provision of health services ultimately depend on the quality of education and training, as well as the numbers and distribution, of the people who render such services.

The more clearly recognized and longer established health professions of medicine, dentistry, and nursing have received serious attention for a number of years. However, only recently has the broad range of other professional and technical functions essential to all types of health services been recognized for its significance and attracted the attention of educators, practitioners, managers of health services, and the consumers of health services. This group of occupations, so essential for the expansion and quality of health services, has been designated as the "allied" health occupations. It includes an extensive range of endeavors for which special training or education is required.

. . . There is a paucity of information about the numbers of people serving in these professions, their distribution, their education and training, the ways in which their skills are used, and the directions that should be taken for better utilization of their skills in the variety of personal and community health services settings which exist or are contemplated for the future. In environmental health services, available information is even more rudimentary. Nonetheless, the experience gained during the initial 2 years of the implementation of the Allied Health Professions Personnel Training Act of 1966 has provided significant information about the education and training of allied health personnel and information which is important for future planning.

. . . The Allied Health Professions Personnel Training Act of 1966 has been effective in providing a focus for the allied health professions. It has enabled junior colleges, colleges, and universities with established training programs in the eligible allied health professions to acquire additional needed faculty and equipment to improve the quality of the programs offered. It has provided opportunities for a limited number of allied health personnel to prepare for positions as teachers, supervisors, administrators, and specialists in their disciplines. It has stimulated innovative thinking in the areas of curriculum development, teaching methods, and the development of new types of health personnel to fill unmet needs. . . .

The enactment and subsequent implementation of the Allied Health Professions Personnel Training Act of 1966 focused national attention on a vast pool of health manpower, which provides a multitude of services associated with the health of people. Administrative responsibility for implementation of the Allied Health Professions Personnel Training Act of 1966 was placed in the Bureau of Health Manpower of the Public Health Service.* . . .

There are more than 100 professional, technical, or vocational specialties which can be identified as components of the general, broad allied health manpower concept. Most of them require some formal post-high-school education. However, the preparation for employment varies from on-the-job training to a few occupations that require formal education at the master and doctoral levels.

The level of education required for employment is influencing the designations attached to job titles. Increasingly, those people trained in formal education programs that include theoretical and practical courses usually leading to a certificate or the associate degree are considered "technicians"; and those who are required to have at least a baccalaureate degree are referred to as "technologists."

. . . Although St. Louis University established its School of Nursing and Health Services in 1929 and offered programs in several allied health disciplines, it was not until 1950 that a second university, the University of Pennsylvania, established a School of Allied Medical Professions. In 1957, the University of Florida established an allied health professions school; and Indiana University followed in 1958. The recognition of increasing needs for allied health workers and the rising demand for health services were factors in the development of at least nine other allied health professions schools in 1963 and 1964. An added impetus was given by the enactment of the Allied Health Professions Personnel Training Act in 1966. Today, about 50 institutions have similar programs at various stages of development.[1]

---

*The Bureau of Health Manpower was established as one of five bureaus of the Public Health Service on Jan. 1, 1967, to provide a central focus for health manpower activities. It was incorporated into the National Institutes of Health agency on Apr. 1, 1968. On Dec. 26, 1968, Secretary Cohen approved a change in title to the Bureau of Health Professions Education and Manpower Training.

Shortages

In 1965, according to an official estimate, there were 2,417,000 workers in all health occupations. By 1975 over a million more would be needed. Professionals judged that substantially greater increases were needed in the number of other health professionals than in the number of physicians, dentists, and nurses (see table 6.1).

There are already sizable deficits in manpower in the allied health occupations. In 1967, the deficit among occupations requiring at least a baccalaureate degree was estimated at 50,000, and for occupations requiring less than a baccalaureate it was 60,000 (see table 6.2). For 1975, the projected deficits are 78,000 and 88,000, respectively, and for 1980 they are 93,000 and 105,000.[2]

Personnel needs in hospitals are outlined in some detail in table 6.3. Personnel are also in great demand in extended care facilities. In 1966 it was estimated that 275,000 workers were employed in these facilities, with 22,520 additional workers urgently needed and 31,900 more required to reached optimum staffing (see table 6.4). In view of the $17 billion being spent in 1971 in Medicare and Medicaid programs and the special place given to extended care

TABLE 6.1 Workers in Health Occupations, 1965 and 1975

Category of Personnel	Number of Workers (Thousands)		
		1975 Needs	
	1965	Professional Judgments	Based on Highest Region
Total	2,417	3,665	3,460
Physicians	289	400	430
Dentists	93	160	140
Nurses	600	920	940
Other professional and technical personnel	764	1,380	1,080
Dental hygienists	15	42	*
Medical record librarians	10	16	12
Medical technologists	32	70	53
Occupational therapists	8	54	14
Physical therapists	12	54	18
Speech and hearing therapists	13	29	19
X-ray technologists	70	100	93
Practical nurses	265	380	311
All other	339	635	*
Aides and attendants	671	805	870
Hospital	460	405	*
Nursing homes and other	211	400	*

Source: HEW, *Indicators,* January 1967, p. 5.

* Not available.

TABLE 6.2   Allied Health Personnel Requirements and Supplies

Occupational category	Item	1967	1975	1980
Total allied health manpower	Supply	653,500	909,000	1,066,000
At least baccalaureate	Supply	229,500	350,000	410,000
Less than baccalaureate	Supply	424,000	559,000	656,000
At least baccalaureate				
Medical allied manpower	Requirements	225,000		
	Supply	175,000	270,000	320,000
	Deficit	50,000		
Environmental health manpower	Requirements	105,000	135,000	155,000
	Supply	54,500	80,000	90,000
	Deficit	50,500	55,000	65,000
Less than baccalaureate				
Medical allied manpower	Requirements	336,500		
	Supply	276,500	400,000	475,000
	Deficit	60,000		
Dental allied manpower	Requirements	165,700	202,000	246,000
	Supply	137,000	139,000	151,000
	Deficit	28,700	63,000	95,000
Environmental health manpower	Requirements	20,000	35,000	50,000
	Supply	10,500	20,000	30,000
	Deficit	9,500	15,000	20,000

Source: HEW, *Report to the President and the Congress, The Allied Health Professions Personnel Training Act of 1966, as Amended* (1969), p. 35.

facilities under these programs, these estimates of 8 percent and 12 percent more workers needed seem low.[3]

Dental allied manpower is clearly inadequate. Shortages varied by categories from one-third to one-fifth of the supply in 1967; by 1980 they were expected to range from one-third to nine-fifths (180 percent).[4]

Estimates of the needs for personnel vary, because bases, coverage, and assumptions vary. It is difficult to get adequate and non-conflicting statistics, because some records are unavailable.

A "numbers game" for health manpower can be confusing and misleading because of the different bases and assumptions used. The Bureau of Labor Statistics estimates 75,000 medical technologists and 100,000 laboratory assistants, for a total of 175,000 in 1975. The American Hospital Association ends up with a total of 120,600 personnel in diagnostic services, for hospitals alone. And the Bureau of Health Manpower, on the basis of "professional judgment," estimates a need for 70,000 medical technologists for 1975, with no estimates for other categories of laboratory workers. The Manpower Administration report of the Department of Labor estimates 160,000 medical laboratory

TABLE 6.3   Personnel Needs in Hospitals, 1966

Category of Personnel	Present Number	Additional Personnel Needed	
		Urgently	For Optimum Care
Total professional and technical	1,380,800	108,600	275,300
Professional nurses	370,200	56,920	83,300
Licensed practical nurses	148,500	14,100	42,800
Aides, orderlies, etc	373,100	14,200	48,700
Psychiatric aides	156,200	7,600	31,300
Medical technologists	52,900	4,100	9,100
Radiologic technologists	23,700	1,000	3,900
Laboratory assistants	14,400	800	2,400
Medical record personnel			
Professional	6,200	600	1,800
Technical	10,000	300	1,800
Surgical technicians	17,400	500	3,800
Dietitians	12,600	1,600	3,600
Food service managers	5,300	100	800
Cytotechnologists	1,600	-	500
Histologic technicians	2,900	-	600
Electrocardiograph technicians	5,900	-	900
Electroencephalogram technicians	1,900	-	400
X-ray assistants	5,700	-	900
Occupational therapists	4,600	1,200	2,800
Occupational therapy assistants	5,600	-	1,500
Physical therapists	8,000	800	2,800
Physical therapy assistants	5,200	-	1,100
Speech pathologists and audiologists	1,000	-	600
Recreation therapists	4,600	100	1,900
Inhalation therapists	5,500	600	2,300
Pharmacists	9,500	600	1,900
Pharmacy assistants	5,500	100	900
Medical librarians	2,900	-	800
Social workers	12,100	2,000	6,400
Social work assistants	1,500	-	600
All other professional and technical	105,900	1,300	15,100
Total other personnel	*	11,700	*
Food service	*	2,600	*
Laundry	*	300	*
Housekeeping	*	2,800	*
Maintenance	*	2,800	*
Management	*	300	*
Secretarial, clerical	*	2,900	*

Source: HEW, *Indicators,* January 1967, p. 7; data based on a survey by the U.S. Public Health Service and the American Medical Association.

* Not available.

TABLE 6.4 Personnel Needs in Extended Care Facilities, 1966

Category of Personnel	Present Number	Additional Personnel Needed	
		Urgently	For Optimum Care
Total professional and technical	275,050	22,520	31,900
Professional nurses	31,030	5,050	6,000
Licensed practical nurses	33,620	7,680	9,400
Aides, orderlies, etc.	177,420	7,230	10,700
Dietitians	4,610	530	900
Occupational therapists	1,590	410	800
Occupational therapy assistants	1,330	50	300
Physical therapists	2,040	660	1,200
Physical therapy assistants	930	20	300
Recreation therapists	2,580	380	900
Medical record librarians	280	30	100
Medical record technicians	760	-	100
Medical social workers	1,160	210	500
Speech therapists	270	130	400
All other professional and technical	17,430	140	300
Total other personnel	140,820	1,750	6,300
Business office	14,650	80	700
Food service	59,320	890	2,500
Laundry	16,380	110	600
Housekeeping	32,190	350	1,500
Maintenance	18,280	320	1,000

Source: HEW, *Indicators,* January 1967, p. 8.

personnel will be employed in the health service industry, and, when an estimated 43,200 projection for those outside the health service industry is added, the total of about 203,200 seems to come nearest to predictions of future needs by those closest to the field.

The "health service industry," as described here, includes private and government-owned hospitals and nursing homes, offices and clinics of private medical and other individual practitioners and groups, and privately operated laboratories. Employment of medical laboratory personnel in these areas, in full-time equivalent terms, and excluding physicians, is given as:

1965	*1970*	*1975*
100,000	130,000	160,000

Of the 100,000 estimated for 1965, the report breaks them down into approximately 80,000 in hospitals and 20,000 in laboratories, private offices, etc. Types of workers are given approximately as follows:

Medical technologists, technicians, scientists: 60,000 (55,000 in hospitals)
Laboratory assistants (certified, semi-skilled): 25,000 (15,000 in hospitals)
Laboratory helpers, orderlies, etc.: 15,000 (10,000 in hospitals)

This study also estimates that there are 27,000 *additional* medical laboratory personnel working *outside* the health service industry (schools, out-patient health centers of government agencies, etc.). This would make a total of 127,000 for 1965. (Although this total is not projected to 1975, if the 60 percent estimated increase noted above—from 100,000 to 160,000—also represented the rate of increase for these 27,000, it would make a total of some 43,200 additional workers in 1975 outside the health service industry—for a grand total of about 203,200.)[5]

Geographic Distribution

There are large differences in the numbers of persons in health occupations in different geographic areas (see table 6.5). The variations are relatively small for physicians compared with most other occupations. For example, the highest state has four times the number of pharmacists per 100,000 population in the lowest state and 270 times the number of osteopaths in the lowest state.

TABLE 6.5   Persons in Health Occupations by Highest and Lowest States, 1962

Occupation	Number per 100,000 Population			
	State with Highest Ratio		State with Lowest Ratio	
Dentists	New York	82.8	South Carolina	22.5
Nurses				
Total	Massachusetts	813.0	Arkansas	178.9
Active	Massachusetts	560.0	Arkansas	123.9
Pharmacists	Massachusetts	105.5	Hawaii	26.5
Physicians				
Total	New York	218.8	Alaska	82.0
M.D.	New York	215.6	Alaska	81.6
D.O.	Missouri	27.0	Alabama	0.1
			Mississippi	0.1
Sanitarians	Hawaii	16.3	New Hampshire	1.9
Sanitary engineers	Nevada	9.1	Louisiana	1.4
			Mississippi	1.4
			South Carolina	1.4
Veterinarians	Iowa	42.4	Alaska	3.7
General hospital beds per 1,000 population	North Dakota	5.5	Alaska	2.3
Effective buying income per capita	Nevada	$2,765	Mississippi	$1,222

Source: HEW, *Health Manpower Source Book,* section 19 (1965), table B, p. 7.

Sources of Increased Supply

To achieve adequate numbers of personnel, training programs must be improved and extended and much better treatment must be accorded to workers in health occupations, including adequate pay and provision for moving up the ladder.

The number of enrollees in health occupations has increased sharply. Vocational students in health occupations rose from 83,677 in 1966 to 178,399 in 1969; in 1965 the health professions accounted for 11,668 baccalaureates or between 2 and 3 percent of the total. [6] And yet the supply is inadequate to meet the needs.

Training goals are shown in table 6.6, and the sources of training are depicted in figure 6.7. Upgrading, postsecondary preemployment programs, and industry training are especially important.

Much manpower now comes from special reserves. For example, from 1950-51 to 1967-68, the percentage of internships and residencies filled by foreign graduates rose from 9 percent to 32 percent.[7]

The number of new workers mobilized in the future depends on improved chances for moving up the ladder (perhaps through a system of national tests), more financial aid by government, and higher pay scales. Although the allied health occupations have

TABLE 6.6   Health Manpower Training Goals

Level of Training	Annual Output (Thousands)	
	1965	1975
Total	124	224
Doctoral (including first professional degree)	11	14
Physicians	7.9	9.6
Dentists	3.2	4.2
Nursing (baccalaureate, diploma, and associate degrees)	34.7	60
Baccalaureate and master's (excluding nursing)	11	20
Pharmacy, optometry, and podiatry	4	6
Allied health professions	7	14
Technical and vocational programs	47	90
Practical nursing	25	40
Other	22	50
Short training	20	40

Source: HEW, *Indicators,* January 1967, p. 7.

FIGURE 6.7   New Technicians, by Source of Training, 1965

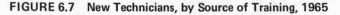

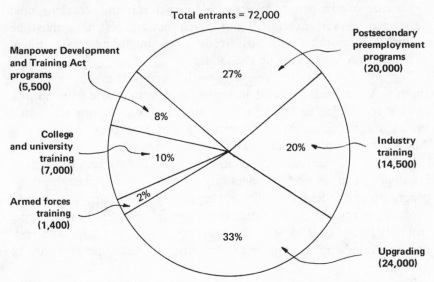

Source: U.S. Department of Labor, *Technician Manpower 1966-1980*, Bulletin no. 1639 (1970), chart 3.

Note: Because of rounding, individual items do not add up to total.

received substantial government outlays, the amounts are rather small in relation to the total budget.[8] The advances made by the government are suggested by figures on the number of institutions awarded basic improvement grants. In fiscal year 1967, 164 colleges and universities and 28 junior colleges received grants; in fiscal year 1968, the numbers were 197 and 33 respectively.[9]

The present pay schedule reflects the preponderance of women in the health work force (80 percent). A ceiling annual wage of $7,500 for high-level personnel is not enough.

Increasing Productivity

Automated procedures will often save manpower. For example technologists spend about one-third of their time on paperwork. But doubts about savings of personnel through technological advances have also been well documented:

Initially it was assumed by many that automation would decrease both the number of personnel needed and the level of skill required in the clinical laboratory. Both these assumptions have proved false. While automation has increased the efficiency and capacity of the laboratory in terms of volume of work and tests performed, as well as in quality control, it has also increased the demand for large numbers of complex tests difficult to perform.

As stated in "Automation in Clinical Laboratories," the report of a 1966 workshop on automation held by the National Institute of General Medical Sciences, "The special problem of automated techniques increases the demand for highly trained scientists who are interested in clinical laboratory analysis. In the future, it will be necessary to distinguish more sharply between training of laboratory scientists and training for the practice of laboratory medicine. Individuals with both types of training are needed desperately."

[In the short term, however,] most medical laboratory personnel will not only have to perform many of the traditional tasks they have always done, but in addition will need to operate, understand, maintain, and adjust complex machines. Laboratorians should be able to recognize significant deviations in the performance of a machine, diagnose problems, and make simple repairs quickly. When a machine cannot be readily repaired, technologists should be able to run the tests manually.[10]

The overall economy of running automated laboratories is still open to question. One study gives the following example of a centralized laboratory and its saving of manpower:

An example of fast, mass laboratory testing has been demonstrated in the Pathology Exhibit Laboratories at the AMA annual meetings for the last 7 years. This June the laboratory offered 21 different blood and urine tests to 800 physicians each day of the meetings. Included were procedures in blood chemistry, hematology and serology, urinalysis, and radioisotope T3. Utilizing $350,000 worth of precision instruments, the laboratory staff of 48 completed approximately 16,800 tests daily. It was estimated that a staff seven times as large would have been needed to do the tests by the usual manual methods. The exhibit laboratory's director, Dr. Vernon Martens, pointed out that the hourly test rate of 2,100, surpassed by 100 the entire daily output of his laboratory at the 800-bed Washington Hospital Center. The principal automated instrumentation consisted of the Technicon Corporation's SMA-12 and SMA-7 Analyzers, Warner-Chilcott's Robot Chemist, and Fisher Auto-Dilutors. . . .

Dr. Martens estimated that as a general, overall average, about three weeks' specialized training would be required to enable a capable technologist to gain adequate proficiency for this type instrumentation. Such instrumentation is, of course, but a beginning stage of advanced centralization and automation of clinical laboratories. . . .

In an article . . . in the May 1967 issue of *Hospitals,* Morris F. Collen, M.D., concluded that an automated multitest laboratory significantly affects the efficiency and economy of health services delivery. He added that such a laboratory operates most efficiently when associated with a medical center offering both in-patient and out-patient services. He stated the opinion, based on the experience of the multitest program operated by the Kaiser Foundation Hospital, Oakland, California, that, in the future, hospitals in communities of 100,000 or more will be affiliated with this type of laboratory. While this "multitest laboratory" is more on the order of a facility for periodic physical examinations than the present concept of a clinical laboratory, the article gives a picture of this possible future development in health care. . . .

It is possible that increased salaries and improved sociological aspects of medical laboratory jobs can be financed by productivity increases from such factors as automation, improved training, and improved manpower utilization. There is little argument that low salaries attract inferior personnel and help account for high turnover, both of which add to the expense of running laboratories.

It has been anticipated that automation would achieve productivity increases of four or five times the manpower investment. An article in the *Wall Street Journal* recently reported that an automatic blood testing and evaluation system from International Business Machines will permit a laboratory technician to perform 50,000 tests a year, 10 times his capacity without the machine. Dr. Arthur E. Rappoport is quoted as saying: "We have two or three technologists doing tests that conservatively would take 13 technologists with old methods." The cost of the system is given as $600 a month rental to IBM. This is considerably cheaper than the cost of salaries of 10 technologists . . . a generous margin for improving economic and sociological aspects of laboratory employment.[11]

Research to date is not conclusive as to the source of the actual cost savings—manpower or other factors. According to Dr. Rappoport, "we do not know, in our system, what part of our increased efficiency is due to improved procedures and equipment and what part is accounted for by linking the laboratory to the hospital's computer," and hence saving manpower.[12]

Automated multiphasic screening of mass populations, which may soon be available for as little as $5 per patient, could be used for both periodic and episodic care.

Adaptation of these techniques to large populations would materially affect health manpower priorities. The most dramatic impact may be the identification of unexpected disease prevalence—i.e., "hidden demand" of considerable proportion. For example, a recent limited pilot study of mass blood chemistry screening in the Varmland district of Sweden (a relatively healthy population) showed a 10 percent incidence of clinically significant, previously unknown chemical changes. The early Permanente Group multiphasic program identified referrable conditions in one of every six participating longshoremen. Episodic screening of children in poverty areas indicates previously unknown or mismanaged conditions in at least one of every three.[13]

Thus, remarkable gains in productivity may be realized from automation and improved training, making additional services available at great savings in costs. But it does not necessarily follow that revolutionary new techniques will cut the demand for personnel, since the demand for medical services itself may grow.

Supply of Nursing Personnel

In 1900, there were but 11,804 professional nurses. By 1960, the number had escalated to 592,000, an increase of forty-nine times (see table 6.8). In that same period the number of physicians rose by less than one time and the number of dentists two times. In the last generation, the number of nurses has moved upward both in absolute terms and relative to the number of physicians, hospital beds, the population, and other variables.

From 1950 to 1967, personnel in nursing and allied services expanded by 138 percent or 3½ times the gain in the number of physicians. Projections estimate a rise of 155 percent more from 1967 to 1980, or about 4½ times that for physicians. According to these projections, the dependence on nurses in relation to doctors will be even greater in the future than it is currently.

The ratio of professional nurses to the national population has been rising (see table 6.9). But the ratios in recent years reflect a jump in

TABLE 6.8   Active Professional Nurses, 1900-60

Year	Number of Nurses
1900	11,804
1910	50,500
1920	103,900
1930	214,300
1940	284,200
1950	405,515
1960	591,829

Source: HEW, *Health Manpower Source Book,* section 20 (1968), table 1.

TABLE 6.9   Ratio of Professional Nurses to Population, 1950-64

Year	Nurses per 100,000 Population
1950	249
1954	251
1958	268
1960	282
1962	298
1964	306

Source: HEW, *Health Manpower Source Book,* section 2 (revised January 1966), p. 37.

the number of part-time nurses: in 1960 there were 231 full-time and 51 part-time nurses per 100,000; in 1964 there were 237 full-time and 69 part-time.

The percentage increase in the nurse-population ratio by decades has tended downward (see figure 6.10). But in absolute numbers the increase has been larger each decade. For example, from 1950 to 1960 the number of registered nurses rose by 129,000; from 1960 to 1969, the number rose by 196,000.[14]

Assuming a 2 percent annual rise in the number of professional nurse graduates and a 4 percent attrition rate among active nurses, the number of nurses will increase from 656,000 in 1969-70 to 724,000 in 1974-75. If we assume a constant 35,000 graduates and the same 4 percent attrition rate, the 1975 total would be only 688,000.[15]

There is an increasing dependence on nonregistered nurses. While all persons engaged in nursing numbered 737,000 in 1950 and 1,767,000 in 1967, the number of registered nurses increased only from 375,000 to 659,000, dropping in proportion to the total.[16]

More economies are expected through this kind of dependence on less costly services. From 1967 to 1980, all health workers will increase 50 percent and all nursing workers will increase 56 percent, but registered nurses will increase only 36 percent and physicians 33 percent.[17]

The trend toward using less costly personnel is also evident in the projections from 1950 to 1980 (see figure 6.11). Registered nurses are expected to increase 138 percent, licensed hospital nurses 393 percent, and nursing aides, orderlies, and attendants 411

FIGURE 6.10   Percentage Increases in Professional Nurse-to-Population Ratios, 1900-60

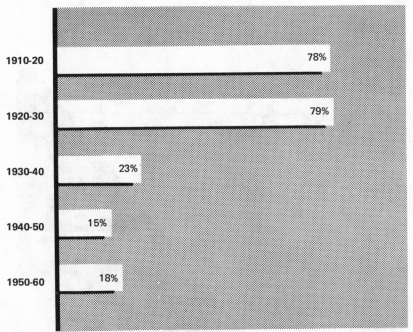

Source: HEW, *Health Manpower Source Book,* section 2 (revised January 1966), p. 5.

percent.[18] The relative growth of these categories and the excess of requirements over supplies are evident in table 6.12.

To solve the problem of inadequate supply there are two approaches: control demand and increase supply. The emphasis has been on the latter, while large resources have also been devoted to improving quality—e.g., training more highly educated nurses. Raising the relative numbers of active and part-time nurses has also improved the supply situation. How many nurses will be available, however, depends first on the number of new entrants for training in relation to the population of the relevant ages. Here the trend has been downward. From 1955-56 to 1963-64, the percentage of students entering nursing schools dropped slightly in relation to the population aged seventeen and dropped substantially (from 6.4 to 5.3 per 100) in relation to the number of female high school graduates.

FIGURE 6.11   Employment in Nursing and Related Services, 1950-80

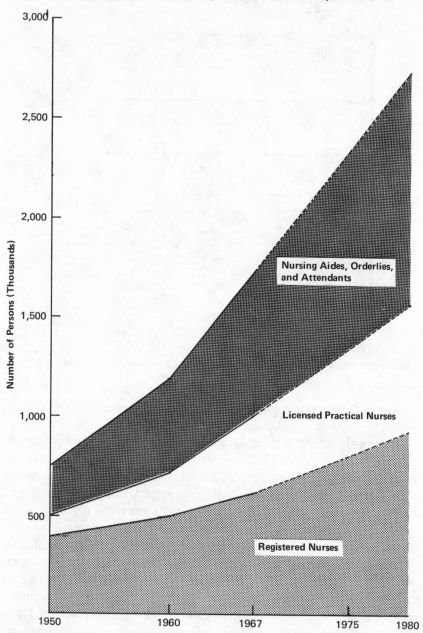

Source: HEW, *Health Manpower Source Book*, section 21 (1970), p. 23.

TABLE 6.12   Nursing Manpower Supply and Requirements, 1950-80

Year	Registered Nurses	Licensed Practical Nurses	Aides, Orderlies, Attendants, and Home Health Aides
Estimated number in practice			
1950	375,000	137,000	225,000
1960	504,000	206,000	475,000
1965	621,000	282,000	625,000
1967	659,000	320,000	775,000
1968	680,000	345,000	*
1969	700,000	*	*
1975	816,000	546,000	1,000,000
1980	895,000	675,000	1,150,000
Personnel requirements			
1967	800,000	375,000	860,000
1975	1,000,000	550,000	1,075,000
1980	*	*	1,210,000

Source: HEW, *Health Manpower Source Book,* section 21 (1970), p. 24.

* Not available.

Another relevant factor is the number of nurses who stay in nursing. The attrition rate is high: apparently only about two-thirds of nursing students complete their training period.

From 1945 to 1963, the number of professional nurses licensed for the first time was reasonably stable (see table 6.13). But note from table 6.7 above that the total number of professional nurses rose from 284,000 in 1940 to 592,000 in 1960. This is a large increase in view of the stability of entrants.

One important source of additional manpower is the influx of part-time nurses, mobilized in part in response to federal policies. The number of general duty nurses working part-time in hospitals is

TABLE 6.13   Newly Licensed Nurses, 1945-63

Year	Number Newly Licensed
1945	30,000
1950	25,000
1955	32,000
1960	32,000
1963	35,000

increasing at a faster pace than the number who are working full-time.[19]

The proportions of active and inactive nurses are, of course, important. In 1949, the number of inactive nurses was 69 percent of the number of active; by 1962, it had gone down to 53 percent. Thus, the substantial increase in the total number of nurses was apparently related to a rise in the proportion of active nurses. Undoubtedly, improved working conditions and higher pay contributed to this result. But it has been argued, by Professor Yett and others, that a federal policy of increasing the number of workers tends to reduce income and hence discourage new entrants to the field.[20]

In general the average age of nurses is moving upward. It was 33.9 in 1949 and 39.2 in 1962. I suspect that productivity is higher at age 34 than at 39. A rise in the proportion of nurses that are married would probably tend to reduce the productivity of nurses. But from 1949 to 1962, the proportion married dropped slightly, from 87 to 85 percent.[21]

Types of Nursing Employment

The number of nursing personnel in hospitals has increased tremendously. In 1941, there were more than 219,000, or 16.5 per 100 hospital beds. By 1966, there were 1,003,000, or 59.4 per 100 beds.[22] From 1956 to 1966 more nurses went into institutional employment and fewer went into private practice. A detailed breakdown of employment situations is given in table 6.14. The trend

TABLE 6.14   Field of Practice of Professional Nurses, 1964

Field of Practice	Number of Nurses	Percentage of Total
Total	582,000	100.0
Hospitals, nursing homes, and related institutions	390,400	67.1
Private practice	66,000	11.3
Office	47,000	8.1
Public health and school	37,200	6.4
Occupational health	18,700	3.2
Professional nursing education	17,600	3.0
Practical nursing education	3,100	0.5
Other fields	2,000	0.4

Source: HEW, *Health Resources Statistics, Health Manpower* (1965) table 80, p. 111.

toward hospital employment and away from private duty is evident from the comparison in table 6.15.

Nursing Education

In providing aid, the government had to decide how much to focus on adding to the supply of nurses and how much to concentrate on improving the education and quality of nursing personnel. The federal government has concentrated on higher education, in part because such personnel as teachers, administrators, and head nurses tended to be undereducated. Yet the pressure to add to the supply was so great that admissions rose especially in diploma programs and associate degree programs, both requiring lower levels of education (see figure 6.16). The largest percentage gains among nurses with various

TABLE 6.15   Type of Position of Active Registered Nurses, 1949 and 1962

Position	Percentage of All Nurses*	
	1949	1962
Hospital	47	67
Public health	9	8
Training	4	3
Private duty	22	12
Office	9	8

Source: Calculated from HEW, *Health Manpower Source Book,* section 2 (revised January 1966), pp. 25, 28.

* Percentages do not total 100 because some categories have been omitted.

degrees were in those holding higher degrees (see table 6.17). But the proportion of nurses holding baccalaureate or higher degrees has to grow more rapidly to meet the needs. For example, projections in 1966 indicated a tremendous spurt would be required to meet 1970 needs (see figure 6.18). In the mid-1960s 77 percent of all nurses had diplomas or associate degrees; hence the small rise in the number holding baccalaureate or higher degrees.[23]

In the past, training of health personnel has largely been tied to hospitals. The federal government sought to offer increased aid, especially in the mid-1960s, and this took the form of training grants, funds for improvement and extension of programs, assistance for providing facilities, and funding for cooperative enterprises with

FIGURE 6.16   Admissions to Schools of Nursing by Type of Program, 1950-74

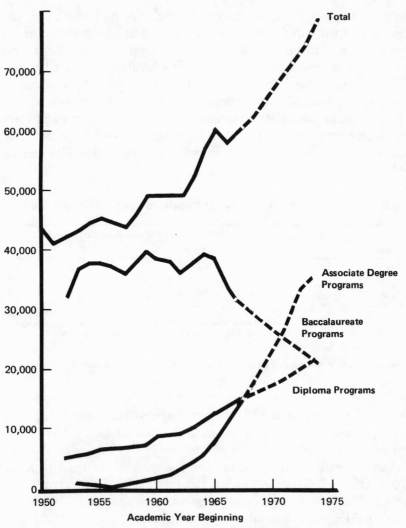

Source: HEW, *Health Manpower Source Book,* section 20 (1968), figure 14.

TABLE 6.17   Academic Credentials of Professional Nurses, 1952 and 1964

Degree Held	Percentage of All Nurses		Percentage Gain
	1952	1964	
Masters or doctors	1.0	2.3	130
Bachelors	7.2	9.0	25
Diploma or associate	91.0	88.7	−3

institutions of higher education. There are present needs for more students, teachers, and facilities.[24]

Geographic Distribution of Nurses

Variations in the number of nurses in different states and regions are large indeed, even in relation to the population of the area (see table 6.19). Of interest is the narrowing of the difference from 1910 to 1960. In the earlier year, the Northeast had 2-1/5 times the number of nurses per 100,000 population in the South, but in 1960 it had less than 1-1/2 times the number in the South. The differences in ratios of nurses to patients are much less than those in ratios of nurses to population. There was a larger relative difference for professional nurses than for all nursing personnel.

The regional variations in nursing education are depicted in figure 6.20.

Seriousness of the Medical Personnel Shortage

In general, most experts feel that serious shortages of medical personnel exist, but there are some who take exception to this view. Professor Victor Fuchs finds there is considerable excess capacity among general surgeons, and Dr. Harry Schwartz, of the *New York Times,* looks to reduction of demand instead of increase of supply:

Millions of Americans would benefit more from changing their dietary habits, losing weight, exercising, stopping cigarette smoking and cutting down or ending their consumption of alcohol and other drugs than from having more physicians and more hospitals available to treat them after their bad habits had laid them low.

Some experts would treat the shortages by increasing the capacity of medical schools, reducing the training period, facilitating the importation of doctors, and relying more on medical assistants.

The financial problems of medical schools interfere with the

FIGURE 6.18   Proportion of Professional Nurses with Baccalaureate or Higher
Degrees

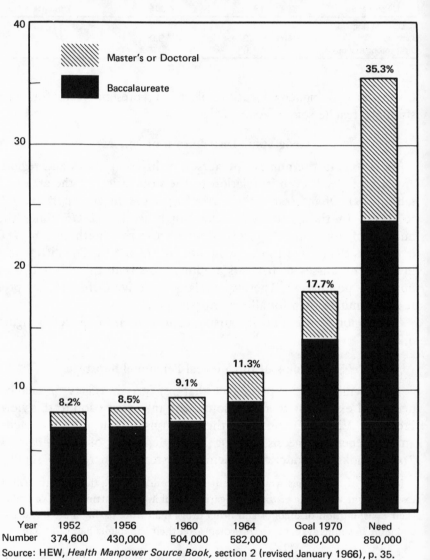

Source: HEW, *Health Manpower Source Book,* section 2 (revised January 1966), p. 35.

TABLE 6.19   Maximum and Minimum Distribution of Nurses

Category of Ratio	Geographic Unit	Maximum		Minimum	
		Place	Ratio	Place	Ratio
Active professional nurses per 100,000 population	Region				
1910		Northeast	75	South	34
1960		Northeast	349	South	245
Active practical nurses per 100,000 population	State	District of Columbia	229	Alabama	52
		Massachusetts	220	South Carolina	68
		Vermont	174	Wyoming	74
Professional nurses per 100 patients, 1959	Region	West	28	South	19
All nursing personnel per 100 patients, 1959	Region	West	85	Northeast	75
Professional nursing graduates, 1960	Region	Northeast	37.1%	West	9.3%
Practical nursing graduates, 1960	Region	South	34.0%	West	14.7%

Source: HEW, *Health Resource Statistics, Health Manpower* (1965), p. 115; *Health Manpower Source Book,* section 2 (1960), pp. 10, 90.

needed expansion. Hence, with rising deficits, and declining federal subsidies, medical schools are seeking other financial resources. New York's Mount Sinai has used the interest from its $100 million building fund to meet expansion needs. The Marquette School of Medicine in Milwaukee liquidated endowments and sold its building for $1.5 million. The New York Medical College sold off endowments of $6 million and mortgaged property to a possible maximum of $10 million. George Washington University uses its unrestricted income, but this causes serious reductions in future income.[25]

The financial problems of medical schools are increasing despite these strong measures. In the last twenty-five years, emphasis has been put on expanding the educational facilities for allied medical personnel. The policy has been to increase disproportionately the number of less costly members of the medical team, stressing not only nurses and allied health workers rather than doctors, but also the less costly health workers, such as hospital aides, rather than registered nurses. Thus, the increase of nurses greatly exceeded that of physicians, while that of nurses' aides exceeded that of registered nurses. Doctors, dentists, and nurses still accounted for a rising share

FIGURE 6.20 Distribution of Nursing Education Among Regions

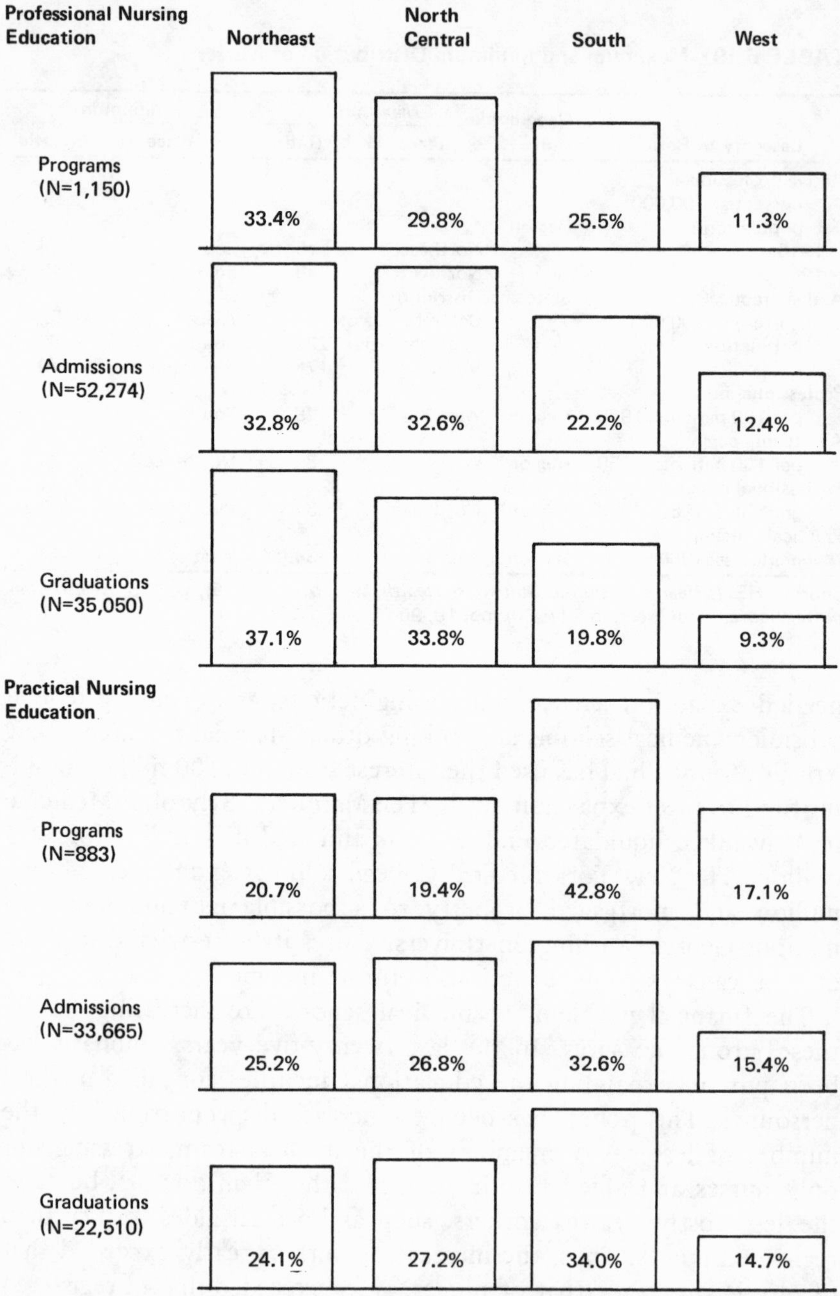

Professional Nursing Education	Northeast	North Central	South	West
Programs (N=1,150)	33.4%	29.8%	25.5%	11.3%
Admissions (N=52,274)	32.8%	32.6%	22.2%	12.4%
Graduations (N=35,050)	37.1%	33.8%	19.8%	9.3%

Practical Nursing Education	Northeast	North Central	South	West
Programs (N=883)	20.7%	19.4%	42.8%	17.1%
Admissions (N=33,665)	25.2%	26.8%	32.6%	15.4%
Graduations (N=22,510)	24.1%	27.2%	34.0%	14.7%

Source: Adapted from HEW, *Health Manpower Source Book,* section 2 (revised January 1966), p. 74.

of medical personnel and of the total number on the labor market, however.

Shortages of skilled personnel call for rising economic status, higher educational achievements, and more opportunities for promotion.

Notes

1. U.S. Department of Health, Education, and Welfare (HEW), *Report to the President and the Congress: The Allied Health Professions Personnel Training Act of 1966, as Amended* (1969), pp. xi-xii, 1-3.

2. HEW, *Health Manpower Source Book,* section 21 (1970), table 4.

3. HEW, *Indicators,* January 1967, p. 8. By fiscal year 1971, Medicare and Medicaid involved almost $15 billion of expenditures annually.

4. HEW, *Report to the President and the Congress: The Allied Health Professions Personnel Training Act of 1966, as Amended* (1969), pp. 27-28.

5. HEW, *Manpower for the Medical Laboratory,* Proceedings of a Conference of Government and the Professions, Washington, D.C., October 1967, p. 117.

6. Ibid., p. 120; U.S. Senate, Committee on Labor, Subcommittee on Public Health and Welfare, *Allied Health Professions Personnel Training* (1970), p. 19.

7. HEW, *Health Manpower Source Book,* section 20 (1968), tables 27, 31.

8. HEW, *Report to the President and the Congress: The Allied Health Professions Personnel Training Act of 1966, as Amended* (1969), pp. 7, 9, 14, 16.

9. Ibid., figure 1.

10. HEW, *Manpower for the Medical Laboratory,* Proceedings of a Conference of Government and the Professions in Washington, D.C., October 1967, p. 77.

11. Ibid., pp. 91, 100.

12. Ibid., p. 77.

13. Ibid., p. 107.

14. HEW, *Health Manpower Source Book,* section 21 (1970), table 10.

15. HEW, *Health Manpower Source Book,* section 2 (revised January 1966), pp. 24, 113.

16. HEW, *Report to the President and the Congress: The Allied Health Professions Personnel Training Act of 1966, as Amended* (1969), p. 22.

17. Ibid., p. 34.

18. Calculated from HEW, *Health Manpower Source Book,* section 21 (1970), p. 24.

19. HEW, *Health Manpower Source Book,* section 2 (revised January 1966), p. 82.

20. D. E. Yett, "Causes and Consequences of Salary Differentials in Nursing," *Inquiry,* March 1970, pp. 95-96.

21. HEW, *Health Manpower Source Book,* section 2 (revised January 1966), pp. 11, 15, 21, 24, 55.

22. HEW, *Health Manpower Perspective: 1967*, p. 8.

23. For the last few paragraphs, see HEW, *Health Resources Statistics, Health Manpower* (1965), p. 113; HEW, *Health Manpower Perspective: 1967*, table 4; HEW, *Health Manpower Source Book*, section 18 (1964), table 35; HEW, *Report to the President and the Congress: The Allied Health Professions Personnel Training Act of 1966, as Amended* (1969), pp. 22, 34; and HEW, *Health Manpower Source Book*, section 2 (revised January 1966), pp. 15, 35.

24. See especially HEW, *Report to the President and the Congress: The Allied Health Professions Personnel Training Act of 1966, as Amended* (1969), pp. xi-xii and chaps. 1-3, for a discussion of supply and demand and federal subsidies.

25. *Business Week*, July 25, 1970; *Los Angeles Times*, August 23, 1970, October 17, 1971; *New York Times*, June 28, 1971.

PART III

Inflation and
Medical Markets

7

Inflation of Prices

Most Americans know there is a "health crisis" in the United States. Medical care costs have soared. Physicians' bills rose 130 percent in the last ten years and hospital costs 217 percent in the same period. In most metropolitan areas, hospital patients can expect to pay at least $100 a day.

All patients do not pay the same price for a given service. For example, the insured patient pays less than the uninsured, because the insurance intermediary intervenes on behalf of its clients and, with its greater market power, bargains for better prices. But as insurance becomes more prevalent, intermediaries have less leverage for reducing prices for their enrollees: the uninsured become a smaller part of that universe. Meanwhile, other discrimination arises as physicians and hospitals raise their charges more because of more extensive insurance coverage.

Some areas have too many hospitals and physicians, while others have too few or none. In the suburbs there is one doctor for every 500 people; in the inner cities and in many rural areas there is one doctor for every 2,000. In Mississippi and Alaska there are only 78 doctors per 100,000 people. Some 130 counties in the United States have no doctors at all.

Medicare and to some extent Medicaid have greatly increased the number of people who can pay directly or indirectly for health care at relatively nonsubsidized rates. That means that more resources become available for others in great need, e.g., individuals not in the labor market.

Discrimination occurs in the hospitals. Hospitals charge competitive prices for room, board, and routine nursing. But, profiting from superior knowledge, they charge more than their costs for ancillary services. Some spirited discussions have taken place between hospitals and government administrators on the issue of costs for patients over sixty-five as compared with those under sixty-five. The hospitals claim the elderly patients require much more care and hence are more costly. The government contends that, since the older patients stay longer in hospitals, the cost of ancillary services per day for them is much lower because the total cost of these services is allocated over longer periods.

Other aspects of discrimination derive from the sliding scales under which physicians and hospitals charge more to the affluent or favor the poor directly. This method of reimbursement becomes less popular as the poor increasingly are financed by the government to cover their needs.

The present inadequate resources in medicine and inequitable distribution of medical services are all the more serious because similar problems are confronted in education and in housing. Moreover, the deficiencies in medicine require advances in education and housing among other things. Recent substantial gains in the education of minority groups suggest what can be done in other fields and to some extent may reduce the damage done by deficiencies in medical care.

Even in education, however, the gains have not achieved equality. For example, in a recent year, nonwhites constituted 12.1 percent of the population, but they accounted for less than 6 percent of freshmen enrolled in institutions of higher learning and only 3 percent of all classes in such institutions. Moreover, almost half go to four-year Negro colleges, which suffer from underfinancing and poor conditions.[1]

Inflation is a serious problem in this country. With medical prices rising twice as much as all consumer goods generally, they accounted for about 0.8 percent out of the 6 percent rate of inflation in 1971, and by 1973-74 inflation had risen to about 8 percent per year.

Comparisons of Medical Care Prices

In the 1950s and 1960s medical care prices increased much more than the cost of living. This had not been true in the 1940s. The erosion of the dollar's purchasing power has thus been felt in a vital area of expenditures in recent decades. That a large part of the additional funds pouring into the medical market is consumed in rising prices or rising incomes is an additional cause of public discontent.

Yet we may be exaggerating the damage done by rising prices. A comparison of the percentage rise of family or per capita income with the increase of medical care prices may suggest another conclusion. For example, if medical prices rise by 100 percent while per capita disposable income increases by 200 percent, the capacity to finance medical care has actually increased. In the last generation, per capita disposable income has increased much more than medical prices. But a consumer who has used hospital services primarily may find his capacity to pay for this type of medical care greatly reduced.

The price of medical care has been rising much more rapidly than the consumer price index (see figure 7.1). In the three periods depicted in the figure, 1946-60, 1960-65 and 1965-68, prices of medical care rose 40 percent, 90 percent, and 76 percent more than the consumer price index.

Figure 7.2 shows the increase in the consumer price index, the medical care component, hospital daily charges, and physicians' fees for 1966, 1967, and 1968. What stands out is the large inflation of hospital charges each year; physicians' fees are also higher than the other indexes. The moderation of fee increases from 1966 to 1967 and 1968 was greater for physicians' fees than for hospital service charges.[2]

From 1959 to 1969, physicians' fees rose about as much as all medical prices, but drug prices rose considerably less than the overall index and hospital daily service charges rose spectacularly more than other categories (see figure 7.3).

Between 1946 and 1966 medical care services more than doubled in price (see figure 7.4). During this period physicians' fees almost doubled; dentists' fees rose by 81 percent; daily service charges at hospitals rose by 359 percent; and drugs and prescriptions rose by 32 percent. The details of increases in the medical care price index

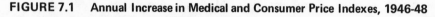

FIGURE 7.1   Annual Increase in Medical and Consumer Price Indexes, 1946-48

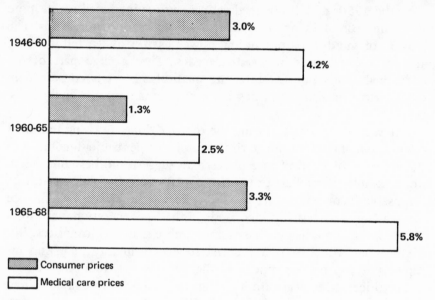

Source: HEW, *The Size and Shape of the Medical Care Dollar: Chart Book* (1969), p. 8.

are given in table 7.5. It is obvious that patients requiring hospitalization found medical care especially burdensome, though the spread of public and private hospital insurance eased the burden to some extent.

Price Measurement

There are several approaches to measuring prices. Samuel Bradbury in 1937 made a study of 1,000 people, with a view to discovering the costs of the diseases and medical procedures likely to arise.[3] He examined the total cost of providing these services over a year, the cost of each kind of service, and the cost per hour of service for each service category. The results are given in table 7.6.

The average cost per illness varied from $508.36 for nervous and mental disorders to $148.60 for heart disease, arteriosclerosis, and high blood pressure, and to $66.10 for ear mastoid infection.[4]

On the basis of his data, Dr. Bradbury estimated the *gross* income

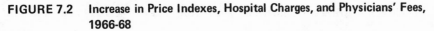

FIGURE 7.2   Increase in Price Indexes, Hospital Charges, and Physicians' Fees, 1966-68

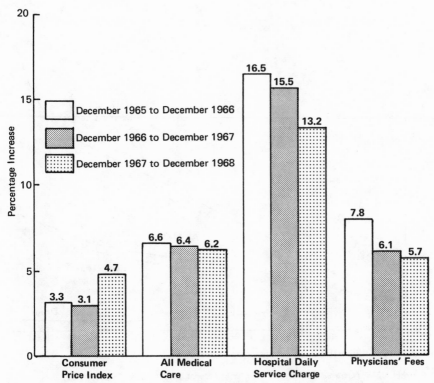

Source: HEW, Office of Research and Statistics, *Medical Care Price Fact Sheet,* Note no. 8 (May 9, 1969).

of specialists in 1929 at $45,285 and of general practitioners at $22,200; these are about 2½ times the actual incomes. The differences result from fees not collected, idle time, and the excess of fees set by the medical society over actual fees collected.[5]

Use of fees as a measure of the price of medical care is replete with difficulties. For one thing, fees are a varying share of total payments. In recent years, for example, capitation payment and salaries have been used increasingly, and prices of physicians' services reflect the use of these methods of payment. Another troublesome problem is discovering what is the customary and reasonable fee. Many doctors

FIGURE 7.3   Rise in Hospital, Physician, Drug, and All Medical Prices, 1959-66

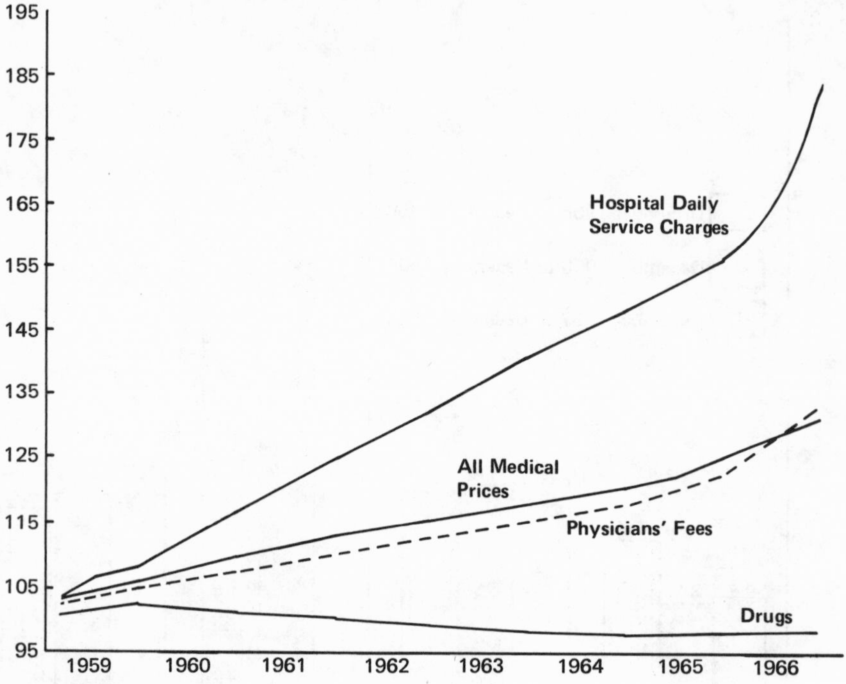

Index: 1957-1959=100

Source: HEW, *National Conference on Medical Costs, Chart Book* (1967), p. 11.

know what they charge but few know what the customary and reasonable fee for a service is.

The number of fees is also significant, for the price is a function of both the level and the number. Fragmentation of care, which increases the number of fees for treatment of a particular condition, has become more popular with physicians. The practice of gang visits to nursing homes—visiting fifty patients within a few hours—is also increasing. Another weakness of the fee indexes is that no allowance is made for free or subsidized services.[6]

The orthodox measure of prices is the consumer price index. For various reasons, however, the accuracy of this index has been

FIGURE 7.4   Source and Amount of Medical Price Increase, 1950-69

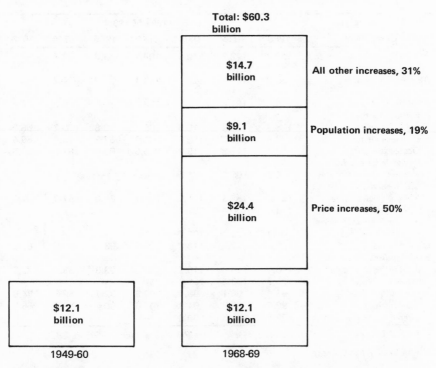

Source: HEW, *The Size and Shape of the Medical Care Dollar: Chart Book* (1969), p. 6.

questioned. One reason it is not a precise measure of changes in prices is that it is very difficult to measure quality changes. A day at the hospital in 1930 is not identical to a day in 1970. The hospital now has many more employees per patient, more expensive equipment, and a larger proportion of newer and better beds.

To some extent the same trends are evident in doctor visits. The physician today has much improved equipment, greater recourse to other members of the medical team, greater access to specialists, and generally better and more extensive training. But there are some offsets: under great demand pressures, physicians have tended to cut the time per visit and have increasingly abandoned home and night visits, forcing patients to use the hospital for treatment. The

TABLE 7.5   Components of Medical Care Price Index, 1946-66

Component	Index (1957-59=100)						
	1966	1965	1964	1960	1955	1950	1946
All medical care	127.7	122.3	119.4	108.1	88.6	73.4	60.7
All medical services	133.9	127.1	123.2	109.1	88.0	71.7	58.4
Physicians' fees	128.5	121.5	117.3	106.0	90.0	76.0	66.4
Family doctor							
Office visits	128.7	121.2	116.8	105.4	90.8	76.2	66.7
House visits	133.4	124.9	119.9	106.9	87.3	75.4	66.4
Obstetrical care	123.0	117.8	115.2	105.0	90.8	67.7	57.5
Pediatric care office							
visits*	114.3	106.1	101.5	–	–	–	–
Hospital services							
Daily service charges	168.0	153.3	144.9	112.7	83.0	57.8	37.0
Operating room charges*	113.7	106.4	101.9	–	–	–	–
X-ray, diagnostic, upper							
gastrointestinal*	105.7	102.1	100.7	–	–	–	–
Dentists' fees	121.4	117.6	114.0	104.7	93.1	81.5	67.0
Examinations, prescriptions,							
dispensing of eyeglasses	116.1	113.0	110.7	103.7	93.8	89.5	79.3
Routine lab tests*	105.7	103.5	101.6	–	–	–	–
Drugs and prescriptions	98.4	98.1	98.4	102.3	92.7	86.6	74.6
Prescriptions	90.6	90.8	91.8	102.6	90.4	82.4	65.9
Over-the-counter items*	102.4	101.3	100.6	–	–	–	–

Source: HEW, *Report to the President, Medical Care Prices* (February 1967), p. 38.

*December 1963 = 100.

patient may gain from access to the hospital, but he accepts higher costs from the transportation and increased waiting time burdens that are put on him.[7]

The weighting in the consumer price index is seriously inadequate, although improvements have been made in recent years. Before 1939, surgeons' and specialists' fees were not included in the index; in mid-1947, in response to budget cuts, the Bureau of Labor Statistics stopped including prices for dentists' services, fees for private nurses, and several other important charges; from 1918 to 1956 the only general item added was insurance; and in March 1960, long after the drug component had become outmoded, the bureau added prescriptions for antiinfectives, sedatives, hypnotics, ataractics (tranquilizers), antispasmodics, antiarthritics, cough preparations, cardiovascular medicines, and antihypertensives. In December 1952,

TABLE 7.6   Costs of Services per 1,000 Persons, 1937

Provider of Service	Number of Annual Services Used	Total Annual Costs	Cost per Service
Total, all services*	17,426	$65,530	$ 3.64
General practitioners	5,150	13,111	2.54
Specialists	1,187	15,575	13.11
Hospital services (days)	1,384	5,537	4.00
Institutional services (days)	2,368	7,103	3.00
Nursing services	3,838	7,760	2.02
X-ray examinations	2,282	5,497	24.08
Laboratory examinations	2,695	5,618	2.08

Source: S. Bradbury, *The Cost of Adequate Medical Care* (1937), p. 19.

*Several small items omitted.

multiple-vitamin concentrates had been added. Thus, a serious lag prevailed here.[8] The unreliability of the old index is illustrated by the fact that the nonprescribed drug component was made up of two items: aspirin and milk of magnesia.

Since 1958, important changes have been made. The former sample was excessively weighted with older physicians; its ratio of general practitioners was too large, and there were too few in places some distance from metropolitan centers. Until 1960, only three prescription drugs were priced: penicillin, a narcotic, and a nonnarcotic. In 1960 the list was increased to sixteen items. By 1967 the health care component included thirty-eight items: eighteen services and twenty drugs (prescription and nonprescription).[9]

The impact of rising collections poses another problem for the consumer price index. When collections jump from 75 percent to 95 percent of charges, the index gives a misleading view of price movements. Inflation of the medical care component is substantially increased as the ratio of collections to charges rises by about 25 percent. This is a rough estimate of the improvement in collections since the 1930s.

Anne Scitovsky, in a pioneering approach, proposed using the costs of diseases as a measure of medical care prices. She suggested that the consumer price index was deficient in numerous ways: tardy adjustment to changes in spending patterns, neglect of high-priced items, inadequate coverage of items, and inattention to changes in quality. Measuring prices against costs of disease would give greatly improved coverage, she argued. In fact, Mrs. Scitovsky found that this measure yielded a much higher rise of prices than the medical component of the consumer price index.[10] Over fourteen years, the cost of treatment rose 87 percent by her measure, compared with a rise of 57 percent in the medical component of the consumer price index. The difference is explained by such factors as the excess of actual charges over customary charges, better treatment (quality changes), and inclusion of a greater number of expensive items.

As the cost of a day at the hospital rises from say $10 to $50, the increase in price is not 400 percent but much less if the measurement is based not on rising charges per day but rather on the increased cost of an entire stay. This is because over the years the average stay has tended to decline. If the hypothetical cost per day rises from $10 to $50 but the length of stay is reduced from thirty to twenty days, the cost of a stay rises from $300 to $1,000, an increase of 233 percent not 400 percent. Concentration on costs per day tends to give an exaggerated view of the inflation.

The American Medical Association estimated that in the late 1920s the average stay of thirty days cost $125; by the late 1950s the average stay had dropped to seven or eight days, costing $250. On a price per day comparison, the rise would be 700 percent to 800 percent; but comparing prices per stay, the increase is only 100 percent.[11] In addition, the patient gains more working income as stays in the hospital are reduced.

Factors in Price Increases

Prices rise as demand expands more than supply. The increase of demand stems from growing income among large segments of the population, greater interest in medical services as a result of more disposable income, growth of the population, rising educational achievement, and a greater availability of medical services. The rising demand for services also feeds on the expansion of intermediaries that can purchase medical services without the usual financial restraints. Blue Shield, for example, spends more freely for health care than the consumer who purchases directly and feels the sting of using up his private resources.

If supply had responded to rising demand adequately, the inflationary impact would have been reduced. But this did not happen for numerous reasons: the market for physicians was restrictive, the flow of funds into health schools was slow, and the gestation period for training a physician is ten years from the time plans for a school are made to the time the first doctors graduate. Provision of more hospital beds is also a slow process, and maldistribution and excessive duplication in some areas have reduced the effectiveness of the country's existing supply.

Inflationary forces are not brought about only by the excess of demand over supply. Economists also watch the impact of cost increases, that is, the cost-push, directly on prices. This is indeed an important factor in medical inflation. Increased charges for services by physicians, hospitals, drug manufacturers, etc., are part of the cost-push pressures. They are not easy to contain.

Tying costs to reimbursements removes the usual control of markets through price movements. Markets for medical services are also unusual in the response of purchases as prices rise. An increase of prices of 10 percent according to various estimates yields a reduction of purchases of only 2 percent to 5 percent. In other words, the inflationary impact is not greatly diluted by a reduction of units purchased as prices rise. The response of expenditures for medical services as incomes rise is greater than the response to price rises.

Thus the estimate of income elasticity of demand for physicians' visits varied from 0.1 to 0.62 in four estimates; and for expenditures for physicians' services, seven estimates ranged from 0.17 to 2.9.[12]

Insurance Intermediaries

Various insurance programs, public and private, have played an increasing role in medical markets. Perhaps the fact that third parties have a less direct interest in the loss of resources, as they spend on behalf of others, also explains their recourse to reimbursement of purveyors on the basis of cost. This is a wasteful manner of spending. The importance of outlays by third parties is illustrated in table 7.7. In 1950, government, philanthropy, and private health insurance accounted for 41 percent of medical care expenditures, but by 1969 they provided as much as 65 percent.

From 1950 to 1970 benefits from private insurance for hospitals rose three times as much as gross enrollment for hospital care. The increase in benefit expenditures for physicians' services over the same period was 2.3 times the rate of increase in gross enrollment

TABLE 7.7 Third-Party and Direct Outlays for Medical Care, 1950-69

Source of Outlay	1949-50 Amount (Billions)	1949-50 Percentage	1959-60 Amount (Billions)	1959-60 Percentage	1965-66 Amount (Billions)	1965-66 Percentage	1968-69 Amount (Billions)	1968-69 Percentage
Total	$12.1	100	$26.4	100	$42.3	100	$60.3	100
Government	3.1	25	6.4	24	10.8	26	22.6	38
Philanthropy and others	1.0	9	2.2	8	3.7	9	4.7	8
Private health insurance	.9	7	4.7	18	8.9	21	11.7	19
Patient outlays	7.1	59	13.1	50	18.9	44	21.3	35

Source: Adapted from HEW, *The Size and Shape of the Medical Care Dollar, Chart Book* (1969), p. 14.

for hospital care. The higher rate of increase in benefit expenditures is due to rising costs of medical care, expansion of benefits, and higher utilization.[13]

In 1970, about 17 percent of the population (31 million) were wholly unprotected by insurance. Children and the poor were disproportionate parts in this group. The percentages of the population lacking specific types of coverage are shown in table 7.8.

Of the population with annual incomes under $3,000, 36 percent were covered by hospital insurance and 35 percent had surgical insurance. Of those earning $10,000 or more per year, 92 percent had hospital coverage and 91 percent surgical coverage. Benefit payments per enrollee for hospital care in 1970 ranged from $18 for individual insurance policies to $66.01 for Blue Cross.[14] The percentage of consumer expenditures for health care that is met by insurance has risen steadily since 1950 (see table 7.9).

The rising scope of the fiscal intermediaries in the field of health care greatly affects price movements, because purchases are increasingly made by agencies that are not directly involved in receiving the services provided. The incentive for providers to economize is absent when recovery of all their costs is guaranteed by Blue Cross, Blue Shield, and other insurance companies. The intermediaries do put some pressure on purveyors of services to keep costs down, because insurance rates rise greatly as costs of services increase. But the availability of insurance encourages physicians, hospitals, and other purveyors to charge more than they otherwise would, since the patient does not bear the burden directly.

TABLE 7.8   Population Uninsured by Type of Coverage

Type of Coverage	Percentage of Population Not Covered
Hospital service	16.5
Surgical service	19.2
In-hospital visits	24.9
X rays and laboratory exams	26.2
Office and home visits	52.0
Dental care	89.7
Prescription drugs	46.5
Nursing home care	85.0
Private duty nursing	46.9
Visiting nurse service	43.5

Source: HEW, Office of Research and Statistics, *Medical Care Costs and Prices: Background Book* (January 1972), p. 96.

TABLE 7.9   Consumer Expenditures Covered by Insurance, 1950-70

Year	Total Expenditures	Percentage Met by Insurance	
		Hospital Care	Physicians' Services
1950	12.2	37.1	12.0
1955	21.7	56.0	25.0
1960	27.8	64.5	30.0
1965	31.8	71.2	32.8
1970	40.3	73.2	48.1

Source: HEW, Office of Research and Statistics, *Medical Care Costs and Prices: Background Book* (January 1972), p. 101.

Demand for dental care is much more responsive to rising income than demand for physicians' services. Yet during recent periods of rising health care outlays, expenditures for dental care have risen less than those for physicians' services. This may be explained by the fact that insurance for dental services is generally unavailable.

One economist seems to deny the positive correlation of insurance and rising expenditures and prices. If insurance accounts for rising prices, he asks, why have prices for surgery, with the largest coverage by insurance, increased the least and those for dentistry, with the least coverage, increased the most?[15]

I am not convinced by some of these arguments. The small rise of prices for surgery despite the heavy insurance coverage may well be explained by other factors, such as the relatively large influx of surgeons or possibly modest rises in the number of surgical procedures. The large increase in prices for dental care may be explained in part by the high income elasticity for dentists at recent high levels of income.

The rising level of insurance indeed tends to give the insured advantages. But to a considerable extent it results in lower *relative*, not lower *absolute*, prices. As demand exceeds supply, prices tend to rise. The intermediaries absorb a certain proportion of the windfalls that arise from greater excess income as insurance spreads. The physicians, operating through associations such as Blue Shield, then try to intercept part of this windfall. The physicians and hospitals who attempt to siphon off some of the excess are accused of indulging in corporate medicine.

Dr. Ray Brown has discussed the impact of the intermediaries on prices:

If the demander is freed of cost considerations the supplier is deprived of price lists that ordinarily guide and control his operations. When cost is used as the basis for reimbursement then price is no longer an independent variable and to that extent loses its effectiveness as a means of checking and controlling the demand for hospital services. Reimbursement means that the provider gets back what he spends. He is not compelled to meet a set of prices or the prices of his competitors. . . .[16]

Insurance coverage is still inadequate in terms of both numbers of people and medical services covered. Moreover, the present system of insurance encourages abuses. Providers tend to waste resources as they call for more services for patients who are insured, and the insurance interests have been most inept or ineffective in checking on the quality of services and the validity of charges. Under Medicare, for example, the net potential contribution in services was greatly reduced as purveyors of services greatly increased their charges. Fear of annoying doctors and hospital administrators contributes to the lack of cost control, and state insurance officials have failed to correct abuses.

Hospital Prices

The largest increase in medical prices in recent years has occurred in hospital charges. Relevant factors include the efforts to correct the low pay of hospital employees, the improvement and extension of services, the rising demand for hospital beds, which is associated in part with the increase of incomes, the spread of private and public health insurance, and the general inflation of the economy. But there is also evidence of inefficiency. The Hill-Burton Act, for example, provided federal subsidies for hospitals, especially in smaller communities. But it soon became clear that what was needed, as large segments of the population moved into metropolitan centers, was more help for urban hospitals. Moreover, the location of hospitals was too often determined by political and other irrelevant considerations. Recourse to hospitals, when less expensive facilities would do, and excessive stays also added to costs and reduced efficiency.

The cost of a day at the hospital varies depending on the patient's use of ancillary services. Hence the daily service charge may be misleading. According to one study, ancillary services accounted for 36.4 percent of the costs when the patient stayed 50 days or more, but they were up as high as 63.2 percent when the patient stayed only one to two days (see table 7.10 and figure 7.11).

TABLE 7.10   Relative Cost of Ancillary Services by Length of Stay

Days of Stay	Percentage of Bill		Number of Cases	Weighted Percentage of General Hospital Sample
	For Accommodation	For Ancillary Services		
1-2	36.8	63.2	2,189	21.9
3-4	48.0	51.7	1,786	21.9
5-6	53.9	45.9	1,585	18.9
7-8	54.6	45.5	1,040	9.9
9-10	54.8	44.2	660	6.0
11-14	54.9	44.2	792	7.2
15-19	55.5	44.3	462	3.9
20-49	59.5	40.4	672	5.6
50 and over	63.5	36.4	71	.6

Source: W. J. McNerney, *Hospital and Medical Economics* (1962), vol. 1, p. 395.

Note: Percentage may not total to 100 because of rounding error.

Insofar as a hospital passes costs on to patients, instead of absorbing them, prices tend to rise. For example, a Michigan study in the late 1950s found that hospitals do not ordinarily have large depreciation funds, since they depend partly on gifts for capital purposes. In a large sample of Michigan hospitals only roughly one-quarter funded their depreciation charges, and 94 percent of these had less in assets than their accumulated depreciation. A small proportion of these hospitals used their depreciation funds to buy equipment, expand, and pay off debts.

Depreciation is an acceptable cost to be financed by patients. The charge should be related to donated value or historical cost of the hospital's capital. But patients should not fund depreciation on rents paid to holding companies that own a hospital and its equipment; nor should they be burdened with interest and rent costs, which would further raise prices. For capital, hospitals should depend primarily on drives, public gifts, and loans.[17]

A case can be made for hospitals passing on their educational costs to patients, because patients profit from them. In a recent year it was estimated that hospitals turned out about 80 percent of the registered nurse graduates. However, government has been financing a rising share of these educational costs.[18]

Research costs present a more difficult problem. The patient surely should not pay for research that is only remotely related to patient care. In view of the difficult financial problems confronting both hospitals and patients, it would be desirable to spare the patients most research costs. Government and foundations should shoulder these costs.

Physicians' Fees

Doctors have the highest earnings of any professional group: their average yearly income seems to range between $40,000 and $50,000 (these figures include interns and residents who make $10,000 to

FIGURE 7.11   Ratio of Ancillary Services to Accommodation Charges by Length of Stay

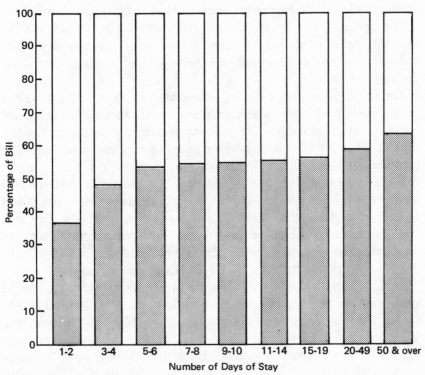

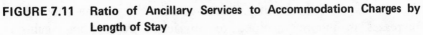

Source: W. J. McNerney, *Hospital and Medical Economics* (1962), vol. 1, p. 395.

$15,000 a year). A recent Maryland study shows that a typical hospital pays its department chiefs $150,000 to $200,000, its chief assistants $65,000, and its "regular" doctors $35,000 to $40,000.[19]

The high level of income of physicians, when compared with the income of the working population, other professional groups, or other members of the medical team, raises serious problems.

It is now a confessed objective of both political parties to tie increases in incomes to overall increases in productivity. It is difficult for government to pursue an effective antiinflationary policy when the practicing physician earns about seven times the pay of the average worker, three times the income of the college professor, and three to four times the income of the average scientist. In the 1960s, large increases in income accrued to physicians even though gains of productivity in medicine were generally held to be relatively small.

The damage done by the rapidly rising income of physicians spills over into other areas, both because other groups seek similar rewards and because the large incomes are then spent, increasing inflationary pressures elsewhere.

For the economy as a whole, physicians' incomes that are far out of line raise problems for any policies that tie incomes to increased productivity. It is difficult to sanction increases of income of 8 percent or more a year when low-income groups are asked to keep their incomes from rising more than 5 percent.

To some extent the Social Security Administration has tried to justify the pricing policies of physicians. The rise in their prices was a product of both the number of doctors who increased their fees and amount of increase demanded. In other words, although prices doubled when Medicare took effect, a large percentage of physicians showed remarkable restraint by not increasing their charges.

There clearly were some excesses in physicians' charges, and a small number of doctors even indulged in fraud. The Senate Finance Committee and Blue Shield, for example, publicized the case of a Michigan physician who received $177,000 in a single year from Medicaid. He apparently practiced for 300 days a year; his daily gross averaged about $540; and at $10 per visit he would see fifty-four patients for twelve to fifteen minutes per service.[20]

This does not necessarily suggest fraud. It might have been smarter, however, for the doctor to cut his fee from (say) $10 to $5 and reduce his working day by one-third. His income then would have been around $54,000, and the quality of service would have greatly improved. He might have been confronted with large unfilled demands for his services, however.

During 1966 the consumer price index for physicians' services advanced more rapidly than the price of any of five procedures for the aged. The implication is that the physicians treating older patients restrained themselves from unduly benefiting from the flow of Medicare funds. But for the thirty-six months ended December 1968, the index for physicians' fees increased 21 percent while increases for the five procedures ranged from 16 percent to 21 percent (see figure 7.12). The conclusion was that "physicians increased their customary fees for services to the aged in line with the upward trend in all physicians' fees."[21]

Drug Prices

Forbes magazine calls the drug industry "one of the biggest crap games in U.S. industry." For over ten years, the drug industry has

FIGURE 7.12   Increase in Physicians' Fees and Prices of Common Procedures under Medicare, 1965-68

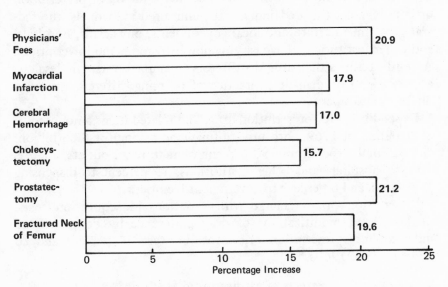

Source: HEW, Office of Research and Statistics, *Medical Care Price Fact Sheet,* Note no. 8 (May 9, 1969).

held either first, second, or third place among all American industries in terms of profitability—outdistancing the cosmetics, aerospace, recreation, and entertainment industries. The highly monopolistic nature of the drug industry makes it a prime example of how excessive concentration brings inordinate profits. Attempts to deal with inflation of drug prices have faced great difficulty. The emphasis by physicians on *proprietary* drugs rather than *generic* names also contributes to uneconomic performance. The federal government is slowly increasing its regulation of drug costs and quality. Stiffer scrutiny of new drugs under a 1962 law caused a sharp drop in the rate at which new products were introduced, and pushed many companies to expand abroad in countries where drug testing and marketing laws are much more permissive.[22]

Improvements in the pricing of drugs, and hence reduction of inflationary pressures in the economy, could be had in numerous ways: for example, insistence upon prescription of generic drugs when no substantial advantage can be shown for a proprietary name; and exclusion of differentiated drugs from the market when they have no advantage, or only a slight advantage, over substitutes.

Drug prices vary greatly, partly because some drugs are patented while others are not. Another factor is that a variety of prescription drug purchasers (insured individuals, uninsured individuals, the federal government, state and local governments, physicians, hospitals, and other institutions) have varying power to command lower prices. A third factor is that drug distributors (manufacturers, wholesalers, and retailers) have made a practice of charging different prices to different customers.[23]

Expenditures for prescription drugs and related items amounted to $8.5 billion in 1969, with private financing paying for $7.8 billion. Of the total expenditure, 58 percent went to retail outlets, 21 percent to hospitals and other institutions, 13 percent to dispensing physicians, and 8 percent to government facilities.[24]

Prescription prices change with variations in acquisition costs, markups, and modifications of drug preference by doctors. Four indexes show prescription prices rose between 17 percent and 26 percent in the 1960s.[25]

Effects of Medicare and Medicaid

With the introduction of Medicare and Medicaid in 1966, inflation in medical markets accelerated. Under these two programs, expenditures ran about $13 billion in 1970. Inflation arose from the classical cause: rising demand. However, the response of supply—particularly supplies of physicians, nurses, nursing homes, and to some extent hospital beds—was slow.

Effect on Physicians

Doctors reacted to rising demand by increasing their prices, although charges did not rise as much as might have been expected under free market conditions before 1960. Hence the shortage proved more troublesome than it otherwise would have been. But over the last thirty years doctors have relied primarily on both increases in fees and rationing of their time to handle the excess demand for their services. On the whole they have tended to rely more on price increases because this was an easier technique to exploit.

The explanation of rising prices also lay in part in what economists call "cost-inflation." Physicians feared that the introduction of Medicare and Medicaid would result in ceilings being placed on their fees. At the same time, they were experiencing the impact of a flood of dollars into the medical care market. They responded by greatly increasing their charges beginning in 1965. Doctors also exploited the fee-for-service reimbursement system and the customary and reasonable fee approach.

Effect on Hospitals

Hospitals in considerable financial trouble before Medicare and Medicaid were able to become viable through these programs. Their revenues rose much more than their costs. Hospitals began to receive reimbursements for services that previously were not paid for or were paid only in part. With the increased resources from insurance, occupancy rates increased. The net result was a large increase in hospital charges. From June 1966 to December 1967, hospitals increased their daily service charges by 18.7 percent. Net revenues of short-term voluntary hospitals rose from $135 million in 1960 to $287 million in 1966 and $399 million in 1967.[26]

Hospital costs and prices respond to economies of scale, the reduction of slack, and hence declining unit costs. They also reflect the burgeoning increase in utilization. Thus hospital utilization rates rose from 3.25 percent in July-December 1966 to 3.88 percent for the calendar year 1968, according to one study, and from 3.73 percent to 4.03 percent according to another study. Annual average daily costs increased in this period from $52.44 to $65.30, according to one source, and from $37.28 to $48.60, according to another estimate.[27] Reimbursement on the basis of costs improved the condition of hospitals.

Measures to Combat Inflation

What therapy is required to reduce inflation in the health care field? Possible measures include improved productivity, attacks on monopoly (notably in the drug industry), improved planning of resource allocation, containment of the rising demand associated with the large growth of insurance not matched by measures to prevent excessive use of services, and increased supplies in markets that are now inadequately provisioned, such as the supply of doctors.

Provisioning the Medical Market

It is necessary to provide for a rise in the number of doctors, with each working thirty to forty hours a week instead of sixty. Productivity could also be increased—for example, through greater use of group practice and of technical aid. A national health insurance program that fixes compensation, as the British system does, is a more drastic approach that can be used if other ways are not found.

Another approach to eliminating the shortage of physicians in certain areas is the National Health Service Corps, which was created under the Public Health Service. Its prime function is to send young doctors to remote regions. Some 500 doctors applied for the initial 220 NHSC positions as an alternative to military service.

Still another plan has been offered by Dr. Samuel Proger of Tufts University. He suggests creating a new specialty of physicians: the primary medical doctor, or P.M.D. These physicians would receive an abbreviated course of the general training now given to M.D.'s. During most of their training, expert diagnosticians would instruct them. The P.M.D.'s would learn to recognize what they do not know and to establish the limits of their abilities to treat patients, beyond which they would refer patients to specialists.

It is also imperative that the number of black and other minority group physicians be increased. The problem is a tough one. Blacks account for about 12 percent of the population, 6 percent of the entering freshman classes, 2½ percent of the college population, and less than 2 percent of the college graduates. General measures by the government to build medical schools and to finance black and disadvantaged medical students would help. In view of the small number of black doctors in the past, the goal should be an output at least equal to the proportion of the disadvantaged in the population. With special aid, this can be achieved. Success is more likely for this minimal objective than for larger goals that are sought immediately. With appropriate aid, the proportion of black medical students may and should rise substantially above 11 percent. Moreover, it may be necessary to introduce incentives or controls—possibly by putting conditions on the financial aid offered—to improve the geographic distribution of physicians.

A related issue is the use of physicians from abroad to achieve an adequate supply. Foreign doctors now constitute about 25 percent of our output, with half of the imported doctors coming from developing countries. This raises an ideological issue: Should the rich United States depend on countries with a third to a tenth of its per capita income for doctors whose education may have cost $50,000 apiece? California, ranked near the top among the states in per capita income, seems to be importing half its doctors, thus exploiting other parts of the country.

Use of Credit

There is much to be said for greater recourse to credit for health care expenses. Why should there be some $600 billion of private credit (excluding farm credit) and no substantial development of medical credit? The availability of credit for nonmedical fields diverts excessive resources to automobiles, television sets, household gadgets, and similar consumer goods. Under good management, incomes should rise by more than 60 percent per family in ten years, while the national income will rise from about $900 billion to $20 trillion in fifty years. This projection reflects the increase from 1961 to 1968 and allows for the rise in population in fifty years. The projected trend greatly strengthens the case for recourse to credit. The burden of financing medicine would be significantly reduced as debts are repaid out of rising income. The gain in purchasing power would be a major factor once the capital market becomes more normal.

Government Controls

The government responded in various ways to the inflation from 1965 to 1970. Although third parties, including government agencies, often rejected charges as arbitrary, Medicare generally accepted these charges. Payments were to be based on the reasonable costs of services actually provided to beneficiaries. Specific items of necessary and proper costs had to be related to services rendered. A limit could be imposed when institutional costs were out of line with those of similar institutions. At one point the government imposed reimbursement ceilings, based on overall trends in fees, and it ruled out increases in fees beyond the overall average rise of fees.

An attempt was made to keep costs down by reducing the appropriations for Medicaid. California, for example, passed legislation that would allow a 10 percent cut in Medi-Cal fees if a deficit seemed likely, although the state had a $97 million surplus of funds at the time. New York proposed a 20 percent slash in the 1966 fee schedule for physicians under Medicaid. Michigan paid only about 80 percent of usual and customary fees, and California paid up to the 60th percentile of fees charged by state physicians in January 1967.

Some government experts recommended capitation payment to organizations that would provide medical and remedial care and services; a prior authorization requirement for all elective medical and surgical procedures; and improved techniques for utilization reviews. They concluded that, even under a usual and customary fee approach, excessive fees were a problem. The emphasis on physicians' fees may be misplaced, however. A New York City study revealed that physicians get only 9 percent of the total Medicare cost of $1 billion.

The government discouraged the practice of compensating physicians in teaching hospitals who did not actually treat patients. It also eliminated the 2 percent compensation originally paid for non-identifiable costs. Nursing homes, growing at an unbelievable rate, were subjected to increased scrutiny of both prices and quality, to eliminate shoddy and high-priced services.[28]

Notes

1. See U.S. Congress, Joint Economic Committee, *The Economics and Financing of Higher Education in the United States* (1969), pp. 181-93, for a discussion of the unsatisfactory conditions under which black people live.

2. HEW, Office of Research and Statistics, *Medical Care Price Fact Sheet,* Note no. 8 (May 9, 1969).

3. S. Bradbury, *The Cost of Adequate Medical Care* (1937), especially pp. 23-29, 40, 71-72.

4. Ibid., p. 40.

5. Ibid., pp. 27-29, 40, 71-72.

6. H. E. Klarman, "Increases in the Costs of Physician and Hospital Services," *Inquiry*, March 1970, p. 25.

7. For a discussion of waiting time for the patient and wasted time for the physician, see R. B. Fetter, J. D. Thomson, and L. P. McCorkle in *Health Services Research* (summer 1966), pp. 66-114.

8. E. A. Langford, "Medical Care in the Consumer Price Index," *Monthly Labor Review*, September 1957, p. 1053; *Consumer Price Index* (December 1960) and (September 1961); U.S. Department of Labor, *Medical Care Average Retail Prices in 20 Cities, 1956-58.* On weighting, see U.S. Department of Labor, Bureau of Labor Statistics, *Relative Importance of Components in the Consumer Price Index, 1967-1968.*

9. E. M. Croft, "Health Care Prices, 1950-1967," *Journal of the American Medical Association*, July 22, 1968, pp. 91-94.

10. A. Scitovsky, "An Index on the Cost of Medical Care—A Proposed New Approach," *Conference on the Economics of Health and Medical Care*, Ann Arbor, Mich., May 10-12, 1962, pp. 133-41; U.S. Senate, Committee on Governmental Operations, Subcommittee on Executive Reorganization, *Hearings on Health Care in America* (April 1968), part 1, p. 308.

11. *A.M.A. News*, September 22, 1958.

12. H. E. Klarman, "Increases in the Costs of Physician and Hospital Services," *Inquiry*, March 1970, p. 33.

13. HEW, Office of Research and Statistics, *Medical Care Costs and Prices: Background Book* (January 1972), pp. 94-95.

14. Ibid., p. 100.

15. J. N. Garbarino, *Health Plans and Collective Bargaining* (1959), pp. 43-45; V. R. Fuchs, "Medical Costs, Why They Are What They Are," *Modern Hospitals*, September 1967, p. 107; U.S. Senate, Committee on Governmental Operations, Subcommittee on Executive Reorganization, *Hearings on Health Care in America* (April 1968), part 1, pp. 295-96.

16. HEW, *Report of the National Conference on Medical Costs*, Washington, D.C., June 27-28, 1967, pp. 280-85.

17. W. J. McNerney et al., *Hospital and Medical Economics* (1962) vol. 2, pp. 940-41, 954-55; also see H. M. Somers and A. R. Somers, *Medicare and Hospitals: Issues and Prospects* (1967), pp. 177-83, 233-34.

18. H. M. Somers and A. R. Somers, *Medicare and Hospitals: Issues and Prospects* (1967), p. 234.

19. See D. Blumenthal and J. Fallows, "Health: The Care We Want and Need," *Washington Monthly*, October 1973, p. 15.

20. *Time*, August 15, 1969.

21. HEW, Office of Research and Statistics, *Medical Care Price Fact Sheet*, Note no. 8 (May 9, 1969).

22. For more information on the drug industry, see Health Policy Advisory Committee, *The American Health Empire* (1970).

23. HEW, Office of Research and Statistics, *Medical Care Costs and Prices: Background Book* (January 1972), p. 59.

24. Ibid., p. 60.

25. Ibid., pp. 66-68.

26. See P. J. Feldstein and S. S. Waldman, "Financial Position of Hospitals in the Early Medicare Period," *Social Security Bulletin,* October 1968, pp. 18-23.

27. HEW, Social Security Administration, Office of the Actuary, *Actuarial Note,* no. 61, by R. J. Myers, September 1969, November 1969; H. E. Klarman, "Increases in the Costs of Physician and Hospital Services," *Inquiry,* March 1970, pp. 27-28.

28. N. I. Townsend, "The New Threat to Usual and Customary Fees," *Medical Economics,* April 28, 1969, especially pp. 23-24; H. M. Somers and A. R. Somers, *Medicare and Hospitals: Issues and Prospects* (1967), pp. 161-69, 182-83; H. E. Klarman, "Increases in the Costs of Physician and Hospital Services," *Inquiry,* March 1970, especially pp. 33-34; U.S. Senate, Committee on Finance, *Staff Report: Medicare and Medicaid, Problems, Issues and Alternatives* (February 1970), chaps. 6 and 9.

8

Physicians

Supply and Demand

Less than 50 percent of the nation's 340,000 doctors are in solo practice. The remainder work in group practices, hospitals, teaching, administration, and research. Only 20 percent of practicing physicians are general practitioners, and with only 2 percent of the medical graduates entering general practice, the number is still falling. Many specialists are tied to hospitals, and their fees are increasingly paid by Blue Shield, commercial insurance companies, Medicare, or Medicaid. Only about a quarter of the nation's medical expenditures goes to private practitioners.

As the number of private practitioners falls, so does their power. The membership of the American Medical Association has declined to less than half of the nation's doctors.

The supply of and the demand for physicians relate, of course, to doctors' productivity and to the total investment in personal health care. Overutilization contributes to a large and rising demand for physicians. One authority puts utilization of physicians' services in this country at 50 percent above that in the United Kingdom. Supply and demand are related to doctors' incomes, and incomes in turn are related to compensation methods, general price movements, and the number of services rendered. Comparing income movements in the 1940-to-1960 period with those in the 1960s, we find substantial differences in the factors creating the rise.

How productive our medical care system is depends on the contribution of medical 'schools and other schools. Hospitals are responsible for a large proportion of medical personnel and promise in the future to assume major responsibility for the second four years of medical training. Adequacy of the supply depends on the attrition rate among students in the medical schools, gains in productivity, and the influx of foreign-trained doctors.

The Demand for Medical Services

Decisions made by physicians largely determine the number of hospital days patients consume each year and determine to some extent the quality of hospital services. It is generally believed that the elasticity of demand for medical services is low. For example, the price elasticity of demand for medical services has been estimated to be as low as 2—that is, when prices go up by 10 percent, demand is cut by but 2 percent.[1] The precise elasticity figure is not available. However, when excess capacity prevails in hospitals, cutting prices drastically does not improve their position much. Very little space is demanded because the prices are reduced. When hospitals are operating at capacity level, they can increase their revenues by raising prices and demand will be reduced only slightly. Physicians are more disposed to recommend that their patients be hospitalized when excess space becomes available, and they reduce the demand when space is is at a premium. Doctors therefore have a cushioning effect: they tend to restrain demand and thus check increases in hospital prices in periods of high utilization, and to increase demand and moderate price declines in periods of excess capacity. Hence hospital prices do not rise or decline as much as they would if doctors' requests for space were not influenced by the supply and demand conditions.

Over a period of twenty-nine years, from 1930 to 1959, the number of visits per physician increased by 100 percent. The increase suggests a rising demand for physicians. The rise of visits may be partly explained by rising productivity, including greater relative use of auxiliary manpower, improved and extended use of plant and equipment, and new ideas. All of these raise output more than input, increasing productivity. But to some extent the increase in visits does not reflect rising productivity: the physician may well reduce his time and use of equipment per visit and may force on the patient the costs of transportation and the burden of waiting, which in the past were borne by the doctor. As pressures on physicians rise, transfer of these burdens to patients becomes more important.

What accounts for the rising demand for physicians? The factors include rising population; increases especially of the old and very young, who need more medical attention than the population in the middle age-groups; greater public awareness of medical needs, as a result of rising educational achievements; large rises of income, especially the excess income after essential needs—food, housing, and clothing—have been paid for; and improvements and extensions of health insurance and medical programs. The large relative rise in the demand for physicians in nonpractice functions is also relevant.[2]

The rising demand for physicians is suggested not only by the rising number of visits per physician but also by their rising incomes, the long queues for doctors' services, the increasing lag between contact of a physician and treatment, the unfilled vacancies in Veterans' Administration hospitals, internships, and residencies, and the shortage of psychiatrists.

The Available Supply of Doctors

A shortage of physicians has troubled the country for many years, due to the American Medical Association's tight control over how many physicians are trained. The unusual advance of demand and the long gestation period required for the output of a doctor help to induce shortages. Increased productivity diminished the shortages somewhat, though the rise in productivity was modest.[3]

The availability of physicians' services is not measured merely by increases in the total number of doctors. In recent years, a rising proportion of doctors has been diverted to nonpractice areas. Thus from 1950 to 1965 the physician-population ratio for private practice dropped from 109 per 100,000 to 97 per 100,000. The rise of graduates was modest indeed from 1960 to 1966: from 7,081 to 7,574. A 1959 report (*Physicians for a Growing America*) set a goal of 11,000 graduates per year by 1975, but on the basis of gains from 1959 to 1966 this goal would be reached only by the year 2008, and the increase is largely due to inclusion of persons formerly excluded.

It is not clear that by 1975 we will have enough physicians. But at least one authority, Dr. C. H. W. Ruhe, is optimistic that the total number of physicians by 1975 will exceed the projections of the Bane Committee (1959) and the United States Public Health Service (1964). He explains his expectations on the basis of anticipated expansion of existing medical schools, the development of large numbers of new medical schools, lower population projections, and a large number of foreign medical graduates who were not previously counted.

The general view is that doctor shortages will persist for many years. In the light of current physician compensation—about $40,000 net income for nonsalaried physicians under sixty-five—the continued shortage is a puzzle. The explanation may be that students are ignorant of the rewards available or are less concerned over compensation than is generally assumed.

Differences of opinion still prevail on the number of doctors needed. Professor Eli Ginzberg, for example, is critical of rising estimates of needs. Besides the usual explanations of assumed needs, he lists other factors stressed by the expansionist groups:

the increasing time that physicians must spend per patient as a result of new medical and surgical procedures and the following desiderata to improve the quality of medical care by increasing the number of younger, better trained physicians, to emancipate the country from reliance on foreign-trained physicians, to enable the United States to contribute more readily to assisting the developing nations, to establish better medical care for many disadvantaged groups, and to reduce the average hours of work of physicians.[4]

A relevant item in assessing the adequacy of the number of physicians is the growth trend in the number of interns and residents. From 1950-51 to 1965-66, the number of internships filled rose from 7,030 to 9,670; residencies rose from 14,495 to 31,898. The percentage of residencies filled tended to move upward. Of special interest is the rising foreign contribution to this supply. Foreign-trained interns increased from 722 to 2,361 (from 10 percent to 24 percent of internships) in these years, and foreign-trained residents rose from 1,350 to 9,133 (from 9 percent to 29 percent of the total). These movements reflect the inadequacy of the supply from domestic sources.

The large drop in the number of general practitioners creates a troublesome problem of mobilizing substitutes. The number of physicians in pediatrics, internal medicine, and general practice dropped from 117,179 in 1931, to 98,109 in 1965, or from 94 per 100,000 to 50. The drop per year was especially large from 1957 to 1965.

The impact of the large rise in nonpracticing physicians is suggested by table 8.1. It is clear that the availability of practitioners is related to the rising drain from such activities as research, education, administration, and training.

Table 8.2 compares the number of physicians, dentists, and professional nurses with requirements for 1960. For example, the actual supply of physicians was 241,000. To meet specified standards of services 263,000 would be needed; to bring all regions of the country up to the 1949 average ratios for New England and the Central Atlantic states and to meet the needs of the armed forces, 292,000 would be needed.

Experience during World War II, however, points to satisfying responses to shortages. At that time 60 percent of the physicians cared for 91 percent of the population (the 9 percent of the population that was in military service required the services of 40 percent of the doctors).[5]

From 1900 to 1950, the response of the supply of physicians to unusual rises of demand was disappointing (see table 8.3).[6]

Use of Auxiliary Personnel

Assistant Physicians

In recent years there has been much pressure to use assistant physicians. Duke University, Colorado University, and Florida University, among others, have been supporting assistant physician programs.

TABLE 8.1 Physicians by Type of Activity, 1950-68

Type of Activity	Number (Thousands)		Percentage Increase
	1950	1968	
Total active	209	286	37%
In practice	158	187	19%
In training	17	32	88%
Other activities	34	67	100%

TABLE 8.2   Supplies and Requirements of Physicians, Dentists, and Nurses, 1960

Measure of Supply	Number (Thousands)		
	Physicians	Dentists	Professional Nurses
1953 estimate of 1960 supply	233	101	415
Supply needed to maintain 1940 overall ratios	227	103	368
Supply needed to maintain 1949 ratios	231	101	406
Supply needed to maintain 1949 civilian ratio, staff new hospitals, and meet projected military and mobilization needs	244	109	475
Supply needed to meet specified standards of services	263	161	475
Supply needed to bring lower areas of country to 1949 average ratios and meet needs of armed forces at present levels	255	117	458
Supply needed to bring all regions of country to 1949 average ratios for New England and Central Atlantic states and meet needs of armed forces at present levels	292	131	529
Actual 1960 supply	241	102	504

Sources: *Building America's Health*, vol. 2, p. 189; HEW, *Indicators*, December 1961, p. 48.

This is an obvious way to improve the use of personnel and raise productivity. The current ten-to-one ratio of medical personnel to physicians suggests promising possibilities. Note, however, that the flow of personnel currently yields a ratio of about five to one. Mobilizing assistant physicians is a problem. How much should they do that doctors now do? Certainly they should not diagnose and prescribe treatments for patients. Licensing rules present another obstacle. How much education should be required? Many physicians are antagonistic because they fear the loss of patients.

The response of physicians to modern technology has likewise been slow. In response to the expanding complexity of medical practice, doctors have increased specialization and centralization of facilities.

With general hospitals' assets rising from $4 billion in 1950 to $15 billion in 1965 and with medical expenditures rising 10 percent a year, one might expect rising productivity. But Dr. Ward Darley and Mrs. Anne Somers commented: "Unless we can succeed in making

TABLE 8.3 Percentage Increases in Manpower Supplies, 1900-50

Type of Manpower	Percentage Increase
Health personnel (1900-50)	370
Physicians	58
Dentists	156
Professional nurses	3,970
Pharmacists	410
Other professional personnel (1940-50)	
Engineers	91
Accountants	71
Chemists	38
Physicians	16
Lawyers and judges	2

better use of the resources we already have—not just money, but brains, hands, technology, organizational and managerial skill, and above all education—the American people most assuredly will not receive a fair return on the money being poured into the national medical establishment."

Other Medical Workers

New technology and mass production in the health sector have created new and more specialized categories of work among allied health personnel (see table 8.4). In their need for decent salaries and job security, hospital workers, who are among the lowest paid in the entire work force, have begun to organize. Some, mostly those in the lower echelons, are now unionized.

Wages for these jobs are scandalous in many parts of the country: $60 a week is still common. Hours are long, duties are dirty and boring, and job security is nonexistent. Anyone who can get out of a

TABLE 8.4 Growth in Allied Health Manpower

Year	Number of Workers
1900	15,000
1950	286,000
1960	515,000
1970	927,000

hospital into another job does so. Turnover rates often approach 90 percent per year.

Local 1199 of the Retail, Wholesale, and Department Store Workers, the Teamsters Union, the Service Employees International Union, and the American Federation of State, County, and Municipal Employees are organizing hospital workers throughout the United States.

The impact of unionization is very important. In New York, for example, wages for unskilled hospital workers have more than tripled in the eleven years since the first major union breakthrough. Paid vacations, health insurance, workmen's compensation, and pension plans have become standard. A training and upgrading program is planned, to permit hospital workers to move up the ladder into more skilled and higher paying positions. Hospital workers are also protected against arbitrary firing, discipline, or reassignment by the hospital administration. Nonetheless, more than 80 percent of the nation's hospital workers are still not unionized.

Other health workers, mainly those doing specialized medical tasks, are organizing into professional associations, which certify members, establish entry requirements, and seek to codify the profession's functions into state law. Since the early 1900s, the allied health professions have proliferated tenfold until there are now over 125 recognized health occupations and 250 secondary or specialist designations. Among the new health job titles in the field of inhalation therapy, for example, are: cardiopulmonary technician, circulation technologist, respiratory technologist, and respiratory therapist. In radiology, we now find the job titles X-ray equipment repair technician, radiation physicist, radiobiologist, radiologic technologist assistant, radiologist administrator, radiologist assistant, and radiology aide.

New health professional organizations follow the leads of their predecessor, the American Medical Association. Each new organization tries to gain power without encroaching on that of the more established and powerful professions. In fact, most are under the indirect control of the AMA, and, on the job, their members are under the control of the doctors themselves.

The allied health profession associations are like the craft unions of the old American Federation of Labor, which organized workers on the basis of particular skills. One result was that workers were set against workers, skills against skills, and the skilled against the less skilled. Already one can see the nurse practitioner vying with the assistant physician, the research technician competing with the lab technician for status, autonomy, and upward mobility. This internal competition directs the workers' attention away from those who set the conditions of hospital employment.[7]

Distribution of Physicians

The distribution of physicians by region, by income level of the population, and by type of community is a troublesome problem. Merely turning out more doctors or raising patients' incomes does not solve the problem. A study of a ghetto area in the Bronx, New York, for example, revealed that in 1938 the area had 25,000 middle-class white persons served by fifty physicians; in 1969 the population was almost double, but there were only five physicians and the physical plant had greatly deteriorated. In the Bronx as a whole the ratio was 700 patients per physician. But in this ghetto area there apparently were 10,000 patients per physician.

Achievement of a viable ratio requires not only more doctors and rising productivity among them but also an incentive system that would attract physicians to ghetto areas. Quality of service is another problem. The best students do not necessarily gain admission to medical school, Dr. Dwight Wilbur of the American Medical Association admits.

A skewed distribution of physicians is found in the United States generally in the ratio of general practitioners in private practice to the population. In 1959, the region with the lowest ratio was the South, with 74 per 100,000; the Northeast had the highest ratio, 118 per 100,000. The difference was about 60 percent. A much smaller difference (15 percent) is found between the lowest and the highest ratios of private physicians engaged in full-time specialties per 100,000 population.

By 1963, Dr. Rashi Fein found the ratio of full-time specialists to population in metropolitan areas was 2-1/3 times that in isolated areas. This difference in ratios is indeed large compared to the 15 percent difference among highest and lowest regions for these specialists in 1959. There was little difference, however, in the ratios of general practitioners from metropolitan to isolated areas, whereas the regional difference was 60 percent.[8]

It is clear that older people require more doctors. Hence the maldistribution worsens as the population's average age goes higher. If the number of visits per person is a reliable indicator, more highly educated people need more physicians. Those with less than five years' education averaged 4.0 visits per year, while those with thirteen or more years' education averaged 5.4 per year (a difference of 35 percent).

Doctors choose their locations for a variety of reasons:

> Among the factors proven to influence the choice of a place of practice are: demand for medical services, location of the medical college attended, place of residence before entering medical college, place where internship and/or residency was served, the method and quality of transportation and community, ready accessibility of hospital and consultation facilities, climate, availability of good schools, and many other personal, social and economic factors.[9]

Small towns suffer sharply from the doctor shortage. In 1959, only 19 percent of physicians practiced in communities of less than 5,000 population, but these communities accounted for 45 percent of the nation's population.

The availability of physicians is clearly related to economic conditions. Table 8.5 shows that distribution of physicians by state mirrors the per capita income. The ten states with the highest physician-population ratios were mainly in the Northeast, including the District of Columbia, plus California. The bottom ten were mainly in the South, plus the Dakotas and Wyoming.

An interesting trend is noted on a regional basis. The South has experienced large increases in the net income for physicians. By 1966, the South had the highest average, 18 percent more than the West, which was the region with the lowest net income for physicians. These figures undoubtedly reflect the shortage of doctors in the South. When allowance is made for the low per capita income in the South,

TABLE 8.5   Ratios of Physicians and Per Capita Income by State

	Percentage of U.S. Average Per Capita Income	Percentage of Physician-Population Ratio
Ten states with lowest per capita income	64	66
Ten states with highest per capita income	128	129

Source: Adopted and calculated from *Medical School Inquiry*, p. 278.

the disadvantage of that region for its population is clearly revealed.[10]

Physicians' Incomes

Confronted with a rising and persistent demand, the physician increases his fees and rations his time, either by refusing to take on new patients or by cutting the time he allots per visit or by depending more heavily on auxiliary manpower and various mechanical aids. Although doctors have increased their incomes greatly since the 1940s, they have not responded to shortages by raising prices as much as other parts of the health care market. Actually price rises were smaller than they seemed to be, assuming there was no deterioration of quality. But this generalization of restraint by doctors may not have held for the 1960s. In the heated discussions in the early days of Medicare (1966-68), doctors claimed, and government officials corroborated, that procedures involving the under-sixty-five population had risen in price as much as or more than the services of special interest to the old.

The rise of physicians' fees from 1940 to 1960 was modest compared to the increases over the last 100 years. Since the 1870s, fees have increased fifteen to thirty times more than prices. In the 1940s and 1950s, they roughly corresponded to the increase in prices. During the 1940s despite large deficits of manpower, prices for physicians' services lagged substantially behind other rising prices.

In the last generation, physicians' incomes have increased much more than the prices charged per service. Doctors have profited from a rise in the number of services they can provide per day, as a result of rising productivity and other factors. In the twenty years from 1940 to 1960, the price of hospital services rose about 3½ times as much as physicians' fees. This was undoubtedly one of the factors cutting the rise of income for the doctor. Counterbalancing this was an increase in the number of fees actually collected by doctors.

In the 1960s rising prices played a much larger role than in the 1940s and 1950s, although, in fact, the increase in prices is less than the index numbers suggest, because the large growth of government-subsidized medicine is not registered in the index number. Had allowance been made for this factor, the price rises indicated would have been less than they now are.

Over a period of twenty-five years (from 1936 to 1961) physicians' incomes increased 475 percent, but increases in the fees charged per service accounted for less than a fourth of this increase. Improved collections apparently were a larger factor, and the rise in the number of services provided yielded about a third of the gain. From 1929 to 1961, physicians' net incomes rose by 371 percent whereas incomes in the labor market as a whole rose by 293 percent. In 1951, physicians averaged $12,518 annual income compared to $3,384 for all workers, $7,743 for dentists, and $9,375 for lawyers. Nonsalaried physicians received about 75 percent more income than nonsalaried dentists.[11]

In 1960, the average pay of faculty members in four-year colleges was $6,810—roughly a fourth that of physicians in private practice. Full professors in universities were then receiving an average of $10,000. In a famous study, Kuznets and Friedman showed that incomes of doctors greatly exceeded the amount justified by their extra costs of education. Another expert felt the pay should be high enough so that an adequate supply of doctors of appropriate quality would become available, but the resources should not go disproportionately to raise fees and prices.

The excessiveness of physicians' incomes is exaggerated if we do not allow for the long hours they put in. In the early 1960s, the average physician's working hours were 50 percent longer than those of the average worker. Allowing for this, the doctor's income ($25,000 per year) was a little more than four times that of the average worker ($4,000 per year), not over six times.

In general physicians receive much higher incomes when paid on a nonsalary basis, especially a fee-for-service basis, than when paid a salary. For example, in 1949, the mean net income for salaried doctors was $8,434, while for nonsalaried doctors it was $11,744, roughly 40 percent more.[12] (For physicians under sixty-five, the average net income was even higher, approximately $40,000.) This difference is explained in part by the shorter hours, more fringe benefits, and less concern for purely financial considerations among salaried physicians.

Comparison of Solo Practitioners and Partnerships

From 1945 to 1966, the net profit for physicians showing a net profit rose considerably (see table 8.6). Net income per solo practitioner rose more than two times; for partners, it rose a little more than one time. Per capita disposable income rose 131 percent. It is

TABLE 8.6   Net Profit of Physicians, 1945-66

Type of Practice	Net Profit		
	1945	1966	Increase
All physicians	$ 8,625	$27,155	219.8%
Sole proprietorships	8,241	25,497	209.4%
Partnerships	15,104	32,701	116.5%

Source: HEW, *Studies of the Incomes of Physicians and Dentists* (1968), p. 31.

striking that sole proprietorships experienced a much greater rise although partnerships had a 28 percent higher income. But from 1962 to 1966, the gain for partners was 33 percent, slightly more than that for solo practitioners, 30 percent.[13]

The average net profit per self-employed physician, combining solo practitioners and partnerships, is shown in table 8.7. Overall, the statistics suggest a higher monetary incentive (net profit) for partnerships, notably from 1945 to 1960. But average net profit per physician from 1960 to 1966 rose somewhat more for solo physicians.

In general, the largest relative rises were in numbers, rather than in income per physician. Total net profits skyrocketed, with the major explanation being the increase in numbers of physicians, especially partners, while average net income per physician rose relatively little by comparison.

An overall view of the incomes of physicians in self-employed practices is given in table 8.8. In general, the number of doctors involved in solo practice is 3½ times as large as that in partnerships, but the business receipts for solo practice are only 2½ times as great. Net profit per physician is almost one-third larger for partnerships.

TABLE 8.7   Net Profit per Self-employed Physician, 1945-66

Year	Number of Physicians	Net Profit for Physician
1945	100,000	$ 8,096
1960	171,000	18,461
1966	197,000	25,186

Source: HEW, *Studies of the Incomes of Physicians and Dentists* (1968), p. 75.

TABLE 8.8   Income of Physicians from Self-employed Practice, 1966

	Type of Practice	
	Sole Proprietorship	Partnership
Number of physicians	152,198	44,671 (14,916 partnerships)
Business receipts	$6,055,000,000	$2,430,000,000
Average net profit per physician	$23,922	$31,357
Net profit as a percentage of business receipts	60.1%	57.8%

Source: HEW, *Studies of the Incomes of Physicians and Dentists* (1968), p. 64.

Incomes vary greatly in both solo practice and partnership arrangements (see table 8.9). The incomes included in the table, from $10,000 to $200,000, account for 82 percent of the solo practitioners and 96 percent of their business receipts. For partners, the respective figures are 73 percent and 49 percent.

Among solo practitioners 97 percent have net profits between $10,000 and $200,000, while 54 percent of partnerships fall in this bracket. Another 34.7 percent of partnerships have net profits in the $200,000-$499,999 class, and 11.8 percent have net profits of $500,000 and over. As might be expected, the average for partners reaches a higher level than for solos.

In 1966, there were 741 sole proprietorships with incomes in excess of $200,000, and three in excess of $1 million. *Medical Economics*

TABLE 8.9   Income Brackets of Solo Practitioners and Partners

Income	Percentage of Solo Practitioners	Percentage of Solo Business Receipts	Percentage of Partners	Percentage of Partners' Business Receipts
$10,000-24,999	19.0	10.2	4.6	0.5
$25,000-49,999	33.7	31.0	5.1	1.2
$50,000-99,999	25.2	42.4	21.0	10.0
$100,000-199,999	4.1	12.9	42.6	37.5

Source: Adapted from HEW, *Studies of the Incomes of Physicians and Dentists* (1968), pp. 68-69.

listed ten physicians with gross incomes from $100,000 to $182,000, and net incomes from $32,000 to $119,000. Of the ten, only three were solo practitioners. Their collection ratios varied from 80 percent to 98 percent, and the percentage of their gross incomes that derived from health plan payments ranged from 2 percent (internal medicine) to 85 percent (general surgery).[14]

It is possible in many states for physicians to incorporate and thus greatly increase their income on retirement. A physician who accumulates savings of $1,665,000 over twenty-three years can increase his retirement income at age sixty-five from $10,000 as a solo practitioner to $100,000 as a corporation.[15]

Medicare Compensation

The Senate Finance Committee staff in 1970 was especially critical of the compensation methods used for physicians under Medicare:

The provisions of the statute and the clear congressional intent that Medicare carriers should not pay physicians more than they would ordinarily pay for their own subscribers has not been followed. Congress said that in paying physicians "consideration" should be given to customary and prevailing fees. In actual practice the Medicare regulations require that payment should be made solely on the basis of customary and prevailing fees and that private insurance schedules should not have any influence on what Medicare paid. As a consequence, Medicare generally allows payments for the aged which are substantially higher than those paid under Blue Shield's most widely held contracts for the working population, and thus physicians' incomes have been inflated.

The failure to maintain detailed data with respect to customary charges for each physician and for prevailing fees in each locality has led to weak administrative practices. . . . Undoubtedly, Medicare's pattern of inflated payments has also served to increase physicians' charges to the general public because a doctor is not permitted to charge more under Medicare (at least theoretically) than he does for his other patients.

The Senate committee recommended that "all Blue Shield plans serving as Medicare carriers be required to limit the physicians' charge recognized as 'reasonable' to not more than the average payment actually made for a given service or procedure under all of its basic surgical-medical subscriber contracts during a reasonably recent prior period of time."[16]

It is not surprising that, in 1968, more than 4,000 physicians received more than $25,000 from Medicare payments. (These constituted between 1 percent and 2 percent of practicing physicians.) In some instances practitioners received $15,000 or $20,000 for laboratory services.[17] One practitioner received almost $118,000 for taking care of 300 Medicare patients. A profile of his services and charges is given in table 8.10. The doctor's gross receipts averaged $400 per patient. For nursing home visits he received $83,020 for 104 patients, or about $800 per patient.

Impact of Medicare and Medicaid on Fees

In the two years ending June 1968, medical care prices increased about twice as much as the consumer price index. Physicians' fees rose by 13.2 percent, while the CPI increased 7.1 percent. From 1964 to 1966, physicians' fees rose by 9.5 percent, and they jumped another 6 percent in the year 1966.

TABLE 8.10   Profile of One Physician's Medicare Reimbursements

Type of Service	Allowed Charges	Number of Patients	Number of Services
Total	$117,824.50	300	14,338
Deductible and coinsurance amounts paid by patients	33,978.14	–	–
Amount reimbursed by Medicare	83,846.36	–	–
Visits			
Office visits	8,167.00	208	1,355
Home visits	1,620.00	29	154
Nursing home visits	83,020.00	104	8,332
Hospital visits	8,509.00	69	1,378
Extended care facility visits	.00	–	–
Outpatient clinic visits	.00	–	–
Surgery			
Surgical service	679.00	19	21
Assistant surgery service	505.00	9	9
Laboratory tests	10,461.00	208	2,136
Diagnostic X rays	714.50	69	76
Therapeutic X rays	.00	–	–
Physiotherapy	.00	–	–
Injectable drugs			
Injection only	3,731.00	158	840
Office visit with injection	188.00	7	19
Home visit with injection	10.00	1	1
Psychiatric counseling	.00	–	–
Other services			
Consultations	15.00	1	1
All other	205.00	12	16

Source: U.S. Senate, Committee on Finance, Staff Report: Medicare and Medicaid, Problems, Issues and Alternatives (February 1970), p. 87.

Undoubtedly the introduction of Medicare and Medicaid contributed greatly to this rise in prices. Anticipating the programs,
doctors sought to protect themselves against a later possible freeze of
charges. Many also envisaged the possibility of imposing usual charges
on those who had been paying less. The rise in prices brought on by
increased demand resulting from Medicare was bound to have an
impact on prices under Medicaid. To justify higher prices under
Medicare, they began raising their regular fees, because they would
not be allowed to charge more under Medicare than they normally
charged.[18]

The 7.8 percent rise of prices in 1966 (Medicare started July 1,
1966), the unprecedented $11 billion increase in expenditures under
the Medicare and Medicaid programs, and the recourse to cost-based
pricing formulas were bound to increase physicians' fees under these
programs. Cost-based pricing was abandoned only in 1969. The 1967
report to the President, *Medical Care Prices,* asserted that Medicare
did not accelerate rising physicians' fees, and noted that prices
charged for treating children's diseases rose more than for five procedures especially common in treating those over sixty-five. I am not
convinced by this argument. The large increase in pediatricians' fees
may relate to previously low incomes among pediatricians.

Disturbed by rising prices and even more by escalating incomes, the
able Commissioner of Social Security, Robert M. Ball, said in 1969:

> For many years before the passage of the Medicare legislation, physicians had
> chafed under what they thought were very restrictive fee schedules imposed by
> third-party payers and had long advocated the development of programs that
> would cover their individual *customary fees for professional services,* limited
> only by prevailing fee levels for similar services in their respective communities.
> The Medicare law basically adopted what the physicians had so long advocated.
> This entire concept and approach is now undergoing a very real public trial.[19]

A peculiarity of the Medicare and Medicaid operations has been
the special dispensation given to physicians by not requiring them to
disclose their payments under these programs to the tax authorities.
Though a $10 interest payment to an investor has to be revealed in
order to discourage tax evasion, physicians' earnings running as high
as $25,000 under these programs were not being revealed to the
Internal Revenue Service. The intermediaries objected to revealing
the payments they made to physicians on the grounds that these

transactions were private. Only in 1969 did the government begin to eliminate this discrimination in favor of physicians.[20]

Rapidly rising physician incomes and prices per service eventually aroused the government into taking various actions. Steps were taken, for example, to improve carrier performance in determining reasonable charges, to establish prevailing charges that were not to be changed for at least a year, to redefine customary charges, to relate physicians' bills for laboratory charges to what laboratories themselves charge, to increase charges that had been restricted from January 1, 1969, to increase customary charges only in unusual situations where equity clearly required an adjustment, to study alternative reimbursement formulas—especially those offering incentives to reduce costs and prices, and to study guidelines by carriers for improving the review of claims.[21]

Shortcomings of The Medical Profession

Unnecessary Services

Much of medical care is a mystery. Dr. Kerr White puts the issue of unnecessary services as follows:

> Only about 10 to 20 percent of the things that physicians and nurses do to patients are based on objective evidence that they are more useful, beneficial, and constructive, than they are useless or harmful. About 20 to 40 percent of what they do is based on the so-called placebo and Hawthorne effects, designed to please and encourage patients, and the other 40 to 70 percent is a mystery and needs to be examined critically. It is this area where much of the opportunity for reducing current high costs is involved and where the opportunity for increasing efficiency exists.
>
> It seems to me three factors discourage improvements in the organization of health services. The first is the categorical approach to the funding of most programs. The categorical approach has served biomedical research very well indeed, although one could raise questions with respect to its adequacy as a means to financing basic scientific research. When it comes to developing informed systems for delivering medical "care" in contrast to medical "cures," we need a more general approach toward the support of personal health services.[22]

It has often been claimed that physicians who are not responsible for budget control embarrass hospital administrations by requesting equipment and supplies not really needed and not fundable.[23]

Fee-Splitting

Incomes of physicians are affected by fee-splitting arrangements. In the last few years, the government has taken an increased interest in fee-splitting and control of kickbacks (from surgeon to primary physician). The arguments against kickbacks are that the primary doctor's choice of surgeon may be determined by the size of the kickback expected, rather than the skill and experience in performing the necessary surgery, and that the expectation of kickbacks may encourage doctors to recommend unnecessary surgery.[24]

Conflicts of Interest

Physicians find themselves in conflicts of interest when they become involved in the control of pharmacies, equipment suppliers, drug manufacturers, and nursing homes. Conflicts of interest raise economic and ethical issues for the physician.

Drug Suppliers. Physician ownership of pharmacies and drug companies has received special attention. By 1969, a Senate subcommittee had identified approximately 100 doctor-owned repackaging and distributing companies involving possibly 5,000 doctors. A survey by the magazine *American Druggist* revealed steady increases from 1950 to 1961. In Texas, for the year ending June 1, 1965, 117 pharmacy permits issued by the state board, or 4 percent of the total, listed doctors as officers, partial owners, or owners. Of the licensed doctors, 259 out of 16,034 practitioners, or 1.6 percent, had an interest in Texas pharmacies. Out of 126 manufacturing permits issued by the State Board of Pharmacy, 26, or 20.6 percent, showed an interest held by doctors.[25] Apparently the Texas Medical Association and the Texas Pharmaceutical Association have been unable to halt the increasing involvement of doctors in ownership of pharmacies.

In the Salt Lake City area a new drug company sold its stock to a limited number of druggists and doctors; in time it was found that these doctors had radically altered their prescriptions, favoring drugs made available by the new company.

After this firm had been in business but a few weeks, many druggists in the area where we worked informed us that they had noticed that the prescribing habits of many medical doctors had changed with the purchase of stock in this new firm. We were told that some doctors had prescribed as many as 20 prescriptions for their patients in one day for products in the firm where they owned stock.[26]

A doctor who purchased $2,000 worth of stock in the company at the outset five years earlier had a stock with a market value of $44,000 as of July 1, 1964, plus his dividends.[27]

The Salt Lake County Medical Society on February 27, 1958, issued a statement on ethics dealing with the situation:

In the opinion of the Medical Ethics Committee a physician should not profit financially from the care of his patients apart from fees for professional services.

In particular we would discourage profit sharing in any pharmaceutical enterprise or medical supply organization. . . . If a doctor holds interests in a drug firm, he can hardly avoid being tempted to favor that firm in handling his patients.[28]

Dr. Charles Edwards, commissioner of the federal Food and Drug Administration, raised some of these ethical problems in his presentation before the Senate Subcommittee on Monopoly on the advertising of proprietary medicines.[29] The FDA estimated that there were between 100,000 and 200,000 drugs sold over the counter. All are formulated from some 250 significant active ingredients designed to alleviate about thirty easily recognized symptoms. Advertising of these drugs is often exaggerated and even dishonest.

Nursing Homes and Laboratories. It is clear that the physician who controls or owns a nursing home or a laboratory may well reap a bonanza. Like the physicians who own pharmacies, these doctors may experience a conflict of interest that leads them to favor use of the facilities they own. Ordinarily physicians should avoid ownership or control of such assets in order to avoid these conflicts of interest.

Another interesting and unfortunate conflict of interest arises when physicians cooperate with the owners of nursing homes for their own gain. The physician greatly increases his number of visits to the nursing home patients and shares the large additional income with the owners of the home. This is the practice of making so-called gang visits, perhaps doubling the number of visits per week and reducing the time per visit by half. A serious deterioration of quality ensues.

The temptation for physicians to exploit the rising demand for nursing home care is great. Table 8.11 shows how rapidly these facilities have grown. Nursing home expenditures rose 20 percent a year from 1960 to 1965, and 18.5 percent a year from 1965 to 1969. In the 1960s expenditures rose about twice as much per year as expenses per patient day.[30]

TABLE 8.11   Nursing Home Expenditures, 1950-69

Year	Total Expenditures (Millions)	Expense per Patient day
1950	$ 187	$ 4.31
1960	526	5.49
1969	2,615	11.83

In addition, there were 333,630 beds in extended care facilities as of July 1970. These establishments required more stringent regulations than nursing homes.

Women in the Health Care System

About 70 percent of all health workers, and 75 percent of all hospital workers, are women. As in almost every American institution, it is men—doctors, medical school deans, hospital directors and trustees, and drug and insurance company executives—who make policy. Men decide which jobs will be available to women health workers, what their salaries will be, and even what kind of uniforms they must wear.

Women health workers generally have jobs that are subordinate to those of men (see table 8.12). Women, and normally not men, are nurses, not because women are more "nurselike" than men, but because women are taught at an early age to aim no higher than nursing. Rarely are women encouraged to enter medical school.

Even when women do more "masculine" jobs, they are not treated equally. Category by category, women earn 10 percent to 15 percent less than men in the same occupation. The few women who become physicians (7 percent of American physicians) are primarily concentrated in lower paying specialties, especially pediatrics, rather than surgery and other more lucrative fields.

For women health consumers, men also decide policies—what form of birth control a woman should use, whether she should have an abortion, what method of childbirth she should use, and how much she should be told about her body, what risks she should take, and what health care options she has. When women enter a hospital or a doctor's office, they encounter a hierarchy dominated by men. Male

TABLE 8.12   Percentage of Women in New York Hospitals by Position

Position	Percentage of Total Employees	Percentage of Total Payroll	Weekly Pay	Percentage Female	Percentage Nonwhite
Management or supervisory	9	13	$200-500	15-20	10-20
Academic	2	5	200-400	20	5
Intern or resident	6	9	180-250	10	8
Staff registered nurse	21	25	155-170	98	40
Lab technician	10	9	135-165	75	40
Licensed professional nurse	7	7	110-130	85	90
Clerical worker	11	8	100-130	85	60
Aide or manual service worker	34	24	95-115	80	80

Source: Health-PAC Bulletin, July-August 1970, p. 6.

physicians assume women are incapable of understanding complex explanations, so they are given none. Women are assumed to be emotional and "difficult," so they are often classified as "neurotic" well before physical illness has been ruled out. Many women hate or fear gynecologists, who play a controlling role in their sexual lives. Middle-class women generally find their male doctors either patronizing or cold and supercilious. Poorer women, using clinics, may encounter outright brutality.[31]

Notes

1. HEW, National Conference on Medical Costs (1967), p. 19.

2. See HEW, Social Security Administration, Sources of Increase in Selected Medical Care Expenditures, 1929-1969 (1970), especially pp. 39-43.

3. See HEW, Physicians for a Growing America: Report of the Surgeon General's Consultant Group on Medical Education (1959), pp. 2-13.

4. E. Ginzberg, "Physician Shortage Reconsidered," New England Journal of Medicine, July 1966, pp. 85-87; C. H. W. Ruhe, "Present Projections of Physician Production," Journal of the American Medical Association, December 5, 1966, pp. 1094-106; M. Cherkasky, Journal of Medical Education, February 1969, pp. 126-31; D. L. Wilbur, "The Professor's View, Medical Manpower—A Contemporary Crisis," Journal of the American Medical Association, September 1967, pp. 845-48; J. Kosa, "The Foreign Trained Physician in the United States," Journal of Medical Education, January 1969, pp. 45-51; W. N. Hubbard, Jr., "The Health Manpower Shortage: The Physician," University of Michigan Medical Center Journal, April, June 1969, pp. 98-100.

5. America's Health: A Report to the Nation by the National Health Assembly (1949), p. 2.

6. Figures are from HEW, *Health Manpower Chart Book* (1957), pp. 1, 4, 5; HEW, *Physicians for a Growing America: Report of the Surgeon General's Consultant Group on Medical Education* (1959), p. 83.

7. See "Fragmentation of Workers: An Anti-Personnel Weapon," *Health-PAC Bulletin*, November 1972.

8. The facts in this section are from Weiskotten et al., *Trends in Medical Practice . . . Medical College Graduates 1915-1950*, pp. 1083-89; *Medical School Inquiry*, p. 33; *Building America's Health*, vol. 3, p. 164; HEW, *Physicians for a Growing America: Report of the Surgeon General's Consultant Group on Medical Education* (1959), pp. 12, 80, 82; HEW, *Volume of Physician Visits, U.S., July, 1966-June, 1967*, Series no. 10, no. 49, p. 9; R. Fein, *The Doctor Shortage* (1967), p. 75; HEW, *Medical Care Financing and Utilization*, Health Economic Series no. 1-A, pp. 68, 217.

9. Weiskotten et al., *Trends in Medical Practice . . . Medical College Graduates 1915-1950*, pp. 1083-89.

10. HEW, *Studies of the Incomes of Physicians and Dentists* (1968), p. 40.

11. *Building America's Health*, vol. 4, p. 251.

12. HEW, *Studies of the Incomes of Physicians and Dentists* (1968), p. 31.

13. Ibid., p. 40.

14. *Physicians' Earnings and Expenses*, based on *Medical Economics' Continuing Survey*, pp. 29, 51.

15. *New York Times*, October 26, 1969.

16. U.S. Senate Committee on Finance, *Staff Report: Medicare and Medicaid, Problems, Issues and Alternatives* (February 1970), p. 10.

17. Ibid., chap. 7.

18. For prices, see *Medical Care Prices, 1967, A Report to the President* (1967); R. M. Ball, "Medical Prices and Their Control," *Social Security Bulletin*, March 1969, pp. 4-9.

19. R. M. Ball, "Medical Prices and Their Control," *Social Security Bulletin*, March 1969, p. 7.

20. U.S. Senate, Committee on Finance, *Hearings on Medicare and Medicaid, 1969* (1970), pp. 58-61.

21. Ibid., pp. 9-29.

22. U.S. Senate, Subcommittee on Executive Reorganization, *Hearings on Health Care in America* (April 1968), vol. 1, p. 182.

23. American Medical Association, *Report of the Commission on the Costs of Medical Care*, vol. 1, p. 19.

24. *New York Times*, January 30, 1972.

25. U.S. Senate, Committee on the Judiciary, Subcommittee on Antitrust and Monopoly, *Hearings on Physician Ownership in Pharmacies and Drug Companies* (1964), pp. 1-5.

26. Ibid., p. 13.

27. Ibid., p. 14.

28. Ibid., p. 316; also see p. 309.

29. U.S. Senate, Select Committee on Small Business, Subcommittee on Monopoly, *Hearings on the Introduction of Analgesics* (1971), pp. 178-79.

30. HEW, Office of Research and Statistics, *Medical Care Costs and Prices: Background Book* (January 1972), pp. 72-73; see also Health Policy Advisory Center, *The American Health Empire: Power, Profits and Politics* (1970), p. 113.

31. See *Health-PAC Bulletin,* March 1970 and April 1972. Also see B. Ehrenreich and D. English, *Complaints and Disorders: The Sexual Politics of Sickness,* Glass Mountain Pamphlet no. 2.

9

Drugs

History of Drug Regulation

The drug industry was first federally regulated in 1906 by the Pure Food and Drug Act. The major drug problem then was the sale of quack medicines, often made of deadly or addictive substances, and ineffective in curing the many diseases for which they were advertised.

However, it took over twenty-five years of pressure for action before Congress passed this law, which required only that drugs not be adulterated or mislabeled with respect to their chemical contents. The act did not regulate the advertising, safety, or effectiveness of drugs. A later amendment, forbidding "false and fraudulent" therapeutic statements, succeeded in making the law unenforceable, because of the difficulty of proving fraudulent intent.

In 1938 a stronger bill was passed after an unsafe drug caused the death of 108 persons. This new bill for the first time required manufacturers to supply the federal Food and Drug Administration with the results of safety tests on new drugs before marketing them in interstate commerce. It also prohibited the use of false or misleading labeling, whether or not fraudulent intent could be proved. But the law did not require that new drugs be proved effective before being placed on the market.

This omission was not altered until twenty-four years later, in 1962, when Congress passed amendments to the Food and Drug Act, popularly known as the Kefauver-Harris Act. The 1962 amendments were passed only after use of the drug thalidomide by pregnant women was related to birth defects in their babies. The bill included sections on the safety, efficacy, and advertising of drugs, supervision of drug manufacturing plants, and decreased patent rights over drugs.

Many powerful interest groups lobbied against the amendments. The American Medical Association opposed the requirement that drugs be tested for effectiveness, as well as most of the other proposed reforms, on the ground that they could achieve the same ends by joint voluntary action between the AMA and the drug industry. The American Bar Association opposed a provision that would have limited patent rights over new drugs. The other major lobbying group was the Pharmaceutical Manufacturers Association, which was willing to compromise on parts of the bill, but would not agree to limiting the industry's profits. The act as finally passed resembles the recommendations of the Pharmaceutical Manufacturers Association.

Even when new laws are enacted, the Food and Drug Administration has been slow in enforcing them. In part this is due to alliances between the FDA and the drug industry. For example, many FDA officials become drug industry executives. Dr. Joseph F. Sadusk, Jr., former director of the FDA Bureau of Medicine became vice-president of Parke-Davis and Company, one of the country's largest drug manufacturers. It was during Sadusk's "reign" that Parke-Davis marketed the controversial antibiotic chloramphenicol, used chiefly to treat infections of the urinary tract. Reports began to appear citing cases of blood toxicity, and linking the antibiotic to deaths from aplastic anemia. Dr. Sadusk prevented the drug's withdrawal and ruled against requiring more precautionary labeling for it. Only after Sadusk's resignation did the FDA demand more stringent warning labels on various chloramphenicol preparations.

Sadusk's successor was Dr. Joseph M. Pisani, who later joined the Proprietary Association, a large trade organization that represents the makers of nonprescription drugs. Pisani's successor was Dr. Robert J. Robinson, who went on to become a top-ranking executive of Hoffman-La Roche, a leading manufacturer of prescription drugs.

Many other FDA officials have gone from the FDA to the drug

industry: Dr. Howard Cohen, former head of medical evaluation for the FDA, went to Ciba Pharmaceutical Company; Dr. Harold Anderson, chief of FDA's division of anti-infective drugs, went to Winthrop Laboratories; Morris Yakowitz, head of case supervision, joined Smith, Kline, and French Laboratories, and Allen E. Rayfied, former director of regulatory compliance, took a job as a consultant to Richardson-Merrell, Inc. From 1959 to 1964, one out of every ten employees (83 out of 813) who left the FDA joined the staff of a company he had previously policed.

The Drug Industry

The ten firms in *Fortune*'s top 500 with the highest returns on invested capital one year included three drug companies. Few if any industries have a better profit record over the years than the drug industry. A survey in the early 1960s revealed the ratios of profits to equity that are shown in table 9.1. This record prevailed into the late 1960s, leading the Federal Trade Commission to cite the drug industry as the most profitable of all industries over the years. Following the reforms of the early 1960s, the industry complained of a decline in the number of new products, which had an unfavorable impact on prices and profits, and of the growing influence of institutional purchasers. But profits in 1969 were still rising, and the *Final Report* by the HEW Task Force on Prescription Drugs found drug profits excessive, given the risks involved.[1]

Concentration of sales volume in relatively few companies reflects the monopolistic aspects of the industry. Thus, in three years the four largest companies accounted for 28 percent, 25 percent, and 27 percent of shipments in the industry; the twenty largest companies handled 64 percent, 68 percent, and 73 percent for the three years.[2]

Higher prices charged by large companies than by small ones are another sign of monopoly. One would expect large companies to have

TABLE 9.1   Drug and Other Manufacturing Industry Profit Ratios

Industry	Profits as Proportion of Equity	
	Before Taxes	After Taxes
All manufacturing	16.7%	9.0%
Drug and cosmetic	35.0%	17.8%

Source: *Quarterly Financial Report for Manufacturing Corporations, First Quarter, 1962*, pp. 10-11.

low unit costs. The price of potassium penicillin G, buffered tablets, 250,000 units packaged in 100s was $2.95 for a small company; but the two largest companies had the highest prices, namely $12.[3]

Monopoly is often the result of collusion. When three major companies submitted identical bids of $17.24 for a government procurement, Senator Dixon of the Kefauver Committee questioned a representative of one of them. He replied: "I had not the faintest idea, Mr. Dixon—it is very easy looking back, but in looking ahead, I had not the faintest idea. Actually, I was astonished that they [two other companies] bid $17.24. I expected someone to bid, with a different situation, $15 or $16. I had no idea what the bids would be."[4]

The absence of competition is marked by variations in prices for institutional and noninstitutional buyers and by prices that are largely unrelated to the magnitude of the transaction. Prices for various volumes, ranging from a low of 250 units to a high of 153,216 tablets, varied by only 8 percent.

The HEW Task Force on Prescription Drugs in its *Final Report* made several recommendations for improvements. It asked for tightened control of quality; more and better instruction in clinical pharmacology; objective, up-to-date information and guidelines from the companies concerning drug therapy; labeling of containers of all prescription drugs with the identity, strength, and quantity of the product, unless waived by the physician; reduction of patent rights; marketing of drugs under generic names; and study of price differentiation. The Task Force also raised questions about excessive profits and improved distribution.

Upon entering private practice, the average physician, knowingly or unknowingly, becomes the key figure in drug marketing strategy. He must choose from a very large number of competitive and often duplicative products. He must deal with a very large amount of advice, biased or unbiased, from detail men, advertisements and other forms of promotion. Substantial efforts are made on his behalf by the drug industry and others to prevent any interference with his right to prescribe as he sees fit. Finally, it is assumed that he has the training, experience and time to weigh the claims and available evidence, and thus to make the proper selection. . . . We find that few practicing physicians seem inclined to voice any question of their competency in this field. We have noted, however, that the ability of an individual physician is now a matter of serious concern to leading clinicians, scientists, and medical educators.[5]

Interestingly enough, the Task Force admits that in comparisons of "two drug products containing essentially the same amount of the same active ingredients, that is two chemical equivalents. . . . in certain instances the chemical effects may *not* be the same."[6]

Cost Structure

The cost structure of the industry resembles that of the soap and tobacco industries. Selling costs are especially large. Whereas, in 1958, wages and salaries were 25 percent of value added for the drug industry, they were 51 percent for all manufacturers. In only 8 out of 436 manufacturing industries and subindustries was the ratio of wages and salaries to value added as low as in the pharmaceutical industry. The Kefauver Committee found selling costs to be 25 percent of prices for twenty-two drug companies. For the corticosteroid Prednisolene V, for example, the production cost to the manufacturer, Schering, was $1.57 per 100; the selling price rose to $29.83 per 100—almost twenty times the manufacturing costs.[7]

Promotion Expenditures

Heavy outlays on advertising partly explain high selling costs. Drug company representatives inundate physicians with vast amounts of literature, to curry recommendations of trademark drugs instead of the less expensive generic drugs. Excessive pushing of patented and trademark drugs as opposed to the generic drugs is one of the most regrettable abuses of the industry.

The markup that ensues from large dependence on selling techniques was noted cogently by Senator Dixon of the Kefauver Committee, addressing Schering's president, F. C. Brown:

You said you thought it was pretty reasonable for a person to pay 30 to 60 cents a day for these pills [Prednisolene] if he was incapacitated. I put this question to you: If you can make the pill for 1.6 cents, do you still consider it pretty reasonable to charge 17.9 cents to a druggist and to fair trade, or rather to suggest that the druggist sell to the public at 29.8 cents per pill? . . . In 1958 you purchased [Estrodiol] from Roussel [a French drug firm] at $3.50 per gram. Your 0.5 milligram tablets in bottles of 60's cost the druggists $8.40. The fair trade price, or suggested price, to the consumer is $14. Thus what goes into this bottle is three one-hundredths of a gram, or a cost to Schering of *11.7* cents. Now the markup from 11.7 cents to $8.40 is 7,079 percent.

The advertising agencies are being asked to sell to the medical profession a whole basketful of sows' ears for silk purses each year. It is no wonder that there are advertising excesses, and that there are so-called product failures and that obsolescence sets in.

One student writes that for the manufacturer the tranquilizers were much more than an important adjunct to the treatment of severe psychotics in mental hospitals. Disregarding their side effects, drug companies pushed them in doctors' offices and private offices. More than half of the $200 million worth of tranquilizers sold annually are bought by normal persons who, whatever their inner tensions, lead humdrum lives.[8]

One physician estimated that he received 1.06 pounds of mail per day from drug companies over a period of two months, implying 80 tons per day were sent to all physicians. The literature is often misleading and frequently fails to give the whole story. In their anxiety to capture a market before a competitor reaches it, drug companies often get doctors to write articles supporting their drugs (the authors are referred to as the "stable"). They frequently advertise references, even though these may be unfavorable or irrelevant. In one instance a major drug company advertised a product called Sigamycin, giving names and cities of residence of doctors approving it. Investigation by the Federal Trade Commission, following a study by the *Saturday Review*, revealed that there were no such doctors. The company promised to mend its ways.

Large drug companies spend four times as much for advertising and promotion as they do for research. In 1966, five drug companies had advertising expenditures above $50 million, and these outlays amounted to 24 percent of their sales. There is a high correlation between advertising and rates of sale and profit. For example, though not a single study has found Panalba therapeutically effective, it is one of the top 200 drugs in sales. Large promotional outlays seriously deter generic drug sales. This factor and the system of patent rights reduce freedom of entry into the drug market. In the mid-1960s brand names accounted for 90 percent of sales. The expansion of brand drugs is related to the impact of detail men, who give doctors only one side of the case for brand names. It would be most helpful if the distribution of unsolicited drug samples were made unlawful. There is a genuine danger of doctors accumulating inventories of sample drugs that have been recalled in large numbers.[9]

Sales of prescription drugs depend on new discoveries and on outlays on advertising and promotion. Expenditures on research in turn induce discoveries of drugs. Research expenditures in the late 1960s were estimated at $500 million. The ratio of these expenditures to sales in the drug industry was three times that of any other industry. For companies making the information available, sales and promotional expenditures amounted to between 15 percent and 35 percent of sales income.

Unnecessary Differentiation of Products

It would be unfair not to acknowledge the contribution of the industry in saving lives, shortening hospital stays, and reducing illnesses generally. With the introduction of sulfa drugs in 1957, deaths from influenza and pneumonia per 100,000 population dropped by about three-quarters. Deaths in childhood declined about 90 percent in ten years and deaths from infectious diseases per 100,000 declined more than 90 percent in fifty years, largely owing to advances in the drug industry.[10] However, not all "new" drugs are true advances in therapeutic technology.

One aspect of monopolistic operations in the drug industry is increasing differentiation of the product as a means of increasing the market. The result is a lower level of output per product and a higher unit cost, generally with little or no improvement of the product and a waste of scientific resources.

Professor Maxwell Finland, of Harvard Medical School, noted that there are more than one hundred mixtures of antibiotics. He was doubtful that all the combinations were justified. Among other disadvantages they encourage "shotgun therapy"; their "implied promise of 'broad spectrum' and 'greater efficiency' engender a false sense of security; [and] they may fail to give the optimum combination for the treatment of any disease."[11]

Another authority commented to the Senate on the dubious practice of combining an effective tranquilizer with an ineffective one, and claiming new effectiveness for the combination—when actually it increased anxiety rather than reducing it.[12]

One observer suggested that very few of the 100 antibiotics (bearing 600 trade names) should be used because "they may cause health hazards and play a part in the development of resistant strains such as those of the dreaded staphyloccocus."[13]

Professor D. C. Brodie estimates the costs of adverse drug reactions at roughly $900 million, excluding the costs of diagnosis and treatment. On an estimate that 25 percent of drugs used are ineffective,

Brodie adds costs of $1 billion to $2 billion. The incidence of complications in drug therapy is put roughly at 10 percent of 500,000 hospital admissions. Drug waste—such as use of drugs when not needed or at the wrong time or place—is a substantial item.

D. H. Knapp has stressed that the supply of drugs is much more responsive to increases in demand than other components of medical care are. For this reason, drugs may well be substituted for physicians' services.[14]

Pharmacists

In 1969, independent pharmacies constituted 79 percent of the country's drug outlets and handled 67 percent of total prescriptions. From 1964 to 1969, total prescriptions rose from 889 million to 1,319 million, but the independent pharmacies' share of prescriptions dropped from 80 percent to 67 percent, whereas the output of chain and other retail outlets rose from 11 percent to 21 percent, and hospital pharmacies' share increased from 8 percent to 11 percent.[15] Hospital pharmacies, which once concentrated largely on inpatient needs, have shifted their interests to outpatient needs, in part because this is one of the few profitable operations of hospitals.

The cost of acquisition and the cost of dispensing are the major components in the price of a drug. Within these costs are innumerable variables, however, such as the source of purchase (manufacturer or wholesaler), the size of the order, the method of payment (cash or credit), the form of dosage, and the potency.

Pharmacists handle many functions, including retail sales of drugs, retail sales of health aids and cosmetics, and sales-related services. Hence it is difficult to isolate the cost of each operation. Overhead costs and joint costs must be allocated among prescription and other sale areas.

Most pharmacists add either a percentage markup or a fee to the acquisition cost of a drug. According to D. H. Knapp, "markups usually vary from 33-50%, with the exact percent determined by costs, competition and desired profit. Use of a straight markup system, i.e., applying the same percentage to all prescriptions regardless of costs, gives small dollar margins on low cost prescriptions and disproportionately high margins on high cost prescriptions." The temptation then is to apply a large markup to low-cost items to increase the return on them and to use a low markup for high-priced items to stimulate sales of these products. Under the fee system, the return the pharmacist sets on an item is independent of its cost.

Pharmacists tend to use hybrid systems, containing elements of a sliding fee or percentage markup, combined with minimums, extra charges, and special prices for highly competitive products. This leaves experts in the dark about prescription acquisition costs.

The division of control between doctors and pharmacists affects the pricing of drugs. Doctors were at first in control, but they increasingly allowed pharmacists to take over; recently, especially with the emergence of group medicine and clinics, doctors are regaining a position of control. Drug manufacturers are seeking to get pharmacists to accept flat fees rather than percentage markups, which are more inflationary.

Drug Prices

The drug industry, unlike the markets for personnel and facilities, contributes to rising prices not through the overall excess of demand over supply but rather through what economists describe as cost-push. High sales promotion costs are an example of the cost-push approach. In 1968, seventeen drug manufacturers revealed that almost 50 percent of their sales dollars went for profits, marketing, administration, and general expenses. Prices in the open market for one product may be five to twenty times as high as for an identical product, judged equal in quality by leading experts. And yet the high-price sellers seem immune from raids by the low-price sellers. Senator Nelson of Wisconsin was one of the leaders expressing concern at this state of affairs. Manufacturers confronted with complaints of excessively high prices have been unable to show corresponding gains of productivity as a justification.

The high prices contribute to spectacular increases in, and levels of, profits in a quasi-public-service industry. Whereas general manufacturing policy has been to contain price increases, in drugs the goals are higher prices and record profits. Another indicator of market imbalance is the pressure mobilized to use trademark and other proprietary drugs in favor of less costly generic drugs. Here again public policy favors high price objectives. Price competition is abandoned for competition in promotion, a factor making for higher prices.

Possibly drug prices have not risen as much as they appear to on the surface. For example, quality may have improved. If so, there is little evidence of it. Indeed, authorities stress the recalls of drugs, the unsatisfactory manufacturing conditions, and similar deficiencies as scarcely proof of a general rise in quality. In fact, the industry gives little helpful material on quality, and even offers misleading information.

Drug Price Indexes

Price indexes reveal both rises and declines for drugs, and questions have been raised on the meaning of these indexes. When prices of drugs rise, some argue that the index number should be corrected to reflect the large saving in hospital costs that antibiotics, for example, yield. The price rises are less than they seem to be, these proponents claim.

At best the index number for drugs is only roughly indicative of price trends. One reason for this is that large changes have taken place in buying patterns. Institutions and government are buying more drugs, while drugstores and dispensaries are purchasing a smaller proportion of the total. Under the old structure of purchases, prices would be higher; they seem to be lower because the major buyers, such as hospitals, are buying for lower, bulk-purchase, prices.

Large purchasers, such as state boards, seek to keep their departments informed of opportunities to buy cheaply through the generic markets, especially in programs for the poor.[16] Prices also depend on the importance of third-party buying. Manufacturers seem to fear the increasing volume of institutional purchases, because they may act as a price depressant. Others anticipate rising prices with the growth of third-party purchases.

In an excellent article, Agnes N. Brewster and Juanita P. Horton show clearly that prescription prices have been rising, not falling as the Consumer Price Index seems to suggest. The authors examined price movements for the 200 leading items, accounting for about two-thirds of the market for prescription drugs. More than half the items had no price change from 1957 to 1965; fifty-seven had higher prices, and twenty-seven had price reductions. Of the 200 top drugs listed, 53 percent had been introduced after 1957. But only 14 percent of the drugs in the Consumer Price Index had been introduced after 1957. A comparison of newly introduced replacements with drugs dropping out of the market showed an upward trend in prices: replacement drugs cost more than their predecessors for the same therapeutic value. For example, the average price of two antibiotic trade name replacements was $25.64, while the average price of three antibiotics dropped from the market was $12.39.[17]

Price index numbers have adjusted only slowly to changing procedures and markets. In 1937, sulfa drugs were introduced; in 1940, penicillin; in 1946, streptomycin; in 1947, antihistamines; in 1950, cortisone, ACTH, hydrocortisone, chlortetracycline (Aureomycin), chloramphenicol (Chloromycetin), and oxytetracycline (Terramycin). No serious notice was taken of these in drug indexes by the Bureau of Labor Statistics until very recently.

An overall examination of the prices of drugs (including prescription drugs) suggests that the rise has been modest compared to other categories of health services. But there is one important reservation. Frequent and substantial advances in chemotherapy bring about high prices at the outset, often followed by large reductions. These declines tend to give a picture of reductions in drug prices that is in fact fictitious. Long-range comparisons reveal large elements of inflation in drug prices. For example, from 1929 to 1960 prescription prices rose by 272 percent, the number of prescriptions rose by 171 percent, and the cost of living rose by 73 percent.[18] By 1967, per capita expenditures for drugs and sundries had climbed to $29, about double the 1956 amount, but these payments were a declining share of private expenditures for health services and supplies, as other costs rose rapidly.

International Price Differentials

Drug prices in the United States tend to be higher than in foreign countries. Higher incomes in this country are part of the explanation. But when one commentator estimated the cost in hours of work of producing V-cillin K (package of ten tablets) in six countries, the lowest was the United States at 1 hour, 52 minutes; the highest was Columbia at 19 hours, 32 minutes.

One aspect of monopolistic pricing is the higher prices of drugs in underdeveloped countries where incomes are one-fifth to one-tenth of those in western Europe. Why should Iran pay three times as much as Germany, and Venezuela pay seven times as much as Argentina, for Meprobamate? Why is the price of Aureomycin in India six times that in Argentina? Why does Japan pay almost four times as much as

England for Prednisone? Price differentials such as these are difficult to explain.

Patents often accounted for higher prices in some markets than in others. The Kefauver Committee found that for twelve major products the average price in countries with patents ranged from 35.5 percent to 118 percent higher than it was in countries without patents.[19] The HEW Task Force on Prescription Drugs, in its 1969 report, recommended substantial curtailment of patent rights.

Brand Name and Generic Drugs

The Dispute over Therapeutic Differences

For years now, especially during the Kefauver Committee Senate hearings in the late 1950s and early 1960s, the most hotly disputed issue in the drug field was cost and quality comparisons of generic and trade name or patented drugs. A widely held view was that trade name prescriptions were much more expensive than generic drugs, without any offsetting gains in quality, and could have side effects that were not adequately publicized.

The National Academy of Sciences and National Research Council compiled a final report for the Food and Drug Administration reviewing the therapeutic claims made for 80 percent of the nation's drugs. They concluded "that manufacturers were unable to provide substantial evidence to back one or more claims for significant proportions of the preparations." Moreover, some combinations were actually harmful:

Five NAS-NRC panels reviewed anti-infective agents that combine one antibiotic with another in fixed ratios, or an antibiotic with one or more sulfonamides. In addition to finding about 40 such products to be ineffective, by reason of being no more effective than their components used singly, the panels judged at least 50 combinations to be dangerous. The hazard was said to be not merely to the individual user, but to the public at large, because these agents can permit resistant strains of bacteria to proliferate. The mixtures held to be hazardous as well as inefficacious are the "pen-streps" (penicillin and streptomycin), the "pen-sulfas" (penicillin and sulfa), and Panalba (tetracycline and novobiocin).[20]

The FDA commissioner told Congress that "one out of every five patients who receives the novobiocin component of Panalba is expected to have an allergic or hypersensitivity type of reaction." The novobiocin component created serious risks without commensurate benefits, according to the FDA.[21] The Upjohn Company countered that 23,000 physicians prescribe Panalba and have a right to do so even if their choice is based on advertising and promotion.

The AMA Council on Drugs condemned fixed-ratio preparations as irrational. In the midst of the controversy, however, the AMA Journal published eighteen full pages of advertising for antibiotic combinations.

Antibiotics account for about 25 percent of total drug volume. In 1956-57, 7 percent of all drug expenditures in Public Health Service hospitals were for tranquilizers (psychopharmacologic medications), which were first introduced in 1953. The changing structure of drugs is suggested by changes in the principal categories of drugs included in the *United States Pharmacopoeia:* from 1916 to 1955 the organics increased from about 10 percent to 60 percent, while the biologicals dropped from about 80 percent to 30 percent. The pharmacist has become a dispenser of prefabricated medicines or prescriptions rather than a compounder of powders.[22]

Drug companies in particular have contended that trademark drugs produce benefits beyond those available in the generic drugs. A leading and able British commentator spoke against the "one name" (generic) approach to drugs, noting that "the active constituent of a medicine to which the official or generic name only refers does not constitute the sole basis for its effect—what may appear to be tiny changes in formulation, well within pharmacopoeial standards, such as particle size, disintegration time, and so forth, may make all the difference to the therapeutic efficiency of the active constituent."[23]

The president of E. R. Squibb and Sons explained the difference in costs largely by reference to variations in quality. Squibb contends that it goes way beyond the requirements of the *United States Pharmocopoeia* and the Food and Drug Administration for testing penicillin G. The company does this "because product uniformity in our judgment is an essential element in assuring product reliability." Choice of drugs should be left to doctors, the Squibb executive said. "I think . . . doctors will continue to prescribe by brand name or by choosing the manufacturer," because the brand name will give the patient "uniform and reliable products."[24]

Price Differentials

Usually official or generic drugs are much less costly than their brand-name counterparts. The differences are of such proportions that they are difficult to explain. The large companies that sell brand-name drugs justify their high prices by citing their high costs, especially for extensive research. They emphasize the association between research outlays and discovery of drugs with high therapeutic value. Undoubtedly large promotional outlays also contribute to high prices, but this source is not stressed by the drug manufacturers.

The Master Drug List compiled by the HEW Task Force on Prescription Drugs contained the 409 most frequently prescribed drugs dispensed to the elderly in 1966. These accounted for 88 percent of all prescriptions dispensed by community pharmacies to the elderly in that year and 88 percent of the prescription drug retail costs. Of the 409, 379 were dispensed under their brand names. These accounted for 90 percent of the total acquisition costs to retailers. For 86 of the products dispensed under brand names, chemical equivalents were available, so that these drugs could have been prescribed under generic names. While 23 were available at the same or a higher cost, 63 could have been obtained at lower cost for a saving of 53 percent.[25] The 86 brand-name drugs accounted for 27 percent of retail costs to patients.

Approximately 50 percent of the total costs to patients were concentrated in the top 53 drugs, which accounted for 49 percent of the acquisition costs to retailers. Of these, 30 could be obtained only under brand names from single suppliers; 16 were dispensed under brand names although chemical equivalents were available; and 7 were dispensed generically.[26]

Acquisition by generic names would yield substantial savings. The Master Drug List shows that among 82 drugs that were prescribed for an average of ninety days or more per year, 11 were dispensed by their generic names, and 16 that were dispensed under brand names were available under generic names from more than one source. It is estimated that there would have been a 28 percent saving at the wholesale level if these drugs had been purchased by their generic names at the lowest available cost.[27] Sizable savings could have been achieved in purchases of drugs prescribed for long-term use in the treatment of heart disease, high blood pressure, kidney disease, arthritis and related conditions, and mental and nervous conditions.[28] The ten most frequently used products, which accounted for 20 percent of the sales total on the Master Drug List, included one oral antidiabetic agent, two tranquilizers, two diuretics, one analgesic, one antiarthritic agent, one cardiac drug, and two sedatives.

Under pending legislation, the Secretary of Health, Education, and Welfare would be required to exclude from the reasonable range of drug prices those significantly higher than the price of the drug sold by its established or generic name. He could recognize a differential price for a brand-name drug, however, if the manufacturer could substantiate a claim that his product possessed "distinct therapeutic advantages" over a generic product.[29]

Some examples of price variations are given in table 9.2.

Third-Party Financing of Drug Costs

Out-of-pocket payments in 1970 accounted for 40.5 percent of personal health expenditures, but the proportion varied from one type of expense to another. The extremes were 13.2 percent out-of-pocket spending for hospital care and 88.9 percent for drugs and sundries. Clearly, drugs are a very heavy burden on out-of-pocket payments. Third-party payments and reimbursements for hospital care equaled 86.5 percent of personal health outlays but those for drugs and sundries were only 11.1 percent of outlays.

The amount of money an individual spends on drugs varies with his or her age, sex, color, region of residence, and disability status. The annual per capita cost for all ages is $15.40; for those sixty-five and over it is $41.40; for women it is $18.60 per capita, while for men it is $12.00. Whites spend twice as much as nonwhites.

TABLE 9.2   Price Differentials between Generic and Brand Names

Drug	Quantity	Price
Brand: Melicorten	30 tablets	$8.50
Generic: Prednisone	30 tablets	2.58
Brand: Serpasil	100 tablets	7.06
Generic: Reserpine	100 tablets	2.91
Brand: Achromycin	16 capsules	5.56
Generic: Tetracycline	16 capsules	3.83

A 1964-65 survey showed that the elderly who had no chronic conditions bought an average of 1.2 prescriptions per year for an annual cost of $3.90 per capita. Those suffering from conditions that were sufficiently severe to limit major activity completely bought an average of 21.7 prescriptions per year, costing an average of $78.80 per capita.

Insurance for out-of-hospital drugs has generally been unavailable. Recently there has been intensified interest in providing this insurance coverage.[30] Hospitals also find that patients accept higher charges for drugs more readily than higher charges for room and board.

Scanty coverage of prescription drugs is suggested by the fact that, in 1969, 15 percent of the total costs of outpatient prescriptions was paid by third parties, as compared with 86 percent of hospital costs and 57 percent of the cost of physicians' services.

In 1970, some 1.4 billion prescriptions were bought at a total cost of $4 billion. According to HEW estimates, per capita expenditures on drugs that year were $19.62, but the over-sixty-five population averaged $50.94 per capita, while the under-sixty-five group averaged $16.29.

Factors affecting third-party reimbursement in general apply to drugs as well. These include eligibility for insurance coverage (for example, by age), scope of benefits, range of covered illnesses or drugs, whether benefits are by service or to a community, and utilization reviews of matters such as physicians' prescribing practices.

Third parties may either provide their clients directly with drugs or drug-related services or merely pay for them. Client payment programs generally include a deductible, which must be paid by the enrollee before coverage takes effect. The objectives of deductible provisions are to reduce the high administrative costs resulting from small claims, to reduce the total amount of claims payable, and to permit lower premiums.

Most third-party programs pay the drug providers—pharmacists, physicians, etc. The client may have to pay a coinsurance percentage to the vendor, who is responsible for accumulating claims and submitting them.

A study on behalf of the drug interests on variations in prescription prices gave rise to "a proposal for a system of reimbursement which is essentially usual and customary charges with a procedure for adapting maximum limits to the specific requirements of each vendor. Each pharmacy would be assigned an index number (termed 'prescription service index' or PSI) based upon self-reported data in 36 categories found in the study to be significantly related to the prescription price." For example, external factors included urbanization and income level of residents in the area, while an internal factor was prescription sales as a percentage of total store sales.

The General Accounting Office was critical of the proposal, however, commenting:

The justification for the wide variances among states in the amounts allowed pharmacies over the cost of the drug products dispensed is not apparent. Although there are undoubtedly some variances in the costs of operations among individual pharmacies and among various states and regions in the United States, it appears to us that such variations would not be of the magnitude comparable with that of the variances inherent in the State pricing formulas.[31]

Coverage of outpatient drugs by third-party programs is expected to grow in the next few years. "During the growth process, particular attention needs to be given to improving the methods of reimbursement used for the drug benefit. Current methods are not related to vendor costs, are not responsive to cost charges which occur over time, and do not discriminate on the basis of quality or cost differences among vendors. In general, incentives to increase quality or reduce cost are lacking." Comprehensive coverage of all costs would remove the incentive to keep costs down.[32]

Group Drug Plans

An interesting experiment is the drug insurance program tied to the Group Health Cooperative of Puget Sound, Washington (see table 9.3). The program provides $8.80 per capita for prescription drugs or 55 percent of the similar costs in the United States. The group plan enables economical purchases and utilization, takes no profits, and seems to be thriving because there are tax savings as well.

Proposals for Medicare Drug Coverage

The financing of outpatient prescription drugs has been receiving increasing attention in recent years. Both the Advisory Council to the Department of Health, Education, and Welfare (in 1971) and the HEW Task Force on Prescription Drugs have urged coverage of these

TABLE 9.3   Puget Sound Group Drug Insurance Program, 1962-66

Item	1962	1963	1964	1965	1966
Number of prescriptions	229,635	253,453	283,576	337,142	414,987
Number of enrollees	63,379	65,791	69,938	79,051	86,141
Prescriptions per enrollee	3.62	3.85	4.05	4.26	4.82
Cost per prescription	$1.50	$1.72	$1.76	$1.74	$1.82
Cost per enrollee per year	$5.44	$6.63	$7.12	$7.44	$8.80
Cost per enrollee per month	$0.45	$0.55	$0.59	$0.62	$0.73

Source: K. M. McCaffree and H. F. Newman, "Prepayment of Drug Costs under a Group Practice Repayment Plan," *American Journal of Public Health*, July 1968, p. 1215.

costs under Medicare.[33] The Task Force attested to the need for a program that would finance a large part of outpatient drug bills. These drug expenditures consume about 20 percent of the personal health expenditures of the old. A large proportion of out-of-hospital drugs prescribed for the elderly are so-called long-term maintenance drugs used primarily for control of chronic diseases.

Costs for out-of-hospital prescription drugs are estimated at $1.5 billion. Insurance coverage, tax relief, free drugs, and public assistance would pay about 20 percent of this total. By tying the program to coverage of serious illnesses, setting ceilings on the expenditures per prescription, and restricting coverage because of administrative problems, the total cost of the program can be kept to $1.5 billion. It was anticipated that the drug program would be financed through the hospital insurance component of Medicare, thus exploiting the revenue to be obtained from payroll taxes levied in periods of high income.

A comprehensive drug insurance program with the enrollee paying 20 percent of the charges for drugs would have cost $1.5 billion in 1971. If the elderly were to receive aid in paying costs they find difficult to finance and would rely to some extent on public assistance programs, the costs would be kept down.

But the HEW Task Force on Prescription Drugs did not support a comprehensive program, which would have covered 1,200 drugs and raised serious administrative problems. The theory behind Social Security is to bestow some responsibility on the beneficiaries to finance part of such programs. The Task Force therefore considered that it would be desirable—at least at the outset—to provide drug coverage on a less-than-comprehensive basis.

It favored coverage under the hospital insurance component of Medicare, rather than the supplementary medical insurance component, because "an individual would pay for the protection during his working years, rather than at a time of life when he may well have low income, limited assets, and large health costs."

For keeping the costs down, the Task Force suggested large deductibles, coinsurance, and concentration on drugs for the treatment of cardiovascular diseases, diabetes, kidney conditions, and respiratory conditions.

It would also be possible to set maximum limits on the reimbursable costs of prescriptions and the reimbursable quantity of drugs per prescription. Depending on the limitations imposed, the program would cost between $405 million and $720 million.

Use of utilization review methods would help control costs in a Medicare drug program. A study by states revealed that, when no dollar limits were set on covered costs, the utilization rate was almost 75 percent, but with dollar limits it was only 50 percent.

In the view of the Task Force, costs could be kept down through coinsurance provisions and restrictions on maximum prescription quantities.[34] Among the methods considered by the Task Force for determining drug acquisition costs for the Medicare proposal were the actual acquisition cost, as verified by audit, the usual and customary charge, the listed wholesale price, and fixed program payments. But the Task Force noted that usual and customary charges may often be greater than the cost to the pharmacist in acquiring the drug. It recommended that reimbursement on the basis of "product cost" use the cost of the least expensive chemical equivalent of acceptable quality that is generally available on the market.

Cost Controls

Effective Price Review Mechanisms

The absence of competitive conditions in the drug industry is reflected in price differentials. Drug companies often sell to the government at relatively low prices and to retailers at much higher prices. Striking differences were found in the prices paid by the state of New York and the city of New York; the city has a strong organization to achieve low prices. In Atlanta, the price of a drug may be twenty or forty times what it costs in New York (see table 9.4).

TABLE 9.4 Drug Price Comparisons by City and County

	New York	Chicago	Boston	Atlanta	Baltimore	Dade County (Miami)	Allegheny County (Pittsburgh)	Multnomah County (Portland)	San Francisco	Erie County (Buffalo)	Nassau County	Onondaga County (Syracuse)
Meprobamate 400 mg. (500)	9.45	10.50	11.30	31.20	10.65	10.70	9.88	20.00	9.50	14.00	9.45	11.80
Chloramphenical 250 mg. (100)	6.73	24.99	8.20	21.00	24.99	15.75	25.50	25.50	25.00	15.43	5.50	25.50
Tetracycline hcl 250 mg. (1,000)	25.95	50.00	47.40	59.00	39.50	34.50	—	52.50	37.50	31.00	36.00	90.00*
Streptomycin Sulphate 5 gm. vial (1)	.24	.37	—	.88	—	.37	.33	.50	.37	—	.37	—
Phenazopyridine hcl 0.1 gm. (1,000)	4.80	—	39.84	48.00	—	39.73	4.75	—	—	39.84	6.00	—
Dextroamphetamine Sulphate 5 gm. (1,000)	.57	—	20.21	22.60	—	19.43	1.50	5.06	1.75	—	.70	2.29
Diphenhydramine hcl 25 mg. (1,000)	3.10	—	10.70	7.00	3.55	10.70	—	5.20	10.50	10.49	10.49	10.70
Prednisone 5 mg. (1,000)	4.58	—	9.80	10.50	5.25	15.00	5.94	8.00	6.00	20.90	6.00	6.75
Sulfadizine 5 mg. (1,000)	5.50	—	—	9.30	10.00	14.40	—	19.20	15.00	9.00	13.60	—
Diphenylhydantoin 250 mg. vial (1)	.95	1.30	1.70	2.27	1.40	1.70	—	1.70	1.37	1.17	1.37	1.70

*Price for tetracycline phosphate.

Much higher prices for drugs are charged to low-income groups than to the affluent.

Use of a Formulary

Many countries have established formularies—compilations of drugs approved for use in hospitals—as a technique for dealing with the rising cost and increasing use of drugs. The HEW Task Force on Prescription Drugs strongly favors use of a formulary, which is finding increasing use abroad and even in this country by government, insurance companies, and hospitals. The general view is that formularies save money and improve the prescription process.

In hospitals, for example, the pharmacy and therapeutics committee can be an effective administrative mechanism for drug utilization control. It formulates broad policies for evaluation of, approval of, procurement of, storage of, distribution of, safety procedures for, and restraints on the use of drugs.

Recourse to formularies has risen in hospitals. Opposition to their use is much greater in government programs and facilities. Dr. D. C. Brodie found "no comparable system in public programs nor is it likely that an effective one can be designed because of the large number of patients and professionals dispersed over wide geographic areas." However, the HEW Task Force noted that

even in those countries with relatively restrictive formularies, [when] the selection of drugs [is] made by expert committees of clinicians and scientists, the utilization of formularies appears to be associated with general acceptance by practitioners, physicians and pharmacists, more intensive competition among manufacturers, relative price control, and few, if any, reported problems related to therapeutic equivalency.

Notes

1. *Business Week*, August 16, 1969, p. 39; J. Stetler, "New Drug Regulations—A Year's Perspective," *New Physician*, March 1969, pp. 75-77; "Senate Subcommittee Hearings about Drug Company Operations," *G.P.*, February 1968; HEW, *Task Force on Prescription Drugs*, Release, September 13, 1968, p. 5.

2. Bureau of the Census, *Concentration Ratios in Manufacturing Industry, 1958* (1962), p. 24.

3. *Administered Prices*, Senate Report no. 488, pp. 84-88.

4. Ibid., p. 91; also see pp. 85, 86, 98; *Senate Hearings on Administered Prices*, part 24, pp. 13671-72.

5. HEW, Task Force on Prescription Drugs, *Final Report* (February 1969).

6. Ibid.

7. Bureau of the Census, *Concentration Ratios in Manufacturing Industry, 1958* (1962), p. 7; *Administered Prices*, Senate Report no. 448, pp. 15-24, 31.

8. *Administered Prices*, Senate Report no. 448, part 14, p. 788; Sanders and Fischer, eds., *The Crisis in American Medicine*, p. 102.

9. R. Burack, *Handbook of Prescription Drugs* (1967), pp. 12-31; U.S. Senate, Subcommittee on Monopoly, *Hearings on Competitive Problems in the Drug Industry* (1967), part II, pp. 818, 822-23; part V, pp. 1588, 1837, 1995, 2047-48, 2056; part XII, pp. 5000, 5132.

10. L. M. Kramer, *Drugs and Medicine*, Public Health Reports (October 1958), p. 929.

11. Sanders and Fischer, eds., *The Crisis in American Medicine*, pp. 179-80.

12. Ibid., p. 178.

13. Ibid., p. 105.

14. D. H. Knapp, *Paying for Outpatient Prescription Drugs and Related Services in Third Party Programs* (1971), pp. 831-34.

15. Ibid., pp. 826-27.

16. W. S. Apple, "Pharmaceutical Statement of the American Pharmaceutical Association on Anti-Trust and Monopoly," *South Dakota Journal of Medicine and Pharmacy*, November 1964, pp. 37-40; W. J. Peeples, "Comparative Price List; Generic vs. Brand Name Drugs," *Maryland Medical Journal*, July 1969, pp. 89-91; "Senate Subcommittee Hearings about Drug Company Operations," *G.P.*, February 1968.

17. A. N. Brewster and J. P. Horton, *American Journal of Hospital Pharmacy*, April 1968, pp. 176-78.

18. HEW, Public Health Service, *Medical Care Financing and Utilization* (1962), p. 70; *Economic Report of the President* (1970); National Bureau of Economic Research, *The Price Statistics of the Federal Government* (1961), pp. 35-38; U.S. Congress, Joint Economic Committee, *Hearings on Government Price Statistics* (1961), p. 787.

19. *Administered Prices*, Senate Report no. 448, pp. 107-12. But compare Pharmaceutical Manufacturers Association, *Prescription Drugs and the Public Health*, pp. 20-21.

20. M. Mintz, "FDA and Panalba: A Conflict of Commercial, Therapeutic Goals?" *Science* 165 (August 29, 1969): 875.

21. See especially ibid., pp. 875-81.

22. L. M. Kramer, *Drugs and Medicine*, Public Health Reports (October 1958), pp. 931-32.

23. Sir Derrick M. Dunlop, "Drug Control and the British Health Service," *Annals of Internal Medicine*, August 1969, pp. 237-44. Also see A. D. Little, *A Report on the Social and Economic Benefits of the Pharmaceutical Industry in the United States* (1961).

24. "Senate Subcommittee Hearings about Drug Company Operations," *G.P.*, February 1968, pp. 163-67.

25. HEW, Task Force on Prescription Drugs, *Final Report* (February 1969), p. 36.

26. Ibid., p. 5; U.S. Senate, Subcommittee on Monopoly, *Hearings on Competitive Problems in the Drug Industry* (1967), part II, pp. 612-16.

27. HEW, Task Force on Prescription Drugs, *Final Report*, pp. 65-66.

28. Ibid., p. 37.

29. Ibid., p. 42.

30. K. M. McCaffree and H. F. Newman, "Prepayment of Drug Costs under a Group Practice Repayment Plan," *American Journal of Public Health*, July 1968, pp. 1212-18; also see M. S. Danian and R. W. Hammel, "Insuring Families against the Cost of Prescribed Drugs," *Journal of the American Pharmaceutical Association*, April 1967, pp. 176-78.

31. D. H. Knapp, *Paying for Outpatient Prescription Drugs and Related Services in Third Party Programs* (1971), pp. 837-51.

32. Ibid., pp. 850-51.

33. See especially ibid., including a valuable bibliography; also see the excellent studies by R. Burack, *The Handbook of Prescription Drugs* (1967); M. Mintz, *The Therapeutic Nightmare* (1964); and HEW, Food and Drug Administration, *Facts About Drugs* (November 1965).

34. HEW, Task Force on Prescription Drugs, *Final Report* (February 1969), pp. 49-69.

10

Hospitals

Financial Overview

Hospitals have been in deep financial trouble. One reason is the rising costs of operating hospitals. Using 1957-59 as the base period index of 100, by 1969 the average daily hospital charge had risen to 250 while all medical care prices were at 150 and physicians' fees were also at 150. From 1950 to 1969, rising prices accounted for 50 percent of the increase in medical care expenditures, and in the last few years medical care prices were rising almost twice as much as the consumer price index. Again in 1968-69, hospitals accounted for 30 percent of the private medical care expenditures and 50 percent of public expenditures.

Hospital finance greatly improved as the economy recovered in the 1960s and the government increased its contribution markedly (see table 10.1).

Another important source of help to hospitals was the rising contribution of insurance. Hospitals gained more from insurance than most other health care components. Insurance, of course, has not been an unmixed blessing. One unfortunate aspect is wasteful spending when a third party pays the bill. Dr. John Knowles comments:

The typical hospital patient interviewed did not seem to care about hospital charges since his first three weeks in semi-private accommodation under Blue Cross cost him nothing.

One man, an elderly bank clerk, said he had two wives who died in hospitals and that he had been in five hospitals because of a stomach ailment.

"I never looked at my bills" he said, "because I did not have to pay them. They were covered by Blue Cross. Sure, I got copies of the bills, but I couldn't care less what the costs were."[1]

Hospitals have operated under adverse conditions. With prices tied to costs, lack of a profit motive, and large cost increases, hospitals were in very bad financial shape during the depression. Low incomes among the population resulted in low occupancy rates and reduced capacity to pay, while the nonpatient income of hospitals was declining. The prosperity of recent years and the growth of prepayment insurance saved hospitals from massive government intervention.[2]

Despite the large contributions of insurance and improving economic conditions, however, hospitals have continued to have their problems. In the 1930s and 1940s, they suffered from the depression, the impact of World War II, and rising competition for the donated dollar. In the 1960s government expenditures became much more important and hence private sources were muted to some extent. But increased utilization—however much it may have helped hospitals that had excess capacity—and rising costs aggravated their financial problems. Government increasingly took over the financial burden, with corresponding relief for private sources.

Early in 1968 the American Hospital Association issued a statement on the *Financial Requirements of Health Care Institutions.* Noting that under Medicare and Medicaid the government had assumed the burden of paying the health care expenses of a large segment of the

TABLE 10.1   Private and Public Financing of Hospital Expenditures, 1966-69

Source	1965-66	1968-69
Private expenditures	64%	50%
Federal government expenditures	13%	32%
State and local government expenditures	23%	18%
Total amount (billions)	$14.2	$22.5

population, the statement warned that this source would not meet the total needs of our health care system, and it emphasized philanthropy as an important alternative source of finance.[3] Five major aims were stated:

1. To set forth the obligation on the part of purchasers of health care services to collectively meet the full financial requirements of the providers of those services.
2. To establish that operating income is an integral part of capital financing for preservation, replacement, expansion and renovation as it is in the other segments of the economy.
3. To recognize the health care system's obligation to the community to expend funds wisely and to expand only in accord with community needs as expressed through the community's appropriate planning mechanism.
4. To establish that health care institutions must have an essential role in the development of areawide health plans and in the designation of the areawide health planning agency.
5. To provide an orderly transitional period during which all of the three parties—institutions, planning agencies and contracting agencies—participate in the development of a mutually acceptable plan of implementation. . . .

The need for discipline in the health care system to assure delivery of high quality health care has a corollary: adequate financing for health care services and facilities. The system has multiple sources of financing—self-pay patients, *contracting agencies,* private insurance, tax levies, governmental grants, donations, grants and endowments. From these various sources must come adequate financing—financing that (1) goes beyond *current operating needs;* (2) is sufficient to permit maintenance and, consonant with community needs, expansion, modernization and replacement of physical plant, and (3) recognizes educational and research programs having appropriate approval. Further, the sources of financing should recognize that health care institutions, as community service organizations, must be financed at a level that supports the objectives of community service, including health services for needy patients.[4]

Prices and Expenditures

The hospital price index has steadily climbed. From 1955 to 1965, the total value of hospital services rose from $3.43 billion to $9.15 billion or 167 percent. The hospital price index increased 44 percent and the deflated value of services per patient-day went up 34 percent.

From 1929 to 1967, the changes outlined in table 10.2 occurred. The daily service charge rose 7 times, while the consumer price index increased by less than 1 time. Even more striking is the increase

TABLE 10.2   Rise in Hospital Costs and Prices, 1929-67

	1929	1967
Hospital expenditures (millions)	$380	$13,287
Daily service charge, consumer price index (1957-59 = 100)	24.2	200.1
Expense per inpatient-day	$4.53	$59.48
Consumer price index, all items (1957-59 = 100)	59.7	116.3

Source: Adapted from H. E. Klarman, "Medical Economics," *Inquiry*, March 1970, p. 28.

of hospital expenditures in these thirty-eight years—a rise of 34 times.

Over this period, expenditures on short-term hospitals rose by 9.8 percent a year and the daily service charge by 5.7 percent. The corresponding rise of expenditures for physicians was 6.3 percent and, for the physicians' fee index, it was 2.4 percent.[5]

Various measures of hospital costs can be compared. For example, expenditures per inpatient-day in short-term general hospitals were $4.53 in 1929, but rose to $59.48 by 1967. For state and county mental hospitals, expenditures per patient per day averaged $6.74. In Alaska, however, they reached a high of $23.02, while Mississippi had a low of $3.18.

Expenses per patient-day rose considerably for various types of hospitals from 1945 to 1960 (see table 10.3). For Medicare and obstetrical care, the average cost per patient-day was $30.92. The average hospital cost per case was $151.52. Regional variations were wide: the minimum per patient-day in the Southeast was $26.66, while in the Far West it was $41.38.[6]

Cost per day vary greatly by type of hospital. Thus, in 1960, the expenditures of voluntary short-term hospitals were 49 percent of

TABLE 10.3   Expenses per Patient-Day in Nonfederal Hospitals, 1945-60

Type of Hospital	1945	1960
Psychiatric hospitals	$1.46	$ 4.91
Tuberculosis hospitals	4.03	13.37
Long-term general and other special hospitals	3.23	12.62

total expenditures, and their share of patient-days was 24 percent of the total (see table 10.4). These figures point to high daily costs for these hospitals. In contrast, nonfederal psychiatric hospitals accounted for 14 percent of expenditures but 48 percent of the patient-days. Another survey showed per diem costs of short-term voluntary hospitals at about 9 times the cost of long-term mental hospitals.

Variations in hospital charges of $40 to $80 per day are not easily explained by capital availability or even variations in efficiency. Wide differences in unit costs are found even where input, prices, and quality of output are similar. Where reimbursement is based on costs there is little incentive to economize. A relevant question is: What cost is to be the target? If it is the cost per patient-day, then we must keep the hospitals full, stress low-cost stays, and close the outpatient facilities. If the target is the number of admissions or cases treated, stays should be shortened and the number of cases increased. The tendency of physicians to seek new services and corresponding equipment in the hospitals they affiliate with also raises costs.[7]

Sources of Rising Costs

What accounts for the rise of operating costs? A Michigan study in the late 1950s revealed inflation as contributing 39 percent and increased utilization 40 percent to the cost increase. Of the latter, 60 percent was associated with population growth. Other factors in higher utilization were the rise in the aged population, the increased availability of services, and the increased capacity of the population to pay for health care through insurance and prepayment plans and because of rising salaries. Rising salaries for hospital workers also contributed to higher operating costs, along with the increases in

TABLE 10.4 Expenditures and Days of Care by Type of Hospital, 1960

| | Percentage of Total | | | |
| | Expenditures | | Patient-Days | |
Type of Hospital	1946	1960	1946	1960
Voluntary short-term	43.2	49.2	20.3	24.4
State and local government short-term	11.6	14.3	7.6	8.0
Nonfederal psychiatric	13.4	14.3	45.4	47.9
All federal	19.1	13.5	14.6	11.1

Source: Calculated from "Hospital Statistics," *Hospitals,* August 1961.

hospital personnel and increasing complexity of medical practice. These in turn lead to more services, more expensive equipment, and more personnel.

One estimate found that "the average employee in a manufacturing industry today must contribute two and one half more hours of wages per year to meet the costs of hospital care than he did a decade ago."[8] Hospital costs have skyrocketed especially since the introduction of Medicare and Medicaid. In 1967 and 1968 average daily hospital costs rose by 11 percent and 25 percent according to one estimate and by 13 percent and 30 percent according to another.[9]

Hospital wages have been low for a long time. Under pressure of the labor shortage in the field, they have been rising in recent years more than wages in the economy generally. A comparison of wages in manufacturing and in voluntary hospitals is given in table 10.5.

Expenditures also depend on the number of patients in relation to the population. In 1967, the average daily number of patients in short-stay hospitals was 3.4 per thousand population. In three states the average was in excess of 4.5 and in nine states it was less than 3. Obviously, in many states the inpatient population might increase greatly.[10]

Operating expenses also relate to the medical personnel required. In 1966, extended care facilities had 275,000 employees. According to two estimates, they were short-handed in nineteen occupations by 29,000 and 32,000 workers.[11]

Cost increases create a domino effect: "Generally as cost per day increases, so do average length of stay, per cent of occupancy, size of hospital, personnel per occupied bed, annual payroll per employee, scope of service, and percentage of suitable beds."[12]

The contribution of rising wages, prices, and input, both labor and

TABLE 10.5   Weekly Salaries in Manufacturing and Hospital Work, 1960-66

Year	Manufacturing	Accredited Voluntary Hospitals
1960	$ 84.36	$ 69.20
1966	101.95	109.87

Source: HEW, *Report of the National Conference on Medical Costs,* Washington, D.C., June 27-28, 1967, p. 118.

nonlabor, to the cost per patient in short-term community hospitals from 1951 to 1970 is shown in table 10.6. The overall rise was especially large in the period following enactment of Medicare, 1966-70. Increased wage rates were two to three times as potent an inflationary factor as price increases.

For the whole period, wages and prices raised the cost per patient day as much as the rise of input; but from 1966 to 1970, wages and prices accounted for 56 percent of the inflation, and increases in input only 44 percent.

Price-setting

In their pricing policies, hospital officials favor daily service charges and overcharge for ancillary services, in part because patients are ignorant of the market values for the latter. One result, presumably, is a stimulus to the use of daily service items rather than ancillary

TABLE 10.6 Increase in Cost per Patient-Day in Short-term Community Hospitals, 1951-70

Item	1951-70	1951-55	1955-60	1960-66	1966-70
Percentage increase	8.6%	8.4%	6.9%	6.9%	13.9%
Increase in wages and prices	4.2%	3.7%	3.8%	3.1%	7.8%
Wage rates	5.8%	5.8%	4.9%	4.1%	9.8%
Price levels	2.1%	.8%	2.0%	1.5%	4.8%
Increase in inputs	4.4%	4.7%	3.1%	3.8%	6.1%
Labor	2.9%	4.4%	2.2%	2.5%	2.8%
Nonlabor	6.4%	4.8%	4.5%	6.0%	11.0%
Amount of increase	$3.38	$1.59	$1.82	$2.66	$8.21
Increase in wages and prices	1.67	.71	1.00	1.19	4.62
Wage rates	1.32	.65	.80	.97	3.48
Price levels	.35	.06	.20	.22	1.14
Increase in inputs	1.71	.88	.82	1.47	3.59
Labor	.66	.50	.36	.59	.99
Nonlabor	1.05	.38	.46	.88	2.60
Percentage distribution	100.0%	100.0%	100.0%	100.0%	100.0%
Increase in wages and prices	49.4%	44.7%	54.9%	44.7%	56.3%
Wage rates	39.1%	40.9%	44.0%	36.4%	42.4%
Price levels	10.4%	3.8%	11.0%	8.3%	13.9%
Increase in inputs	50.6%	55.3%	45.1%	55.3%	43.7%
Labor	19.5%	31.4%	19.8%	22.2%	12.1%
Nonlabor	31.1%	23.9%	25.3%	33.1%	31.7%

Source: HEW, Office of Research and Statistics, *The Effect of Changing Technology on Hospital Costs* (February 23, 1972).

services. This may be a desirable result if ancillary services are less available than hospital beds in relation to demand. In view of the striking rise of demand for ancillary services, my guess is that the administrators' policy is a step in the right direction. Dr. J. H. Knowles has written:

The rapidly rising cost of hospital care is due to the "professional care" element (those things and people one needs in a hospital but not in a hotel) and not to the hotel function. . . . At [Massachusetts General Hospital] in 1964, 11.6 per cent of the dollar was spent on the hotel function and 88.4 per cent on the professional or medical function, as contrasted with 28 per cent and 72 per cent respectively in 1952.[13]

Since the hospitals depended heavily on payments from private sources—though less so than five or ten years ago—the manner of rate-making is important. The Committee on Financing Hospital Care put the principles of hospital rate-making this way:

The first and primary objective in rate making is to obtain revenue which will be sufficient to finance the costs of care. All other rate making objectives must be subordinated to the necessity to meet payrolls and to pay bills.

The second objective is to make payments by patients and collection by the hospital as convenient as possible.

The third objective is to promote maximum needed utilization of hospital personnel and facilities since this will mean lowest unit costs, and therefore the lowest possible rate level.

The fourth objective is to set rates in a manner which is considered "fair" and necessary by the community serviced, since the existence of the hospital depends on community support.[14]

In September 1953, the Board of Trustees and the House of Delegates of the American Hospital Association approved certain principles of reimbursement. These were published in 1954 under the title *Principles of Payment for Hospital Care*. In general, rates should reflect overall costs for the hospital as a whole and for each department. The relation of charges to costs varies among hospitals and among services. The rate should reflect allowances for uncollectible bills, overhead, and financing improvements in services. Apparently, the fixing of rates on the basis of costs was far from universal practice, as a study by W. J. McNerney noted:

(1) At present, the rates for individual hospital services are not closely related to the inclusive costs of providing these services.

(2) The absence of refined cost analysis precludes hospitals from determining inclusive costs by departments to provide a basis for scientific rate making.

(3) Hospitals are inclined to price routine care charges below costs and to make up losses sustained from profits earned in specialized departments.

(4) Rates charged for routine care vary by accommodation occupied and by size of hospital. The absence of a cost analysis which computes cost of routine care by type of accommodation precludes hospitals from establishing these rates scientifically.

(5) Charges for special services are uniform for all types of patients.

(6) Hospitals have relatively less control in establishing rates for pathological and radiological procedures than for other services because, for both inpatients and outpatients, radiological charges are paid by the Michigan Blue Shield according to a fee schedule; and for outpatients, laboratory charges are paid in the same way. . . .

Hospital rates for various services should be established in direct relationship to the inclusive cost of each service as determined by periodic cost analyses, prepared on a basis sufficient to pay for the total costs, including overhead, of each service provided the public. . . .

Rates for routine service should be based on cost for each type of accommodation as determined by cost analyses. Charges for special services should likewise be based on cost. All charges should be adequate to provide a margin over cost sufficient to absorb bad debts and allowances and to produce some income for other legitimate purposes, such as support of community service programs. The practice of adopting the reimbursement schedules of Michigan Medical Service (Blue Cross) as a matter of expediency should be discontinued, as should overpricing in one area to offset losses incurred in another.[15]

A study of the Michigan experience throws some light on the inadequacies of cost accounting in the medical sector. For example, only 10 percent of the hospitals in the study used budgets (see table 10.7).

It has generally been assumed that hospitals should not pass depreciation charges on to patients, although this is done to some extent. There are also serious differences in views on the responsibility for financing educational services given by hospitals. Blue Cross now seems to allow hospitals to include remuneration for interns and residents in its bills for reimbursement. Supervisory physicians, under the umbrella of Medicare, have increasingly been submitting bills for their supervision tasks even when no service has been given (see the discussion in chapter 8).

This issue is part of a more general problem: Who is to finance the educational services provided by hospitals? At present it is ultimately

TABLE 10.7 Use of Management Tools in Hospitals, by Size

Management Tool	All Hospitals		500 Beds or More		100-499 Beds		Under 100 Beds	
	Number	Weighted Percentage	Number	Percentage	Number	Percentage	Number	Percentage
All hospitals	33	100	8	100	12	100	13	100
Organization chart								
Have	13	23	6	75	6	50	1	8
Do not have	20	77	2	25	6	50	12	92
Policy manual								
Have	5	13	1	12	3	25	1	8
Do not have	28	87	7	88	9	75	12	92
Budget								
Have	9	10	6	75	3	25	0	0
Do not have	24	90	2	25	9	75	13	100

Source: W. J. McNerney, Hospital and Medical Economics (1962), vol. 2, p. 1217.

the patient who pays. Obviously he derives some benefits from the educational contribution of the hospital. With increasing government aid, some part of the education outlay has been transferred from the hospital. But there is little guidance on how these charges should be allocated.

After a survey of the problem, the staff of the Senate Finance Committee concluded "that there is no justification under the present Medicare statute for reimbursement of supervisory physician services to an institutional patient in a teaching setting and there is no legal obligation on the part of the patient to pay [the supervisory physician] for those services."[16]

Sources of Payments

Sources of payments for patient services varied according to income, liquid assets, and insurance coverage of the patient (see table 10.8). In the early 1950s one study revealed that in half the hospitals patients paid at least 95 percent of the charges, in 31 percent of the hospitals they paid less than 90 percent of the charges, and in 16 percent of the hospitals they paid 100 percent of the charges. The unemployed and those on relief were unable to pay large parts of their bills.[17]

TABLE 10.8   Sources of Payment for Hospital Bills

Source Category	Percentage Paid by That Source
Individual with income under $1,650	
Family funds	69
Outside source	12
Unpaid (still owed)	4.5
Individual with income over $1,650	
Family funds	53
Outside source	16
Unpaid (still owed)	9
Large bills	
Savings	27
Installment or postponed payments	29
Borrowed funds	33
Surgery bills	
Patient's funds	36
Blue Cross-Blue Shield	42
Patient and third-party payment	44
All other resources	40

Source: W. J. McNerney, *Hospital and Medical Economics* (1962), vol. 1, pp. 189, 237, 423.

Effects of Medicare and Medicaid

Utilization

In the first year of Medicare, July 1966 to June 1967, hospital revenues rose more than expenses; hence net revenues increased, particularly for small and medium-sized hospitals, which care for the largest proportion of aged persons. But it should be noted that the gains of revenue are related not only to the rise of income and spending under Medicare but also to the increase in operations. With more funds available to purchase hospital services, the costs per service rose. Thus, Bureau of Labor Statistics studies reveal that over the initial eighteen-month-period of Medicare, from June 1966 to December 1967, hospitals increased their daily service charges by 28.7 percent, their operating room charges by 18.7 percent, and their X-ray diagnostic and upper gastrointestinal service charges by 9.5 percent.

Another factor pushing prices up was the rise in the proportion of services that had been provided by hospitals without charge or at subsidized rates and that became subject to charges or an increased share of costs through Medicare. In the year ending September 1967, expenses per patient-day increased by 12.3 percent compared with an average annual rise of 6.9 percent in the corresponding years from 1960 to 1966.

The aged accounted for 32 percent of hospital days in 1967. This breaks down to 41 percent for hospitals with 6 to 24 beds and 26.1 percent for those with 500 or more beds. Increased utilization tended to increase occupancy rates of short-term hospitals.

In Medicare's first year, the financial position of hospitals improved considerably as a result of increases in occupancy rates, reimbursements for services to some aged patients that were previously provided free or at reduced prices, reduction of losses from uncollectible bills to aged patients, and receipt of additional revenue from higher charges.[18]

Revenue, net revenue, and net revenue ratios (net revenue as a percentage of total revenue) are shown in table 10.9. All three increased greatly in 1966 and 1967 compared to the 1960-65 period. The large rise in total revenue suggests an increase in operations. Net revenue in 1967 was roughly three times that of the 1960-65 average. The small and medium-sized hospitals improved their positions

TABLE 10.9   Hospital Total and Net Revenues, 1960-67

Year	Total Revenue (Billions)	Net Revenue		Net Revenue Ratio
		Total (Millions)	Per Patient-Day	
1960-65 (average)	$5.8	$136	$ .92	2.3
1966	8.3	287	1.74	3.5
1967	9.9	399	2.31	4.0

Source: P. A. Feldstein and S. Waldman, "Financial Position of Hospitals in Early Medicare Period," *Social Security Bulletin*, October 1968, p. 22.

more than others, because they had a higher proportion of aged patients and therefore enjoyed relatively greater increases in occupancy rates after Medicare began. Hospitals with 500 beds or more operated at a deficit before Medicare and continued to incur deficits afterward.

Reimbursement Policies

Under the Medicare and Medicaid legislation, hospitals were initially to be reimbursed for all costs incurred. It was generally realized that the financial results might well be disastrous, but the Social Security administrator insisted that the law required full recovery of costs. Some restraints were nevertheless imposed, however. For example, formulas that would provide incentives to reduce costs were introduced: where the same reimbursement rates were provided, a more efficient hospital would cut costs and thus obtain larger revenues. It was argued that hospitals would not automatically obtain full recovery of costs. Rather, negotiations with hospitals should consider what services were given and the quality of those services, and hospitals of similar size and services should be grouped together in these negotiations.

This cost-plus formula compels us to reimburse hospitals for whatever costs they incur, regardless of the quality of their management practices. This open-ended mode of reimbursement contains no incentives whatever for hospitals to operate efficiently. We have developed reimbursement criteria that would build in incentives to hold hospital costs down . . . [but] we are not permitted to use them because of Federal reimbursement requirements.[19]

The act originally provided generous depreciation allowances, giving incentives to overcapitalize and sell facilities at highly inflated prices. Under the reasonable and customary charge reimbursement policy in the Medicare law, it was made clear that Medicare should not pay in excess of the minimum paid for major contracts under Blue Cross or Blue Shield. But Medicare payments were generally in excess of rates the Blues charged to their private customers. In fact, Medicare was ignorant of the charges made by Blue Cross-Blue Shield. One important result of the requirement that Medicare pay the minimum charge was that other markets revised their prices upward to preclude Medicare from paying more than they were. Eventually, limits were introduced on what constituted reasonable charges.

To conform present medicare practice to the congressional intent . . . the staff recommends that all Blue Shield plans serving as medicare carriers be required to limit the physician's charge recognized as "reasonable" to not more than the average payment actually made for a given service or procedure under all of its basic surgical-medical subscriber contracts during a reasonably recent prior period of time. Thus, for example, if Blue Shield in Massachusetts under all of its various subscriber contracts actually paid an average of $250 for removal of cataract (excision of lens) during 1968, medicare would not recognize charges above $250 as "reasonable" for purposes of reimbursement.

For those services which medicare covers but which Blue Shield does not, maximum allowances could be calculated on a basis relative to the average actual payments which Blue Shield made on the services it does cover.

Additionally, to avoid, at least to some extent, costly and often medically unnecessary "gang visiting," amounts allowed should be reduced for multiple visits, on the same day to patients in the same facility. Similarly, limitation on amounts allowed for "injections" and routine laboratory tests should be established and applied.[20]

Over the years, third parties have set ceilings on reimbursements. But this has had the unfortunate result of penalizing the hospitals that offer more expensive and extensive services. The Medicare administration tried to cope with the dangers of recovery of full costs in various ways. In July 1966, the cost-plus provision was dropped.

A controversial issue was the extra 2 percent payment made under Medicare to hospitals in place of reimbursement for more identifiable costs. Under the pressure of rising costs and deficits, this seemed an unwise way for the government to provide hospitals with capital, and this bounty was abandoned.

In the late 1960s, particularly in relation to Medicare and Medicaid legislation, the tax-exempt status of hospitals, which was justified in part by their services to the poor, was questioned again.[21] The issues are suggested in a letter from Charles A. Byrley of the National Governors' Conference to Senator Russell Long as chairman of the Finance Committee, in 1969:

I understand that the Senate Finance Committee will soon be considering in Executive Session a section in the Tax Reform Act of 1969 that provides that private, non-profit hospitals can no longer be challenged to defend their tax exempt status in terms of the amount of charitable services they provide. This provision, as contained in the House passed bill, HR 13270, and in a recent Internal Revenue Service ruling, could result in hospitals refusing to serve Medicare and Medicaid patients or limiting their services to such patients unless the state meets the hospitals' demands for a certain level of payment.

I urge you, as Chairman of the Senate Finance Committee, to provide in the Tax Reform Act of 1969 for some means for states to control levels of payment to hospitals without endangering the availability of services for Medicare and Medicaid patients.

States have found it necessary to place some control on levels of payments to providers under the Medicaid program. Unless this control on the costs of Medicaid is maintained, states will be faced with an even greater financial burden under Medicaid, as will the Federal government.

Governors of states that have recent experience with freezing of levels of payment to hospitals and with challenges to the tax exempt status of hospitals will also be contacting you on this matter.[22]

Quality

In the gestation period of Medicare, Congress was concerned about the possibility of deteriorating quality. The law specifically provided for utilization reviews and tied them to quality considerations. By 1968, government officials were expressing much interest in, and perhaps excessive optimism about, the contribution of this legislation to the protection of standards.

One major contribution of medicare . . . has to do with raising the quality of care provided older patients.

Providers of service have been required to meet specified standards. For extended-care facilities and home-health agencies, these standards were the first to be nationally recognized.

Professional organizations such as the Joint Commission on Accreditation of Hospitals and the American Osteopathic Hospital Association have been stimulated to reconsider their own standards with the aim of raising them.

States are reviewing and strengthening their licensure programs in ways closely akin to the certification process under medicare.

A special effort is being made by the Social Security Administration to assure the quality of performances by independent clinical laboratories through raising their personnel standards.

Medicare standards have provided benchmarks for determining the adequacy of care now provided by our health resources.

For example, the survey of hospitals—including both participants and those denied participation—showed that 46 percent had some deficiency and that 89 percent of the extended care facilities needed to improve their operations to meet medicare's quality goals.

With this information in hand, we developed a program of consultation and training for State health departments to assist them in their facility certification process and to equip them with sufficient technical and program know-how so they can, in turn, assist the operators of facilities in their efforts to achieve the standards.

For the elderly patient and his family, these standards and our efforts to improve them mean a growing confidence in the quality of care purchased. . . .

Medicare has also made available insured alternatives to hospital care. These include: hospital outpatient service where that is appropriate for diagnosis or treatment; and posthospital extended care and home health care, where further stay in a hospital is not the most appropriate level of care. Also included is the coverage of physicians' services for home and office visits.

From a hospital administrator's viewpoint also, the progress was heartening: . . . Part A of title 18 has been the most successful component of this multi-faceted program. Hospital care is being rendered to the aged as a right, and has relieved those persons from a terrifying burden. On the whole, hospitals are now on a firm, viable financial footing for the first time in their history. The program has had a salutary effect on standards of hospital care, especially in its insistence on utilization committees and review. . . .

Among other long-range dividends expected from medicare are: (1) medicare will more clearly show the need for, and hasten the development of, area-wide community planning of all health, medical, and manpower resources, (2) more doctors may be encouraged to specialize in geriatrics, and (3) the requirement that participating medical institutions conform to title VI of the Civil Rights Act is intended to give members of minority groups access to high-quality care. . . .

Just about every witness who directed the subcommittee's attention to possible shortcomings in medicare prefaced his remarks by saying that he emphatically supported the program and wanted it to increase or improve its coverage, rather than to withdraw it.[23]

It is not easy to define or measure quality. In their thoughtful book, *Medicare and Hospitals,* H. M. Somers and A. R. Somers express some optimism.

> Real progress has been made . . . in the development of objective criteria that may be identified and measured. Medical science, technology, and analytical techniques have advanced to the point where particular segments of quality, specific diagnostic and therapeutic procedures, as well as physical facilities and institutional arrangements, can be and are being subjected to increasingly reliable analysis, measurement, evaluation, and control. Increasing acceptance of epidemiological concepts, progress in biostatistics, and the accumulation of data on patients, diseases, therapeutic procedures and facilities, in aggregates large enough for valid interpretations, have helped facilitate the technical development of quality indicators.[24]

Occupancy

In most hospitals an increase in occupancy rates helps to stabilize expenses per patient day, since the hospital's fixed expenses are allocated among a larger number of patients. But, for some hospitals, increased utilization may bring higher costs, especially in wage payments.

Table 10.10 reveals the occupancy rates and variations in costs for different types of hospitals. Nonfederal short-term hospitals accounted for about one-third of the beds. Expenses per day for these were nine times those of nonfederal psychiatric hospitals—$32.23 compared to $3.45. One reason for the discrepancy is the variation in personnel per hundred patients—226 compared to 35. But occupancy rates were much higher for the nonfederal psychiatric hospitals.

TABLE 10.10   Hospital Occupancy, 1960

Type of Hospital	Average Daily Census (Thousands)	Expenses Per Day	Personnel Per 100 Patients	Occupancy Rate
All United States	1,402	$16.46	114	84.6%
Nonfederal short-term general and other special	477	32.23	226	74.7%
Nonfederal psychiatric	672	3.45	35	93.1%
Nonfederal tuberculosis	39	8.92	99	75.4%
Nonfederal long-term general and other special	58	12.82	95	86.9%
All federal	254	16.34	120	87.2%

Source: "Hospital Statistics," *Hospitals,* August 1, 1961, pp. 394-95.

A key factor in occupancy rates is length of stay. In a Michigan study, 876 patients were surveyed about why they stayed in the hospital the length of time they did, rather than a longer or shorter period. The results are shown in table 10.11. More patients found no special reason for the length of their stay than any other response to the question.

The rise in hospital rates could be reduced by offsets in productivity. But hospital service is a personal relationship, which does not easily yield increased productivity—an increase of output in relation to input—without offsetting declines in quality.

Waste results from many sources. Failure to use hospitals on weekends is one. An excessive number of beds and more beds used than needed are other sources. Here a conflict emerges between the interests of society and of the hospitals. When there is an excessive number of beds using up the nation's medical resources (fixed costs run about 75 percent of all costs), the sensible procedure from society's viewpoint is to close down the hospital. But the hospital's commitments to personnel and capital investors lead it to strive for higher occupancy by encouraging more admissions and longer stays. The increased number of patients then reduces fixed costs per patient-day.

Estimating the total need for beds and the allocation by type of hospital is full of difficulties. For example, the rise in the number of beds in the last generation does not reflect the increasing importance

TABLE 10.11   Reasons for Length of Hospital Stay

Reason	Percentage of All Hospital Stays
Stayed a shorter time because:	
Had limited or no coverage	1
Hospital costs were too high	1
Was needed at home or at work	1
Stayed a longer time because:	
Could convalesce better in hospital than at home	1
Health insurance was paying bill	0
Followed doctor's orders	38
Liked the hospital; didn't like the hospital	2
Other reasons	3
No special reason for length of stay	40
Reason not ascertained	14

Source: W. J. McNerney, *Hospital and Medical Economics* (1962), vol. 1, p. 138.

of degenerative diseases. These now account for more than two-thirds of deaths; cancer, stroke, and heart disease alone account for 70 percent. Long-term hospitals suffer from inadequate resources. Short-term costs per day are nine times long-term psychiatric costs, suggesting that the long-term hospitals are underfinanced.

How many beds are needed? Prices charged, financing methods, age, sex, and distribution of the population, structure of diseases, economic conditions, impact of insurance, public attitudes toward hospitals, skills used in economizing on hospital beds are all relevant.[25]

The cost of a hospital bed depends on the capital invested in and the operating costs of the hospital, which are related to the size of the facility and the range of services it offers. Generous depreciation allowances under Medicare and Medicaid legislation tended to increase capital costs and operating expenses.

Capital Financing

The Need for Capital

The hospital industry appears to be greatly undercapitalized: according to a *Fortune* survey in 1966, there were $12,642 of assets per hospital employee, while the 500 largest industrial firms had assets of $22,921 per employee.

From 1960 to 1965, hospital assets rose by about 38 percent, but the number of beds rose by only 3 percent. In these years, the average amount of assets per bed rose by $148,100. These figures suggest problems of obsolescence and large future needs.

Over most of the years that the Hill-Burton Act was in operation, it provided only 10 percent of the total hospital construction costs and nothing for land and working capital. Large amounts of capital were lost in write-offs of bad debts without replacement from operating expenses. From 1960 to 1965, capital investment in United States hospitals increased from $17.9 billion to $24.8 billion, a gain in excess of 40 percent (see table 10.12). The years 1966 to 1975 are estimated to require a 100 percent increase in investment, if the gains from 1960 to 1965 are projected. Accounts receivable averaged 67 times the daily cash flow of hospitals.[26]

With an increase of 22 percent in employees during these years, the average amount of hospital assets per employee rose by 14 percent. If the ratio of employees to patients had remained the same, the increase in capital requirements would have been over 35 percent

TABLE 10.12   Capital Account of All United States Hospitals, 1961-65

Item	Amount (Millions)		
Capital at beginning of period			
Capital added			
Federal funds	$1,020		
State and local gov't	1,330		
Philanthropy	2,620		
Proprietary equity	26		
Hospital indebtedness	1,284		
Hospital operations	2,746		
Gross capital added		9,026	
Capital consumed (deducted)			
Unfunded depreciation	$ 641		
Asset write-off	1,507		
Total capital consumed		2,148	
Net capital added			6,878
Capital at end of period			$24,774

in these years. These statistics reflect the increasing scope and intensity of hospital service.

Increasing use of group payment from both private and public, insurance and tax, sources affects the uncertainty of medical and hospital outlays. In the last forty years, the number of hospitals has remained remarkably stable at around 7,000 despite a population rise of about 60 percent, a 90 percent growth in bed capacity, a tripling of ambulatory services to 150 million visits annually, and a fifteenfold increase of operating expenses and capital investment.

Long-term nonfederal facilities are concentrated in 300 state-operated psychiatric institutions with a total capacity of nearly 600,000 patients. They account for 14 percent of all hospitals, 42 percent of bed capacity, 2.3 percent of admissions, 15 percent of annual expenses, and about 25 percent of estimated investment in plant assets.

Community hospitals in 1967 numbered 5,850 or 82 percent of all hospitals. The average size was 135 beds. Voluntary community hospitals were 70 percent of the total, governmental 24 percent, and proprietary 6 percent. Replacement costs are estimated at $44 billion for all hospitals, or twice the current book value. Replacement value is substantially less than 200 percent for government hospitals.

In 1966-67, 59 percent of hospital operating expenses were financed with private funds, and 41 percent with public funds. Private funds financed 10 percent of research and 56 percent of medical facilities construction.

In both 1960 and 1967, hospital operating expenses were roughly one-third of national health expenditures. But whereas national health expenditures rose by about three-quarters, hospital plant assets increased by only one-half.

A tough problem is the extent to which one group of patients should finance services to another group—specifically, whether services to the needy should be part of the costs reimbursed by third-party agencies. In recent years reimbursement for welfare patients amounted to only half to three-quarters of costs.

Financing capital costs (interest, amortization, depreciation, and replacement) will help determine the adequacy of payments to hospitals. Is the objective to restore the original investment, and, if so, what about future needs? Capital cost requirements, of course, should be tied to future capital needs. Allowances accumulated on the basis of a hospital's own services seldom are adequate to finance major capital expenditures. Increased funds are required for modernization of plant and equipment to provide for additional outpatient services, extended care for the old, and services stimulated by technological advances and patient demands.

Medicare provides funds for capital costs, depreciation, interest, and replacement. Private and public health insurance programs and government purchases of services for the needy are becoming the major sources of funds for hospital capital projects. The general public provides funds through Blue Cross and Medicare, and others purchase tax-supported care from private or public institutions.

It is expected that capital financing will become more regular especially as price adjustments in insurance finance a contribution to replacements. Dr. C. R. Rorem anticipates development of more community financing of hospital care, by universities, industrial firms, labor unions, Blue Cross, commercial insurance carriers, local governments, and others. Philanthropy will be selective, in his view, concentrating on research, education, and experimentation.[27]

Dr. E. J. Connors stresses that sources of financing will be pluralistic, "but reliance on the ability of the individual hospital to accumulate its capital through unregulated charging mechanisms seems out of step with the times and no longer viable." Control of use of depreciation funds is far from settled.[28]

Depreciation

The medical field needs capital. Since gifts are declining, greater dependence must be placed on other sources. Under the Medicare legislation, the government encouraged accelerated depreciation and high capitalization of hospital facilities, so that larger amounts of capital funds became available. The Senate Finance Committee staff commented:

The liberal depreciation allowances payable under Medicare—including accelerated depreciation—may well be causing the sale and resale of proprietary facilities at inflated prices. The objective of such reductions should be to repeal the write-off of the facility and its equipment through accelerated depreciation and thereby realize inordinately high and duplicative cash payments from the government.[29]

The government later revoked some of its concessions on capital financing.

Depreciation funds seem to be inadequate. In 1960, for example, with gross national product in excess of $500 billion, medical care depreciation funds amounted to only $32 million. Medical care expenditures were around $25 billion or 5 percent of GNP. Yet medical depreciation funds were a mere 1.3 percent of total medical care expenditures. This meant that capital was being used and not being replaced by new funds. The damage was especially serious because replacement values are much higher than previous costs. One estimate puts the replacement value at 160 percent of historical costs.

Failure to build up depreciation funds, especially when other sources of capital—loans, grants, etc.—are drying up, may be extremely costly. The government may indeed help. Dr. John Knowles of Massachusetts General Hospital has stressed the danger of inadequate depreciation. From 1940 to 1964, that hospital had a deficit every year save two. In 1956 the hospital began earning and funding depreciation funds. Without adequate depreciation, Knowles warned, plant and equipment would crumble. By 1964, earned depreciation had risen to $1,218,000.[30]

There is disagreement on the depreciation issue, however. In the depression years, with most hospitals experiencing deficits, it seemed unwise to set aside depreciation funds that would merely increase deficits. In later years, support for these funds grew, as failure to provide funding for depreciation resulted in use of depreciation to finance current operations. Part of the support for a no-depreciation policy rested on the argument that gifts and taxes had previously provided the capital. If capital was needed again later, recourse to loans and gifts could be had. A United Hospital Fund statement in 1963 expressed this view:

> This decline in value (depreciation) is a current expense and is continuous throughout the useful life of the property. But as applied to hospital buildings it is an expense which has to be paid only once in—say a generation. Inasmuch as most hospitals are, in reality, nonprofit organizations finding it difficult and often impossible to obtain sufficient current income to cover current expense, and therefore ending the fiscal year with a deficit, *it is not desirable nor necessary to increase the deficit* by appropriating any part of the current income as provision for replacement of buildings when they shall have worn out or become obsolescent. As past and present generations have provided existing hospital buildings, it is both fair and financially sound to let following generations make similar provision. It is difficult enough for hospitals to provide for current needs without being further handicapped by providing for future needs.[31]

One authority, E. Barbartelli, strongly supports depreciation "as a period allocation of the cost of an asset spread ratably over the expected useful life of the asset." He gives estimates of the average composite rates on buildings at 2.0 percent using an index of 100 for historical annual depreciation and 194 for cost of reproduction.[32] R. M. Sigmond estimates that nonprofit hospitals provide 35 percent to 40 percent of their capital funds out of their own resources including depreciation.

Construction

Sources of Funds

Hospital construction expenditures nearly doubled between 1969 and 1970. This has occurred because of new changes in the way hospital construction is financed. Money comes from three sources: philanthropy, government grants, and sources internal to the hospital, such as borrowing or the use of cash reserves.

In the early 1900s, nearly all hospitals were built as well as operated by philanthropic organizations, but this phenomenon has changed in the last thirty years. While the amount of philanthropic funds for hospital construction has gone up, relative to other sources, it is a declining proportion of the total funding. Philanthropic support varies according to the type of hospital and where it is situated.

Contributions supply as much as 57 percent of voluntary hospital capital construction funds in the Northeast, and as little as 6 percent in the Mountain and Pacific states.

In 1957, hospitals and other health care institutions received 14 percent of the philanthropic dollar; in 1967 it was 18 percent. Philanthropy provides most of the seed money and a considerable part of construction funds for hospitals. Seed money is important because it enables hospitals to qualify for governmental grants and long-term loans. In 1957, philanthropy provided $202 million for hospital construction; in 1967, $969 million. In 1967, of a total of $14,569 million in philanthropic funds for all uses, hospitals and other health care institutions obtained $2,610 million or 17.9 percent and education 17.4 percent. Religion with $6,839 million or 46.9 percent was first.[33]

Direct government financing of capital construction reached a peak shortly after World War II, when it provided nearly two-thirds of all hospital construction funds—most of which went into Veterans' Administration hospitals. By 1970, governmental sources provided only 17 percent of voluntary hospital construction money and 56 percent of construction funds for public (nonfederal) hospitals.

The Hill-Burton program has been the primary source of federal grants for voluntary hospital construction. However, Hill-Burton money provided only 13 percent of the cost of voluntary hospital construction from 1946, when the legislation was enacted, until 1967. In the past, the Hill-Burton program has strongly favored rural and suburban areas. All federal grants together total only 16 percent of all (public and voluntary) hospital construction funds. State and local (county) governments contribute another 7 percent, most of which goes to public hospitals.

Most recently hospitals have been financing themselves—through loans and their own reserves. The growth of Blue Cross, Medicare, and Medicaid have helped to stabilize hospital income and thus enabled this financing. Not only have insurers made hospitals financially viable, but most also include specific allowances for construction costs in their payments to hospitals. These take the form of depreciation on hospital plant and equipment and interest cost on loans acquired to finance hospital construction.

But the single largest source of construction financing is borrowing. It provides 41 percent of the construction funds for voluntary hospitals, 25 percent for public hospitals, and 64 percent for proprietary hospitals.

Contribution of the Hill-Burton Program

Objectives of the Hill-Burton program for increasing the number of hospital beds are stated succinctly in a report by the Assistant Surgeon General:

Over the past 19 years, the Congress has appropriated from $65 million to $220 million annually for distribution among the States and Territories on the basis of population and relative per capita income. Not only have additional hospital beds and health centers been provided as a result of the Hill-Burton program, but there also has occurred: (1) systematic statewide planning for hospital facilities; (2) development of standards of need; (3) development of standards for evaluating the condition of the physical plant; (4) achievement of better distribution of facilities; (5) improvement of hospital design; (6) improvement in hospital operation; (7) effective cooperation between government and voluntary health agencies; (8) improvement of medical care in low income States and in rural areas; and (9) aid to teaching centers for training physicians and nurses.[34]

Despite federal hospital expenditures of $7½ billion from 1947 to 1965, and outlays in excess of $3 billion by 1969, serious shortages still persist. Too much was spent on small communities, while largely obsolete facilities in big cities were not corrected adequately. Communities with populations of less than 50,000 obtained 64 percent of the beds. Other criticisms of the program were its inadequate planning and integration, its high costs in construction of too many small hospitals, and its neglect of beds for long-term care. While 34 percent of all beds in the country were for long-term care, only 16 percent of the beds furnished under the Hill-Burton program were for long-term units. By 1969, the program had approved 442,965 beds, with general hospitals accounting for four-fifths and long-term care facilities only about one-fifth. The expenditures for short-term beds were seven to eight times those for long-term (see figure 10.13).

Favoring the smaller communities raised further problems. An excessive number of small hospitals were built with high unit costs: 12 percent of the new beds were in hospitals with fewer than fifty beds, and 28 percent were in institutions with fewer than one hundred beds. Meanwhile there was an increasing backlog of hospitals in large communities needing additions, renovations, and replacements.

FIGURE 10.13   Types of Facilities Financed under the Hill-Burton Program, 1965

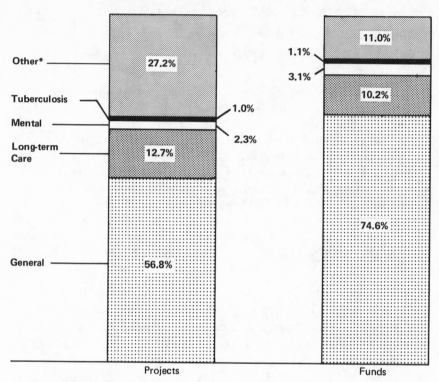

Source: HEW, *Hill-Burton Program Progress Report, July 1, 1947-June 30, 1965,* p. 17, chart 1.

*Includes diagnostic and treatment centers, rehabilitation facilities, public health centers, and state health laboratories.

Large hospitals provide more extensive services, but they also contribute to high costs. Such independent variables as per capita income of the population, population density of the community, and availability of medical personnel determine costs. A strong case is to be made for large hospitals even though unit costs tend to be high. Emergency needs and convenience justify some small hospitals, but large hospitals can offer many more services (see table 10.14).

The Michigan survey found that many respondents were satisfied

TABLE 10.14   Services Available in Michigan Hospitals by Size, 1958

Services Available	Hospital Size	
	Under 50 Beds	50 Beds and Over
Blood bank	37%	100%
Radioactive isotopes	0%	100%
X-ray therapeutic care	12%	100%
Postoperative recovery room	11%	88%
Number of hospitals having all services	0	13

Source: W. J. McNerney, *Hospital and Medical Economics* (1962), vol. 2, p. 788.

with the current situation, perhaps excessively so (see table 10.15). Nearly half the short-term hospitals have fewer than 100 beds. The general view is that this is a high-cost situation. Some indication of the coverage of services and their absolute and relative rises in cost is given by tables 10.16-10.17.

To put the Hill-Burton program in perspective, it furnished roughly 20 percent of the total bed capacity of recent years. Federal facility beds constituted 10 percent of the recent totals. Although the programs favored general short-term hospitals, an allowance should be made for the reduced need for long-term facilities as a result of improved treatments and shorter stays. Nevertheless, in 1969 the shortages were estimated at 164,000 long-term and 85,000 short-term beds.[35]

In a recent year, private hospitals and institutions spent $1,372

TABLE 10.15   Satisfaction with Status of Michigan Hospitals

Aspect of Operation	Percentage of Respondent Hospitals Satisfied with Aspect
Size of hospital	47
Existing wage scale	82
Amount of equipment	84
Quality of plant	86
Number of personnel	87
Quality of equipment	95
Caliber of personnel	99

Source: W. J. McNerney, *Hospital and Medical Economics* (1962), vol. 2, p. 1225.

TABLE 10.16   Services Available in Nonfederal Hospitals, 1948-58

Service Available	1948		1958		Increase in Percentage from 1948 to 1958
	Number of Hospitals	Percentage of Hospitals	Number of Hospitals	Percentage of Hospitals	
All hospitals reporting	4499	100.0	5086	100.0	—
Basal metabolism	3551	78.9	4606	90.6	11.7
Blood bank	1374	30.5	2781	54.7	24.2
Clinical laboratory	3661	81.4	4860	95.6	14.2
Dental	811	18.0	1171	23.0	5.0
Electrocardiograph	3039	67.5	4755	93.5	26.0
Electroencephalograph	375	8.3	668	13.1	4.8
Medical records	3100	68.9	4577	90.0	21.1
Medical staff library	2150	47.8	3538	69.6	21.8
Occupational therapy	367	8.2	487	9.6	1.4
Outpatient department	2136	47.4	2842	55.9	8.5
Pharmacy	1859	41.3	2124	41.8	—
Physical therapy	1523	33.8	1966	38.7	4.9
Social service	656	14.6	821	16.3	1.7
X-ray, diagnostic	4002	89.0	4877	95.9	6.9
X-ray, routine chest	354	7.9	1898	37.3	29.4
X-ray, therapeutic	1631	36.2	1881	37.0	0.8

Source: W. J. McNerney, *Hospital and Medical Economics* (1962), vol. 2, p. 767; adapted from J. R. Griffith, "Hospital Care Is Still a Bargain," *Hospitals,* November 16, 1960, p. 55.

million for new construction—six to seven times the Hill-Burton expenditures per year. Public hospitals spent $634 million, or three times the Hill-Burton spending. The comparison of these expenditures corrected for price rises by using 1957-59 prices is given in table 10.18. Private new construction has made relatively larger gains since 1950. The inflationary component is substantial in the new construction figures, as a comparison with table 10.19 shows. From 1929 to 1950, public spending for medical facilities increased by four times, while private spending rose by only a little more than one time. But from 1950 to 1969 the respective increases were roughly four-fifths and more than six times. The greater recent rises for private expenditures are related to federal legislation.

By 1969, $3,408 million had been made available under Hill-Burton auspices. General hospitals accounted for $2,449 million and long-term facilities $455 million. The 1971 totals of Hill-Burton spending are shown in table 10.20.

From 1960 to 1971, the rise in privately funded construction costs

TABLE 10.17   Common and Less Common Services in Short-term Hospitals

Type of Service	Percentage of Hospitals
Commonly found	
Clinical laboratory	96.5
Delivery room	91.0
Electrocardiography	94.5
Emergency room	91.0
Medical library	84.0
Medical records	96.5
Operating room, major	96.5
Pharmacy	73.5
X-ray, diagnostic	98.0
Less commonly found	
Blood bank	66.7
Dental department	18.0
Occupational therapy	9.5
Physical therapy	41.0
Postoperative recovery room	45.0
Premature nursery	57.0
Radioactive isotopes	21.0
Social service	15.0
X-ray therapy	44.5
Educational programs	
Intern training	20.7
Residency training	23.7
School of nursing	7.5

Source: W. J. McNerney, *Hospital and Medical Economics* (1962), vol. 2, p. 787.

was especially large: from $500 million to $2,500 million (or a 400 percent increase). Federal costs and state and local costs rose from $300 million to $500 million (a 67 percent increase).

Alternative Facilities

Extended Care Facilities and Nursing Homes

Nursing homes have become a booming industry, partly because of the impact of Medicare and Medicaid. Before Medicare, extended care facilities were virtually unknown. In 1967, Medicare introduced coverage of inpatient services in participating extended care facilities. The program paid reasonable costs for all covered inpatient services received during the first twenty days, if the patient was admitted within fourteen days after a hospital stay of three or more days. After the twenty days, Medicare paid for up to eighty additional days if the patient paid coinsurance of $5 a day.

TABLE 10.18   New Construction by Private and Public Hospitals, 1950-67

Type of Ownership	Construction Expenditures (Millions of 1957-59 Dollars)		
	1950	1965	1967
Private hospitals and institutions	$470	$1,142	$1,032
Public hospitals	682	434	477

At least 3.6 million people were hospitalized at least once in 1967 and 354,000 or 9.8 percent used extended care facility services at least once. Among whites, the percentage of hospitalized persons who went to extended care facilities was 9.9 percent; for other races, it was 4.8 percent. Women used more extended care benefits than men: of 2.6 million women hospitalized in 1967, 11.6 percent were reimbursed for extended care facility services; only 7.7 percent of the men used this benefit. At ages sixty-five and sixty-six, 3.4 percent of hospitalized persons used reimbursed extended care services; at age eighty-five and over, it was 22.2 percent.[36]

The expansion of nursing homes from 1960 to 1969 is suggested by table 10.21 and figures 10.22-10.24. Expenditures for care in current dollars rose by 432 percent; the number of beds rose by 90 percent—from 500,000 to 950,000.[37] From 1966 to early 1970, the number of nursing homes increased from 12,000 to 24,000. By 1969, nursing home revenue had soared to $2.5 billion.

With such rapid growth and with a shortage of needed personnel and facilities, abuses were bound to escalate. Most of the employees did not have the needed training. It was not easy to provide adequate services for the million or more old people in nursing homes. Once

TABLE 10.19   Medical Facilities Construction, 1929-69

Year	Amount (Millions)	
	Public	Private
1928-29	$105	$ 102
1949-50	522	215
1959-60	578	524
1968-69	940	1,535

Sources: Compiled from *United States Statistical Abstract, 1968,* and "Social Welfare Expenditures," *Social Security Bulletin,* December 1969, pp. 6, 12.

TABLE 10.20   Facilities Funded under the Hill-Burton Program, 1947-71

Type of Facility	Total Grants Amount (Millions)	Percentage
Total	$3,718	100
General hospitals	2,635	71
Long-term care	523	14
Outpatient	204	6
Other	356	9

Source: *Study of Health Facilities Construction Costs by the Comptroller General of the United States* (December 1972), pp. 14-15, 121.

the government included nursing homes under Medicare and Medicaid, these facilities proliferated. Chain operations estimated revenues of $1,000 per bed. The charge was made that one physician submitted bills for patients who had been dead for a year, and gang visits by doctors to twenty patients in twenty minutes were not unknown. Prices rose and standards deteriorated. Average charges were estimated at $30 per day ($10,000 to $12,000 a year) with one chain estimating daily rates from $15 to $35. Conflicts spread between the Department of Health, Education, and Welfare, which was responsible for administration, and the operators and their clients. Facilities were accused of having food budgets of only one dollar per day per patient and nursing far below acceptable standards.[38]

Under the law, if one bed was occupied by a Medicare recipient, it was possible to impose responsibility for payment for all empty beds upon Medicare, not just responsibility for the proportion of beds occupied by Medicare.[39]

TABLE 10.21   Growth of Nursing Home Expenditures and Facilities, 1960-69

Expenditure or Factor	Number or Amount 1960	1969
Establishments	16,400	20,500
Beds	500,000	950,000
Employees	227,000	480,000
Expenditures for care		
1960 dollars (millions)	$526	$2,200
Current dollars (millions)	$526	$2,800

Cost of extended care facilities by 1967 had risen to ten times the 1965 estimates (see table 10.25). The Senate Finance Committee staff claimed that the promised utilization reviews were virtually nonexistent, that chain operations with rising capital costs were growing, and that provision of unnecessary services was increasing.[40] Extended care facilities responded inadequately to the rising demand (see table 10.26). About two-thirds had not attained the required standards, and in two years the number in substantial compliance

FIGURE 10.22   Gains in Nursing Home Establishments, Beds, Employment, and Expenditures for Care, 1960-69

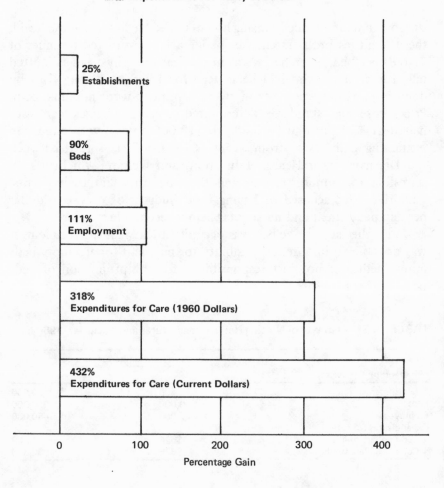

25%
Establishments

90%
Beds

111%
Employment

318%
Expenditures for Care (1960 Dollars)

432%
Expenditures for Care (Current Dollars)

0   100   200   300   400

Percentage Gain

FIGURE 10.23   Types of Employees in Nursing Homes, 1968

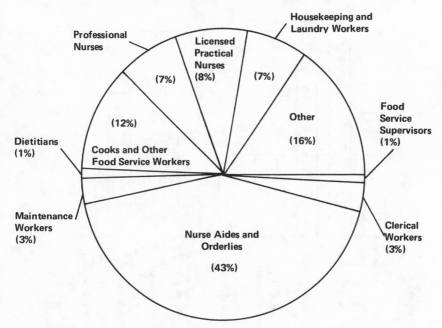

Note: Percentages do not add to 100 due to rounding.

rose by only 200. The Senate Finance Committee recommended that facilities with deficiencies—other than insignificant and minor ones—not be certified.

The fact that the majority of extended care facilities are proprietary explains in part the complaints about prices and quality. The average monthly charge in May-June 1964 was $205 for proprietary homes but only $154 and $157 for homes with other types of ownership.[41]

Medicare legislation offering care up to 100 days following acute illness bestowed virtually a guarantee for the construction of extended care facilities. A study of New York City from October 1, 1964, to June 30, 1967, showed that proprietary hospital construction projects were providing more than two-thirds of the net expansion but less than 40 percent of the total cost. Planned costs were $141 million, of which voluntary hospitals contributed $85 million and

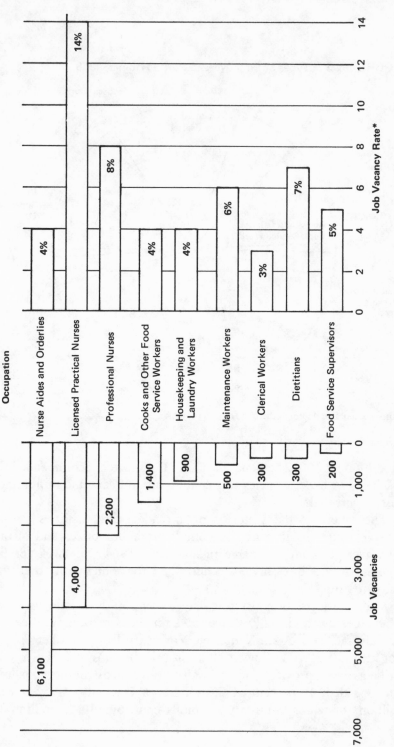

FIGURE 10.24   Job Vacancies in Nursing Homes, 1968

*Job vacancy rate is the ratio of vacancies to all positions (filled and vacant).

TABLE 10.25   Rise in Extended Care Facilities Costs, 1965-67

	1965 Estimate	1967 Actual Figures
Daily cost	$11	$18
Days per beneficiary	0.16	1
Cost per beneficiary per year	$1.80	$18

proprietary hospitals $56 million. In all, seventeen voluntary hospital projects incurred costs of $22,670 per bed. For proprietary projects the cost per bed was $9,706. Again, costs for projects adding 200 or more beds ($23,549) were 1.3 times the mean costs for smaller projects ($18,231).[42]

Some details on the residents of different types of extended care facilities are given in table 10.27.

Aside from exorbitant prices and low standards, the market suffered from maldistribution among geographic areas. Thus, for the country as a whole in 1967, there were 15.2 skilled nursing facility beds per thousand enrollees, but the extremes were a low of 3.7 in Mississippi and a high of 40.7 in Connecticut. For the East South Central states the figure was 9.5; for the Pacific states, 30.5.

One expected relationship is a direct correlation of costs per resident and size of the extended care facility. In California, in 1966, operating costs of nursing homes with fewer than eleven beds were $9.03 per patient; for those with sixty-six to ninety beds, the cost was $11.11 per patient, and for those with one hundred or more beds, it was $10.74.[43]

TABLE 10.26   Compliance of Extended Care Facilities with Federal Standards, 1967-69

Degree of Compliance	July 1967	July 1968	July 1969
In full compliance with the standards	740	1,350	1,374
In "substantial compliance" with the standards	3,210	3,340	3,402
Certified despite failure to obtain qualified charge-nurses for each tour of duty	210	10	—
Total certified	4,160	4,700	4,776

Source: U.S. Senate, Committee on Finance, *Staff Report: Medicare and Medicaid, Problems, Issues and Alternatives* (February 1970), p. 95.

TABLE 10.27   Characteristics of Extended Care Facility Residents, by Ownership of Facility, 1964

Type of Ownership	Percentage of All Residents	Number of Females per 100 Males	Median Age of Residents	Percentage of Residents in Nursing Homes	Average Monthly Charge
All types	100	186	80	68	$186
Proprietary	60	195	80	78	205
Nonprofit	24	280	81	40	154
Other	16	91	76	70	157

Source: HEW, Office of Vital and Health Statistics, *Charges for Care in Institutions for the Aged and Chronically Ill, United States, May-June, 1964,* table D, p. 6.

But the structure of spending varies according to the size of the
nursing home. Thus, administration cost per patient-day rises from
$.66 to $1.30 as the size increases; property costs and related expenses rise from $1.57 to $2.01; and (for California) food costs drop
from $1.57 to $.83.[44]

Home Nursing Services

An important objective in recent years has been to increase home
care facilities and personnel. As of January 1, 1966, there were 124
million people, or almost 70 percent of the total population (179
million) living in areas with some type of organized service providing
necessary care for the sick at home. The largest proportion of the
population, 40.7 percent, live in cities of 25,000 and over that have
home nursing services. Over 60 percent of the population without
these services (55 million total) live in rural areas.[45] Of the communities with populations of 25,000 and over, 82 percent had home
nursing services; of those with populations ranging from 2,500 to
25,000, 52 percent had the services; and only 29.5 percent of communities under 2,500 in size had them. The variations by states are
large (see figure 10.28).[46]

From 1959 to 1966 the number of large cities with services almost
doubled. By 1966, services were available to 15 percent more people
than in 1963. One nurse per 2,500 people had been considered necessary to provide high quality public health nursing services, including
care of the sick. No agency approaches this. The average reported was
only one nurse per 9,452 population.[47]

Possibilities for Improvement

A primary objective of the economics of medical care is to save on expensive hospital beds. Dr. Cherkasky of New York City estimates daily home care costs at $10 and daily hospital care costs at $100. The savings are less than $90, however, because home nursing and other services that might cost $70 are performed by the patient's family. Recourse to group practice yields cost reductions of 20 percent or more and savings in utilization. As the number of staff members per patient almost doubled from 1940 to 1966, rising costs appeared to be associated with increased use of labor.

Government hospitals, relatively few in number, provide more patient-days than voluntary and private hospitals, and their costs per patient-day are considerably lower. They generally provide only custodial care, in part because cures are unavailable. But general short-term hospitals have assumed increasing responsibility for mental patients.

Despite recent legislation supporting planning and integration of health facilities, hospitals tend to be built, expand, and operate with little regard for the community's overall needs. Dr. Sigmond has well put the case for planning and integration. He would even pool depreciation funds as a mechanism for adapting resources to needs. He claims that as conditions change, some hospitals would then shut down, and depreciation funds would be diverted to others that merit stronger support in the particular situation.

Often there are local pressures to create numerous and duplicative facilities. In recent years, for example, despite persistent advice from relevant government agencies, military powers pressed for two new hospitals in the San Francisco area, although all the experts supported a single large hospital. The two hospitals would bring capital losses of around $10 million, cost $8 million extra annually, and face large shortages of medical personnel.[48]

The operating costs of many hospitals equal their initial construction costs every one to three years. In 1970, these operating costs (federal and nonfederal) amounted to over $25 billion or about 38 percent of total health care expenditures.[49] Construction costs could be cut by reducing demand for health facilities or by increasing productivity through various means: programs for the prevention or early detection of illnesses and injuries; treatment of patients in the most appropriate,

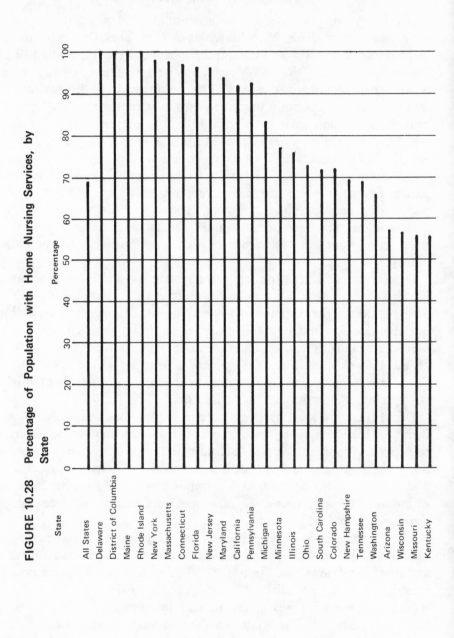

FIGURE 10.28 Percentage of Population with Home Nursing Services, by State

Oregon
Virginia
Hawaii
Iowa
Arkansas
Indiana
Idaho
North Carolina
Alabama
Vermont
Oklahoma
Utah
Georgia
Texas
New Mexico
Nevada
Kansas
West Virginia
Louisiana
Nebraska
Wyoming
Montana
North Dakota
Alaska
Mississippi
South Dakota
Guam
Puerto Rico
Virgin Islands

Source: HEW, *Services Available for Nursing Care of the Sick at Home* (1966).

least costly facilities; alternative medical care delivery systems that reduce the use of hospitals; utilization review programs to cut down hospital admissions and lengths of stays; revised insurance benefit structures to avoid favoring hospital use; sharing of hospital services to reduce underused duplicative facilities; and establishment of regional hospital systems to use existing facilities more efficiently.[50]

Many experts hold that hospitals cannot be expected to cut down or cut off their revenues by voluntarily keeping people out of their beds—whether this is done by serving them as outpatients or referring them to nursing homes or caring for them at their own homes. As one expert, W. J. Rome, noted, "the spontaneous, voluntary efforts of many hospitals in recent years to join in such movements as accreditation, area-wide planning, medical audits, utilization reviews, uniform accounting and pricing policies, and joint ventures and shared services of all kinds" suggest the possibilities for cooperative hospital policies.[51]

A consensus of health care authorities has estimated that 25 percent of patients are treated in facilities excessive to their needs. "This is due to the health care system being oriented towards treating the acute phase of illness rather than offering a complete spectrum of health care by providing available alternatives to acute care, financing the alternatives, and educating physicians and patients in the acceptance of alternatives." A 1968 cost-effectiveness analysis by the Department of Health, Education, and Welfare projected that better matching of hospital patient needs to facilities' services could transfer 81.7 million days of care from short-term general hospitals to alternative health facilities, and save $3 billion in 1970 health system operating costs.

Per bed construction costs for general acute-illness hospitals range from $14,000 to $72,000; for nursing home beds, the figure is $25,000. In 1970, the average expense per patient day was $81 in an acute general hospital but only $24 in an extended care facility.

In 1970, according to a report from the Department of Health, Education, and Welfare, about 20,000 beds could have been saved through effective home care programs, and about 17 percent of days used in acute short-term general hospitals were for cases that could have been handled in long-term care facilities. This would have reduced the need for acute care beds by about 126,000.

In summary, health care programs should be concerned about the quality, availability, accessibility, adequacy, effectiveness, and economic use of the health care services. Many people are not being cared for in appropriate types of facilities because of undue emphasis on acute inpatient care, inadequate alternative facilities, services and reimbursement mechanisms, and physician and patient reluctance to make use of available alternatives.[52]

Medical care costs are considerable greater than they would be if "various types of health facilities were appropriately used."[53]

The General Accounting Office expressed the view that, unless the medical profession and individuals give more attention to preventing illnesses and injuries, the present health care delivery system may become overburdened and not be able to meet future health care demands.[54]

Sharing services among hospitals could free existing facilities to meet other needs for space without requiring new construction. One of the obstacles, however, is that physicians are reluctant to share their hospital staff privileges. Authorities consider regional hospital systems to be an effective way of organizing and utilizing scarce medical skills and facilities and of curbing rising costs. But communities, hospital officials, and physicians resist the development of these systems because they want complete autonomy.[55]

Functional planning consists of assessing the unmet health care needs of the population, the health care services that will satisfy these needs, the types and sizes of the facilities to house the services, and the number and types of personnel to staff the facilities.[56]

Notes

1. J. H. Knowles, ed., *The Teaching Hospital* (1966), p. 113.

2. See E. Ginzberg, *A Pattern for Hospital Care*, pp. 132-41.

3. W. J. McNerney, *Hospital and Medical Economics* (1962), vol. 2, p. iii.

4. American Hospital Association, *Financial Requirements of Health Care Institutions* (1968).

5. H. E. Klarman, "Medical Economics," *Inquiry*, March 1970, pp. 28, 30.

6. HEW, *Medical Care Financing and Utilization*, Health Economics Series no. 1, pp. 35, 129; H. E. Klarman, "Medical Economics," *Inquiry*, March 1970, p. 28; HEW, "State Data and State Rankings," part 2 of *1966-67 HEW Trends*, pp. 5-15.

7. M. V. Pauly, "Efficiency, Incentives and Reimbursement for Health Care," *Inquiry*, March 1970, pp. 124-28.

8. W. J. McNerney, *Hospital and Medical Economics* (1962), vol. 2, pp. 849-55.

9. R. J. Myers, *Hospital Utilization and Average Daily Hospital Costs*, American Hospital Association Actuarial Note no. 61 (September 1969), table 2.

10. U.S. Senate, Committee on Finance, *Hearings on Medicare and Medicaid* (1970), vol. 1, p. 159.

11. HEW, *Indicators*, January 1967, table 9.

12. W. J. McNerney, *Hospital and Medical Economics* (1962), vol. 2, p. 775.

13. J. H. Knowles, ed., *The Teaching Hospital* (1966), pp. 111-12.

14. Committee on Financing Hospital Care, *Financing Hospital Care in the United States* (1955), vol. 1, p. 235.

15. W. J. McNerney, *Hospital and Medical Economics* (1962), vol. 2, pp. 924-25.

16. U.S. Senate, Committee on Finance, *Staff Report: Medicare and Medicaid, Problems, Issues and Alternatives* (February 1970), pp. 71-79.

17. Committee on Financing Hospital Care, *Financing Hospital Care in the United States* (1955), vol. 3, pp. xv-xviii, chaps. 3-5.

18. P. A. Feldstein and S. Waldman, "Financial Position of Hospitals in Early Medicare Period," *Social Security Bulletin*, October 1968, pp. 18-23.

19. U.S. Senate, Committee on Finance, *Staff Report: Medicare and Medicaid, Problems, Issues and Alternatives* (February 1970), p. 51.

20. Ibid., p. 67.

21. For material in this section see especially ibid.; U.S. Senate, Committee on Finance, *Hearings on Medicare and Medicaid* (1970), vol. 1, pp. 3-9, 125, 138-43; *Medical Care in America*, vol. 1, pp. 17, 82, 170, vol. 2, pp. 658-59; U.S. Senate, Special Committee on Aging, *Hearings* (1968), pp. 311-13; Senate Report no. 91-375 (1970).

22. U.S. Senate, Committee on Finance, *Staff Report: Medicare and Medicaid, Problems, Issues and Alternatives* (February 1970), p. 57.

23. *Hearings on Health Care in America* (April 1968), vol. 1, pp. 70-71.

24. H. M. Somers and A. R. Somers, *Medicare and the Hospitals* (1967), p. 76.

25. See Cronin, Reed, and Baney, "Hospital Beds in the United States, 1950," *Public Health Report*, November 10, 1950.

26. I have found most helpful a symposium printed in *Hospitals*, the October 16, 1968, issue, with articles contributed by R. E. Brown, C. R. Rorem, E. J. Connors, J. M. Stagl, R. Williamson, and R. A. Dobbins; and American Hospital Association, *Statement on the Financial Requirements of Health Care Institutions and Services* (1969).

27. C. R. Rorem, "Changing Needs Are Dictating New Capital Approaches," *Hospitals*, October 16, 1968, pp. 48-54.

28. E. J. Connors, "Adequate Financing Demands Astute Planning," *Hospitals*, October 16, 1968, pp. 57-62.

Hospitals 307

29. U.S. Senate, Committee on Finance, *Staff Report: Medicare and Medicaid, Problems, Issues and Alternatives* (February 1970), p. 8.

30. J. H. Knowles, *The Teaching Hospital* (1966), pp. 108-10.

31. Quoted in W. J. McNerney, *Hospital and Medical Economics* (1962), vol. 2, pp. 935-36.

32. E. Barbartelli, "Using Depreciation to Provide for Future Hospital Financial Needs," *Hospitals*, July 16, 1967, pp. 46-49.

33. R. A. Dobbin, "Philanthropy Attracts Other Capital Sources," *Hospitals*, October 16, 1968, pp. 71-72, 76.

34. HEW, *Hill-Burton Program Progress Report, July 1, 1947-June 30, 1965*, p. iii.

35. S. Sweeney, "Health Programs and the Nixon Administration," *Hospitals*, May 1, 1969, p. 24g.

36. HEW, Office of Research and Statistics, *Utilization of Extended Care Facilities, 1967* (April 1, 1971).

37. U.S. Department of Labor, *Nursing Home and Related Health Care Facilities* (1969), p. 3; also see National Center for Health Statistics, *Charges for Care in Institutions for the Aged and Chronically Ill, United States, May-June, 1969; Health Manpower Act of 1968*, Senate Report no. 1307.

38. See especially *New York Times*, February 16, 1970.

39. U.S. Senate, Committee on Finance, *Staff Report: Medicare and Medicaid, Problems, Issues and Alternatives* (February 1970), p. 52.

40. U.S. Senate, Committee on Finance, *Hearings on Medicare and Medicaid* (July 1968), pp. 23-37.

41. HEW, *Nursing Home Utilization and Costs in Selected States*, Health Economics Series no. 8, p. 6.

42. C. Muller, E. Gerber, and P. Worthington, "Planned Capital Formation Nursing Homes in New York City," *Inquiry*, December 1969, pp. 12-25.

43. HEW, *Nursing Home Utilization and Costs in Selected States*, Health Economics Series no. 8, p. 19.

44. Ibid.; also see pp. 3-9, 17-18.

45. HEW, *Services Available for Nursing Care of the Sick at Home* (1966), pp. 3-5.

46. Ibid., pp. 8-9.

47. Ibid., p. 27.

48. W. J. McNerney, *Hospital and Medical Economics* (1962), vol. 2, pp. 762-69, 847, 853; U.S. Senate, Committee on Government Operations, *The Federal Role in Health*, Federal Report no. 91-809 (1970), pp. 25-30, 166-69, 202-3.

49. *Study of Health Facilities Construction Costs by the Comptroller General of the United States* (December 1972), pp. 12-13.

50. Ibid., pp. 93-94.

51. W. J. Rome, "What Is Management Effectiveness in a Small Hospital?" *Hospitals*, June 1969, pp. 57-59, 111.

52. *Study of Health Facilities Construction Costs by the Comptroller General of the United States* (December 1972), p. 98.

53. Ibid., pp. 98-101.

54. Ibid., p. 3.

55. Ibid., pp. 4-5.

56. Ibid., p. 175.

11

Utilization and
Quality Control

Utilization

Overutilization of health services is one of the most troublesome aspects of American medicine. In a market where demand is insistent and rising while supply remains unresponsive, overutilization brings inflation and serious bottlenecks.

Utilization of short-term voluntary hospitals generally rises with age and varies with sex (see table 11.1). Length of stay is longer for patients whose stays end at death than for those discharged alive. Sexual variations in the percentage discharged alive are not large. But the discharge rate per 1,000 population is 264 for those sixty-five and over and 141 for those under sixty-five. These figures reflect the greater utilization by the older group.

The percentage discharged alive is naturally much greater for the group under sixty-five than for those sixty-five and over. Average length of stay is almost twice as great for the older group. Daily hospital bed usage rate per 100,000 population is more than three times as much for the older group. Hence there is rising utilization with advancing age.

Nonobstetric discharge rates per 1,000 population are given by

TABLE 11.1   Hospital Utilization by Patients Over and Under Sixty-five, by Sex, 1965

	65 and Over			Under 65		
Utilization Measures	Total	Male	Female	Total	Male	Female
Number of discharges (thousands)	4,601	2,114	2,474	24,377	9,188	15,152
Percentage discharged alive	89.5%	88.3%	90.5%	98.5%	97.9%	98.9%
Discharge rate per 1,000 population	263.9	276.3	252.9	141.4	108.9	172.2
Days of care (thousands)	60,035	26,070	33,752	167,343	68,999	98,088
Average length of stay (days)	13.0	12.3	13.6	6.9	7.5	6.5
Daily hospital bed usage rate per 100,000 population	943.4	933.4	945.2	266.0	224.1	305.3

Source: HEW, National Center for Health Statistics, *Utilization of Short-Stay Hospitals by Characteristics of Discharged Patients, U.S. 1965*, p. 3.

Note: Totals include patients for whom sex was not stated.

age and sex in table 11.2 (newborn infants are excluded). Especially striking are the differences by age. The combined discharge rate for the middle-aged and the elderly groups was double that for persons under forty-five years of age (202 per 1,000 to 94 per 1,000). Discharge rates were much greater for females than for males; but if adjustments are made for pregnancies and related conditions the differences are largely eliminated.

Hospital discharges per 1,000 population in 1965 also varied by region from 138 per 1,000 in the Northeast to 159 in the South. The Northeast accounted for 11 percent fewer short-stay discharges than the rest of the country. But, owing to a longer stay per discharge,

TABLE 11.2   Nonobstetric Discharge Rates by Age and Sex, 1965

	Discharge Rate per 1,000 Population		
Age	Total	Male	Female
Total	126.5	121.3	130.8
Under 15	71.3	79.1	63.0
15-44	112.7	97.7	125.9
45-64	174.0	169.2	177.9
65 and over	263.9	276.3	252.8

Source: HEW, National Center for Health Statistics, *Utilization of Short-Stay Hospitals by Characteristics of Discharged Patients, U.S. 1965.*

the rate of total inpatient days in the Northeast was 7 percent above that in short-stay hospitals in other regions. The South and North Central states showed the largest relative discharges and utilization.

Hospital utilization is related to the type of disease. The government has classified diseases into eighteen diagnostic categories. Discharges from short-stay hospitals in 1965 were highly clustered among certain categories (see table 11.3). Diseases of the digestive and respiratory systems together accounted for 32 percent of the nonobstetric discharges. Five categories accounted for 65 percent of the discharges—the above two classes, plus injuries, diseases of the

TABLE 11.3   Discharges from Short-Stay Hospitals by Disease Category, 1965

Condition and ICDA Codes	Number of Discharges (Thousands)	Percentage of All Discharges	Discharge Rate per 10,000 Population	Average Length of Stay (Days)
Malignant neoplasms (140-205)	1,002	3.5	53	14.8
Diabetes mellitus (260)	342	1.2	18	12.4
Psychoneurotic disorders (324)	292	1.0	15	10.9
Vascular lesions, CNS (330-334)	370	1.3	19	16.5
Arteriosclerotic heart disease (420)	845	2.9	45	13.6
Respiratory diseases				
Acute upper respiratory infections (470-475)	502	1.7	26	4.9
Pneumonia, all forms (490-493)	875	3.0	46	9.0
Hypertrophy of tonsils and adenoids (510)	1,193	4.1	63	1.9
Digestive diseases				
Ulcer of stomach and duodenum (540-542)	478	1.7	25	9.6
Appendicitis (550-552)	358	1.2	19	6.4
Inguinal hernia (560-561)	496	1.7	26	7.2
Gastroenteritis (571)	543	1.9	29	5.0
Cholelithiasis and cholecystitis (584-585)	500	1.7	26	11.4
Disorders of menstruation (634)	372	1.3	20	4.0
Obstetrical conditions (640-689, Y06-Y07)	4,793	16.6	253	4.0
Symptoms (780-789)	794	2.8	42	5.9
Injuries				
Fractures, all sites (800-826)	995	3.5	52	11.9
Sprains and strains of back (including neck) (846-847)	327	1.1	17	7.9
Head injury (excluding skull fracture) (850-856)	300	1.0	16	5.2
Laceration and open wound (870-898)	324	1.1	17	5.5

Source: HEW, National Center for Health Statistics, *Utilization of Short-Stay Hospitals by Characteristics of Discharged Patients, U.S. 1965.*

genitourinary system, and diseases of the circulatory system. The highest number of discharges per 10,000 population was 253 for obstetrical conditions. By contrast there were only 63 per 10,000 for hypertrophy of tonsils and adenoids. The average length of stay was 4.0 days for obstetrical patients and 1.9 days for tonsillectomy and adenoidectomy patients. But patients with malignant neoplasms stayed an average of 14.8 days, and those with arteriosclerotic heart disease averaged 13.6 days. Thus, hospital utilization is greatly increased by a rise in the incidence of cancer and heart conditions.[1]

Utilization of hospitals increases as greater use is made of hospitals by patients with long-term chronic diseases and as the number of people surviving to advanced ages rises. Because insurance coverage is concentrated on hospital bills, while visits to physicians, recourse to nursing homes, and outpatient and ambulatory services are not as fully covered, recourse to hospital care is increased. Technological advances often place rising dependence on hospitals, and physicians rely increasingly on hospitals for services they previously performed themselves, merely because the hospital is convenient. As hospital financing practices are improved and hospital administration made more efficient, utilization may be expected to rise even more.

Large differences in the utilization of hospitals are found by comparing population incomes and hospital beds (see table 11.4). Clearly there is a great deal of maldistribution. Differences in utilization are especially large in the mental hospitals, suggesting some underutilization in those hospitals. The number of patient-days per 1,000 ranges from 2,250 in New York to 216 in Utah. The relative differences are even greater for tuberculosis treatment facilities. Wide variations in costs are also found. Long-term hospital costs per day range from $46.49 in Idaho to $8.13 in Tennessee.

TABLE 11.4   Variations in Use of Hospital Beds, 1965

	Patient-Days per 1,000 Population	
	General and Special Hospitals	Mental Hospitals
United States average	1,357	1,257
Average of top three states	1,784	2,192
Average of bottom three states	918	291

Source: Adapted from *State Data and State Rankings, 1966-67*, part 2, pp. S-12, S-13.

Utilization rises with income. For instance, the number of physicians per 100,000 population by regions parallels the population income level by regions. The Middle Atlantic, New England, and Pacific states average 123 physicians per 100,000, while the three southern regions average 80.

If differences in utilization can be explained to a considerable degree by differences in income distribution and educational achievement, and distribution of medical care is badly skewed, the inference may be drawn that income and educational differences contribute to overutilization. A Michigan survey found that 73 percent of the people with annual incomes of less than $1,650 had at least one doctor's visit during the year, but 84 percent of those with incomes above $1,650 had a visit. The differences are greater than suggested here, for the health needs of low-income groups are greater than those of the well-to-do.[2]

How much overutilization occurs depends partly on the type of practitioner the patient sees. For example, there may be overutilization of specialists and underutilization of general practitioners. The results of a Michigan survey of physician-patient relationships by specialty are shown in table 11.5. Specialists seen only in a hospital were included if they submitted bills separate from the hospital's bill. A higher percentage of patients saw specialists than general practitioners.

The doctors' services that a patient receives vary in character. About two-thirds of the patients in the Michigan survey received

TABLE 11.5   Practitioner-Patient Relationships

Type of Practitioner	Percentage of Relationships
Total number of physician-patient relationships	4,935
General practitioners	24
Specialists, seen in hospital or elsewhere	34
Clinics (outpatient, joint practice, school, company)	10
Dentists (including orthodontists and oral surgeons	27
Osteopaths	8
Chiropractors	2
Chiropodists	1
Type of practitioner not ascertained	5

Source: W. J. McNerney, *Hospital and Medical Economics* (1962), vol. 1, p. 157.

some services from physicians: 6 percent received surgery, while 53 percent received treatment for disease or injury, treatment for fracture, or maternity care (see table 11.6). The distribution of doctors' services may reflect underreliance on checkups and diagnoses and overreliance on treatment etc.

From 1945 to 1960, the average length of stay in hospitals moved downward, a trend reducing utilization. But overutilization is suggested by the rise in the average number of hospital personnel per 100 patients in these years: from 155 to 226. In the same period, admissions rose by 90 percent, average length of stay was reduced by 21 percent, and number of patient-days rose by 51 percent.[3]

Hospital use varies with the population's income, race, education, and type of community (rural or urban) as well as other factors. In 1945, 79 percent of all births occurred in hospitals; in 1966, almost 97 percent. Does this indicate increasing overutilization or a change in health care standards? The rise in hospital utilization among the more highly educated population, however, seems to have slowed in recent years.[4]

Remedies for Overutilization

It is well known that excessive surgery is sometimes performed. Professor Paul Lembcke, for example, noted: "In one hospital audit it was found when an all specialist medical staff was paid salaries, the gynecologists did about 26 hysterectomies per audit period, but

TABLE 11.6   Types of Doctors' Services Received by Patients in Hospital

Doctors' Services Received	Percentage of Patients
Number of cases	3,516
Received no services from doctors	31
Received doctors' services	69
Injection only	27
Checkup, diagnosis	35
Surgery	6
Treatment, fracture, maternity	53
Other services	2
Service not ascertained	1

Source: W. J. McNerney, *Hospital and Medical Economics* (1962), vol. 1, p. 162.

Note: Percentages of services add to more than subtotal of services received because many patients received more than one type of service.

later on a fee-for-service basis, they did 130 per audit period." A study of five Baltimore hospitals similarly revealed that only 55 percent of appendectomies involved diseased tissues.[5]

Duplication of equipment is common and costly. Martin Cherkasky noted that New York City was providing fourteen to sixteen different data-processing programs. Had a planned centralized program been introduced, the city would have had a much more sophisticated and effective system, with large savings in space, scarce personnel, and money. Similar excesses are to be found in other equipment. For example, 30 percent of the 777 hospitals equipped to do closed heart surgery had no such case in a year; 548 had some use of the equipment; 87 percent had fewer than one case a week; and 41 percent had fewer than one a month.[6] And yet the trend is to increase the amount of specialized equipment in each hospital (see table 11.7).

When comprehensive benefits are made available, utilization tends to increase. When benefits are greatly restricted, utilization declines. On the whole, physicians have not favored comprehensive benefits. They are fearful that the high utilization it brings would put great strains on them. They expect that utilization will respond excessively to rising benefits. Insurance, with its emphasis on hospital care, has contributed to expensive benefits and hence to overutilization. The intermediaries, confronted with excessive use, might have sought to control it, but they have not. By failure to exercise control, they have tended to price themselves out of the market. The cure seems to be governmental measures to reduce costs and subsidize insurance programs.

TABLE 11.7 Specialized Services Available in Voluntary Short-Term Hospitals, 1960-66

	Percentage of Hospitals	
Service Available	1960	1965-66
Pathology laboratory (with pathologist)	60.5	71.3
Premature nursery	61.0	60.5
Intensive care unit	11.1	32.5
Electroencephalography	17.7	31.7
Rehabilitation unit	*	9.3
Dental facilities	30.6	36.8

Source: American Hospital Association, *Hospitals,* August 1961 and August 1967.

*Not listed.

Various approaches to treating overuse have been tried. Under Medicare, utilization reviews and certification of hospital stays were required. But they have not been as successful as proponents had hoped. Hospitals and doctors have not made great efforts to curtail overuse. Hospitals, in particular, seek business when they have excess capacity, in order to improve their financial position.

Increased costs and prices may be expected to curb overutilization to some extent. Yet insurance costs rose from $3 a month in 1950 to $6.35 a month in 1960, while the demand for insurance continued to skyrocket. In 1967 and 1968, average daily hospital costs rose by 14.3 percent and 12.5 percent according to one index (17.9 percent and 14.9 percent according to another), yet the hospital utilization rate for persons aged sixty-five and over rose by 3.60 percent and 3.88 percent (3.88 percent and 4.03 percent according to the second index).

Utilization may be reduced if hospitals avoid increasing their bed capacity beyond that needed currently. Economical use of hospitals is stimulated when substitutes, such as nursing homes and effective drugs, are provided, better financing of substitute services is made available, and reasonable criteria for hospital admission and length of stay are applied.

The chairman of Aetna Life and Casualty Company, the largest insurer in the country, urged greater use of diagnostic and preventive medicine as a weapon to cut overutilization and excessive fees.

In an effort to control excessive physicians' fees the health insurance industry asked the American Medical Association to consider the feasibility of encouraging local medical societies to establish review committees to advise insurance companies on the appropriateness of physicians' and surgeons' fees. AMA saw the value of such a service and urged state and local medical societies to cooperate. When fees are judged by a review committee to be unreasonably high, they are adjusted by consultation between the insurance company and the doctor involved. These committees render remarkably fair decisions, especially after gaining experience.[7]

The Medicare and Medicaid Experience

In the Medicare and Medicaid programs, the federal government required utilization reviews and stressed audits in a fundamental attack on overutilization. But in the first five years of these programs overutilization continued.

On July 1, 1969, Undersecretary of Health, Education, and Welfare, John Veneman acknowledged:

The audit reports revealed . . . that systematic review of services is not being made. I think one of our requirements in the title XIX [Medicaid] program is that there be an accurate and specific procedure for utilization review as part of the State plans.[8]

Officials in the Department of Health, Education, and Welfare stressed the potential of prior approval of certain services for cutting over-utilization.

States should adopt procedures for prior independent professional approval of elective surgery, dental care (except for minor procedures), eye care, and hearing aids.

The experiences of several States indicate that a system of prior approval for selected types of costly health care can be an effective method of controlling utilization and costs as well as avoiding the exposure of recipients to unnecessary hazard and pain.

The New York City "Medicaid Watchdog System" . . . is a prototype for this kind of activity. Under that system, dentists are hired by the health department to review plans of treatment and give their approval or disapproval. The administrators of the system claim savings of $26 million in 1968 in dental care costs alone. Comparable savings were experienced under the prior approval system as applied to optometrists, chiropractors, and podiatrists.

Since the medical or dental procedures involved are not those which generally need to be performed on an emergency or immediate basis, patients should not suffer from the short delay involved in securing the necessary professional approval. A requirement that the review be performed by qualified medical or dental professionals in the health care fields involved would avoid charges of lay interference.[9]

Undersecretary Veneman recommended that permission to raise fees be refused in the absence of effective utilization reviews.

In both Medicaid and Medicare, we feel that much more can be done with utilization controls than has been accomplished to date. Peer group review must become widespread not just in hospitals but also for other medical services. But peer group review alone is obviously not enough to control abuses and escalating costs. We have issued regulations for Medicaid which provide that, starting July 1, 1970, no state may raise fees without demonstrating to the Secretary that its utilization review is effective and that it has effective measures to control fraud by practitioners and facilities. We need new machinery for this purpose—"self-control" by the providers of service is being given a chance, but by itself is inadequate. Too often "peer review" is simply "peer justification". The public and patients both deserve better.[10]

In several situations, the Department of Health, Education, and

Welfare denies benefits if the carrier has not complied with the provisions for utilization reviews or certifications of need. For example, one regulation states:

> Hospital insurance benefits can be paid for up to 100 days of post-hospital extended care services during each benefit period. However, the number of days payable in a particular care facility may be limited if:
>
> A. At the time of the patient's admission, there was in effect a decision that the extended care facility was not making timely utilization review of long-stay cases. In this case, benefits may not be paid beyond a prescribed length of stay; or
>
> B. The extended care facility receives notice of a finding by the physician members of the utilization review committee that the patient's further stay is not medically necessary. In this case, benefit payments will be limited to services furnished before the fourth day following the day the extended care facility receives the notice.
>
> Extended care services count toward the 100-day maximum in a benefit period if benefits are paid for the services, or benefits would be paid if a request for payment were properly filed and the services were certified by a physician to be necessary.[11]

Use of Professional Standards Review Organizations

The Professional Standards Review Organization (PSRO) program was enacted by Congress in 1972 as a national effort at utilization review. It will hold 335,000 physicians and osteopaths and 170,000 other health professionals accountable for the billions of dollars' worth of care they render annually under federal programs.

The PSROs will set standards for treatment, and local boards of physicians will review their colleagues' work for deviance from the local standards. Violators will be liable for nonpayment of the fees they charged or for fines of up to $5,000. The reviewing bodies are part of an attempt to get health costs under control before a program of national health insurance is instituted.

Enactment of the PSRO program has touched off one of the biggest battles between organized medicine and the federal government since the enactment of Medicare in 1965. Dr. Malcolm C. Todd, president of the American Medical Association, told the 1973 AMA convention that "the [PSRO] law poses the greatest threat to the private practice of medicine of any piece of legislation ever passed by Congress." The basis for AMA opposition is a fear among physicians that free enterprise in private practice is threatened by government interference through PSROs.

One of the most difficult and most important parts of the PSRO program will be setting standards for physicians to follow in administering quality care. The Office of Professional Standards Review in the Department of Health, Education, and Welfare wants PSROs to set standards for the most common diagnoses and treatments in their areas. Those standards could cover about 350 treatment procedures and would affect close to 44 million Medicare and Medicaid patients, including 11 million a year who receive hospital care.

Dr. Jay A. Winsten of the Harvard Medical School described the operation of the review boards:

Each PSRO will be responsible for developing guidelines which, for a given illness, injury or health condition, provide answers to the following questions:

Should the patient be hospitalized, or treated on an outpatient basis? (The patient's age and complicating medical conditions will be taken into account.)

If hospitalization is necessary, what is the probable length of stay required for proper care? (At specified times after admission of a patient, the attending physician will be required to certify the medical necessity of continued hospitalization and to justify his decision to the satisfaction of the local PSRO.)

What are the specific health care services required for proper diagnosis and treatment of the patient's complaint? (Recognizing that alternative methods of treatment may be equally efficacious, PSROs are directed to specify alternative modes of treatment whenever appropriate.)[12]

The Office of Professional Standards Review operated in 1973-74 on a $34 million budget. Acting Director Simmons estimated that the office will require $100 million a year when all 182 PSROs are in operation, but he said that this is "a purely hypothetical figure." Former Director Bauer felt that $50 million a year was too low a budget. He said it was based on the assumption that physicians would volunteer their time to set standards and norms for their regions, but "as soon as you start funding you stop volunteering. Doctors figure, 'If we have to do it we will ask for money.' It took our Colorado foundation 18 months to debate criteria and set standards. So I think it will be more expensive than they think it will be."

The only organized nonmedical opposition to the PSROs comes from the Consumer Clearing House for PSRO Action, an ad hoc group affiliated with Ralph Nader and made up of about 100 schools of public health, local health care groups, and regional comprehensive health planning agencies. The Clearing House considers the PSRO legislation significant, but feels it does not provide for enough public input. "It sets up a review mechanism that is the fox guarding the henhouse," said Robert E. McGarrah, Jr., of the Health Research Group—the Clearing House's parent organization. "There is no evidence to show that is on the decline."

A Clearing House report by McGarrah and Leda R. Judd of the National Urban Coalition predicted:

Denials of Medicare claims probably will be rare . . . since rotating panels of PSRO members will conduct the review. Thus a doctor who has difficulty getting a claim approved by his peers will later be in a position to review their work when his turn comes to sit on the PSRO panel. This will result in typical medical society backscratching. . . . Consumers are completely excluded from any involvement in local PSROs, just as they are excluded from participating in local medical societies.[13]

The PSRO law provides for public access to only the PSROs' standards and norms of care and the national council's report to Congress. Senator Bennet, the father of the PSRO legislation, responding to the consumer issue, said: "I don't think consumer pressure can improve the practice of medicine; only doctors can."

Quality

Problems of Measurement

In assessing the costs of medical care, allowance must be made for variations in quality. Especially in periods of shortages, purveyors may try to keep costs down, while they respond to deficiencies of supply, by tolerating a deterioration in quality. The measurement of quality is beset by many problems, however.

A report by the Veterans' Administration on measurement of quality in the field of health care stressed the relevance and significance of the caliber of personnel, facilities, and procedures in determining quality. It is possible to evaluate good medicine, the VA concluded, but it cannot be measured by any average yardstick.[14] The report described

a variety of methods and techniques which permit continuous and direct appraisal of medical care in all its aspects. These procedures do not directly measure the quality of medical care, but do greatly contribute to high level performance. . . . Opportunities for consultants to participate in direct patient care as well as to evaluate the quality enhances the level of performance. Direct observations are discussed with the Manager, Director, Professional Services, and staff, and written reports to the Area Medical Director contribute to improvement of patient care. . . . Reviews of records, checks on laboratory proficiency, comparisons of clinical and laboratory findings, and studies of suicides are devices to continuously evaluate the quality of medical care. In themselves, or in composite, they are not a measurement of the quality of medical care. They do contribute to improvement of patient care. . . . Review of various administrative practices, problems of coordination of inpatient and outpatient medical care, efficiency of admission procedures, and problems of intrahospital communication are under continuous scrutiny at the hospital level. Such activities enhance the quality and efficiency of care, but are not measurements.[15]

The recent history of nursing homes provides an example of deterioration of quality. Standards of quality had been set at unrealistically high levels, considering that the personnel to staff these facilities were just not available. Certification and acceptance of too many low-quality nurses explain in part the rise of expenditures for nursing homes.[16]

Under Medicare, providers were to charge customary and prevailing fees that were consistent with local charges. Physicians are not allowed to charge more under Medicare than they do under other programs. Though the doctor is supposed to recover his full costs, charges do not always equal costs. For example, the aged who incur long hospital stays have low per diem use of ancillary services and may well be charged more than their costs. Physicians do not always exercise sufficient restraint in billing. Hence, it may be necessary to negotiate charges as a means of keeping costs down.[17]

There was much discussion of the items of cost that could be included in the purveyors' charges under Medicare. Interest on capital and depreciation charges, for example, were allowed. But capital funds were to come from private or public gifts or loans.

The *Report of the National Advisory Commission on Health Manpower* (November 1967) analyzed some aspects of the quality problem. The commission noted the danger of overemphasizing a single control such as formal education or licensure. It is necessary for the physician to continue his education throughout his career, to keep abreast of new discoveries and treatments.

Progress in medical science and technology has increased our ability to prevent and cure illness but, at the same time, it has greatly increased the difficulty of assuring that practice fully exploits the potential of current knowledge.

Reliance on quality controls in formal education and licensure have been the primary means of assuring that physicians use the best techniques and information available. But with the increasing pace of medical advances, these "one-time" controls are not enough; the physician's education must be continued as long as he practices. Greatly improved methods of diagnosis and treatment can be developed after he completes his training and, if he is unaware of the new developments, he will continue to use outdated and far less effective techniques and remedies.

Moreover, although the physician remains the central figure in the provision of medical care, he must increasingly rely upon others to assist him. The tests performed by medical laboratories, the medicines produced by drug companies, and the services provided by other professionals and by allied health personnel are all an essential part of today's health care. Not only must the physician apply current knowledge and techniques, but the essential services complementing his own work must meet equivalent modern standards.[18]

The physician needs the cooperation of high-quality laboratories, X-ray technicians, and similar auxiliary services if he is to give optimum quality care to his patients.

One proposal for improving quality called for periodic relicensing of physicians as a means of keeping the physician (and other members of the medical team) abreast of new developments. But there are many obstacles to introducing relicensing, not the least of which is the unavailability of educational facilities for retraining.[19]

To achieve high quality, adequate standards must also be established for graduates of foreign medical schools who wish to practice here. The National Advisory Commission on Health Manpower noted: "On examinations which were passed by 98% of the graduates of U.S. medical schools, only 40% of the foreign medical graduates achieved a passing score."[20]

Deficient quality in community hospitals is suggested by the much better postoperative evaluation record of two major teaching-affiliate hospitals in a study in New York City. Evidence of excessive surgery is one indication of inadequate quality.

An evaluation of all major female pelvic surgery performed during a six-month period in a community hospital revealed that only 30 percent of the operations which resulted in castration or sterilization were justified in the opinion of expert consultants. This compared with a justification rate of 76 percent in two teaching hospitals.

The medical records of a random sample of 430 patients admitted to 98 different hospitals in New York City during May 1962 were reviewed by expert clinicians. In the opinion of these medical reviewers, only 57 percent of all patients and only 31 percent of the general medical cases, received "optimal" care. In voluntary hospitals affiliated with medical schools, 80 percent of all patients received optimal care, compared with only 47 percent of patients in proprietary hospitals.[21]

A commission of the American Medical Association has criticized the medical cost index because it fails to allow for changes of quality.

The failure to take full account of quality changes is the most important and serious defect of the CPI, resulting in a discrepancy between the intent and definition of the Index—measurement of pure price change—and what actually is measured. Many economists believe that since quality changes have generally been quality improvements, a systematic upward bias in the CPI exists. Some persons feel that the "importance of this problem tends to be exaggerated in some quarters, particularly as it affects month-to-month, or even year-to-year changes in the Bureau of Labor Statistics price indexes. Over the long run, however, if real quality changes continue to be made in the same direction, their effects may tend to accumulate.*

Although the importance and degree of overstatement is not a matter of universal agreement, it is likely that the extent of upward bias in the medical care component is greater than for other parts of the CPI. An article in the *Monthly Labor Review* stated:

"... It is probable, however, that the medical care price index reflects more quality changes than do the price indexes for the non-service items, because the 'quality' of a service is necessarily affected by intangibles, such as the fact that doctors' services are generally adapted to the needs of the patient."†

In summary, it is contended that: (a) the Medical Care Price Index does not account for quality changes in medical care; (b) the narrow definition of quality does not adequately describe or include the significant quality features of medical care; (c) present techniques are ineffective means to hold quality of the units constant or to account for quality changes; (d) the units priced, primarily the physician visit and hospital day, do not remain constant over a period of time; and (e) by not defining or adjusting for quality improvements, the Medical Care Price Index and the indexes for the individual items overstate the true price change.[22]

---

*Chase, A. E. Concepts and uses of price indexes. Paper presented at American Statistical Association meeting, August 25, 1960. BLS 61-0336). Washington, D.C.: [1961]. p. 12. Arnold E. Chase, Assistant Commissioner, Prices and Living Conditions, U.S. Bureau of Labor Statistics.

†Langford, E. A. Medical Care in the Consumer Price Index, 1936-1956, Monthly Labor Review, 80:1056, September 1957.

The Columbia University School of Public Health and Administrative Medicine conducted a helpful study dealing with quality problems in New York State.[23] The report acknowledged much that had been done to improve the quality of American medical care:

The reader should not conclude that nothing has been done to upgrade medical care in the United States. The Flexner report, which led to the closing of substandard medical schools early in the century; the development of the specialty Boards; the standard promoting activities of various professional organizations, such as the American College of Surgeons and the American Academy of Pediatrics; the examination required of all foreign-trained physicians, and given by the Educational Council for Foreign Medical Graduates; the policy initiated by the Veterans Administration, which provides that the medical staff of its hospitals shall be nominated by local medical schools; the policy of the Children's Bureau to pay for services only if they are furnished in institutions, and by physicians, that meet professional standards; the standards enforced by the New York State Health Department and by the New York City Departments of Health, Hospitals, and Welfare for special services; and the national impact of the Joint Commission on Accreditation of Hospitals are all examples of national or local influences which have placed a quality of medical care within the reach of many people in the United States which is denied to most of the rest of the world. Yet, within the United States, there are wide discrepancies, and New York State is no exception—in fact, the New York City metropolitan area poses some of the worst unresolved medical care problems in the country.[24]

California Quality Control Experience

The California Hospital Association and California Medical Association have taken some measures to try to assure delivery of high-quality medical services under Medi-Cal, the state's Medicaid program. The associations consider adequate quality "the most important component to effective hospital service." Their program calls for contracting carriers to review claims for service for conformity to prevailing standards of practice and Medi-Cal regulations and, when the justification for a series of claims is questionable, to have their staffs collect information needed to clarify why the services were performed. Members of the two associations are chosen for a peer panel to review quality problems. At least two physicians and two hospital administrators serve on the panel. The associations expressed the purpose and methods of the program as follows:

Aim

To provide Medi-Cal with a system of safeguards in the utilization of hospital services; and to assist hospitals to maintain and strengthen standards of care.

Need

Providers of health services have a responsibility for assuring that the public interest is being served in the delivery of hospital services for persons covered by the Medi-Cal program.

Quality is the most important component to effective hospital service. Standards of quality can be best judged by professional peers, functioning expressly to review patterns of hospital practice.

Methods

In cooperation with the California Hospital Association and the California Medical Association and under the provisions of their agreements as the contracting carriers with the State of California, Hospital Service of California and Hospital Service of Southern California will organize and implement the following procedures for reviewing irregular patterns of practices by hospitals participating in the Medi-Cal program:

1. *Screening for irregularity*

In the conduct of its customary and routine procedures, provider claims for service are reviewed by the contracting carrier for conformity to prevailing standards of practice and Medi-Cal regulations. This work is performed by staff with proven skills for discerning presumptive irregularity. All questionable claims are referred to a special unit of the contracting carrier's organization where specially-trained staff carry out further analyses.

2. *Detecting irregularity*

When there is reasonable question about the justification of a series of claims, contracting carrier staff collects information needed for clarification. If, after this further evaluation which frequently involves field data collection and direct contact with the provider, questions about suspect patterns are not satisfied, the provider institution is placed under special review. A record of the provider's pattern of practices is developed. Should the record reasonably convince the contracting carrier about provider irregularity and subsequent efforts with the provider fail to correct detected patterns, the contracting carrier, with notice to the Office of Health Care Services, shall ask for the establishment of a peer panel to review the problem.

3. *Referring for peer review*

(a) *Panel designation*—Upon request from the contracting carrier, the designated officer of the California Hospital Association and the designated officer of the California Medical Association will appoint appropriate persons from among their respective memberships who agree to function as peer review panelists. Each panel shall consist of at least two hospital administrators and two physicians with a chairman designated by mutual agreement of the respective designated officers. Panel members will serve without compensation but shall receive from the contracting carriers reasonable reimbursement for travel and living expenses. The contracting carrier will serve as staff and attend all meetings of the panel.

(b) *Referral to committee*—The contracting carrier shall make a written report to the panel, informing them of the nature of the matter to be considered, summary of data collected, and history of efforts to resolve issues presented. At the time of referral, the contracting carrier shall advise the panel members that their findings and recommendations will be reported to the Office of Health Care Services. One of the primary aims in activating a peer review panel is to counsel providers on ways for correcting patterns and irregularities and for improving their services and economic practices, regardless of sources of payment.

(c) *Notice of hearing*—The provider shall be given written notice of any meeting at which the peer review panel will receive evidence on the matter submitted. This notice shall be given by the panel no less than 10 days prior to such hearing. The notice shall state the nature of the matter under submission. If particular cases are to be discussed, the provider shall be furnished information needed for identification. If the matter under submission involves a pattern of conduct or if it is impractical to list specific cases, the provider shall be given information sufficient to enable him to identify the period involved and the nature of any procedures in question. The contracting carrier will provide the panel with the facts in support of any alleged irregularities.

(d) *Attendance by the provider*—The provider shall be entitled to attend any panel meeting while evidence regarding him is received. The provider shall have the right to see any documentary material received by the panel. The provider shall be accorded adequate opportunity to present evidence on his own behalf, or to rebut any evidence offered against him, or to offer any explanation to the panel. The provider shall have the right to be accompanied by counsel but counsel shall not be entitled to participate in any hearing unless the chairman or a majority of the panel determines that his participation would be of assistance to the panel. These hearings shall be informal and the rules of courtroom evidence do not apply. Failure of the provider, without reasonable excuse, to attend scheduled meetings shall not preclude the panel from carrying out its proceedings.[25]

In testimony before the Senate Subcommittee on Health of the Elderly, Blue Cross enumerated its goals for and contributions toward providing high-quality medical care under Medi-Cal:

The Blue Cross goals in its fiscal intermediary role under Title 19 [Medicaid] . . . are:

1. To handle, process and pay claims and to pay them on the same basis as in all other sectors of Blue Cross operations;

2. To interpret correctly and carry-out governmental objectives to the satisfaction of both the government and the contracting parties;

3. To recognize problems and areas of potential problems in providing services and to communicate such knowledge to the government as needed. This, of course, requires Blue Cross to represent two parties—the providers—hospitals, nursing homes, extended care facilities, rehabilitation centers, home health agencies, and others—which offer the institutional services, and the government, which provides the benefits to the ultimate recipient, the public.

4. To assist the providers of the service—the institutions concerned—to operate in an optimal manner in all specific and collateral services rendered.

5. Finally, in the administration of the program, to make Blue Cross responsive in seeing that the public's right to good health is recognized and respected.

These goals are consistent with the services Blue Cross provides to the public and to the institutions with which it works. They are also consistent with Blue Cross' major corporate goal, which is to provide all segments of the population with the means of obtaining the highest quality of medical care in the most effective and economical manner with continued dedication to the preservation of the voluntary health care system.

What Blue Cross Provides

The State Government was able to take maximum advantage of Blue Cross' capabilities and unique services. These include:

1. *Experience* in private, prepaid health care programs, particularly in those providing service benefits;

2. *Existing facilities* with related equipment and trained personnel;

3. *Experience* in cost-related reimbursement programs;

4. *Long-established relations* with providers of covered services;

5. *Experience with the coordination* needed for the requirements of both Medi-Cal and Medicare;

6. *Long history of cooperation* with Blue Shield (physician prepayment agency similar to Blue Cross' role in providing prepaid hospital care);

7. *Control mechanisms,* i.e. fiscal claims and utilization of review procedures and systems.

Blue Cross helps to safeguard the tax dollars of the public. It does this in the course of its normal procedures in its review and audit activities. There are two broad categories of this activity:

The first is preventive and is covered by carefully detailed individual billing instructions with on-the-scene visits to smooth out eligibility and processing problems and also various group educational programs, institutes and seminars.

The second could be called correctional, i.e., the creation of safeguards against abuse and follow-up regarding appropriateness of activities in connection with the Medi-Cal program, through audits and utilization reviews.

These two categories of activity are carried out by the seventy-six Blue Cross field people who routinely and regularly visit all hospitals, nursing homes, home health agencies, and other providers. These are trained representatives who are specialists in professional relations utilization review and reimbursement. Their primary purpose is to help the facilities concerned comply with the operational requirements of Medi-Cal.

It is clear, however, that in the process of doing this they create a network of communications and a clearing-house for interpretation and cross-reference which helps prevent and/or correct potential abuses under Title 19.

There are 566 acute care facilities, 1,215 nursing homes, and 122 home health agencies and free-standing clinics, for a total of 1,903 providers in California. These are furnished information regarding the Medi-Cal program through Blue Cross bulletins, workshops, routine and special visits, provider visits to the intermediaries' office, telephone communications, individual letters, and participation by the intermediaries in regional and State provider association meetings.

Since the inception of Medi-Cal, March 1, 1966, Blue Cross has an increasingly intensive utilization review and audit program to safeguard against abuses while at the same time assuring that eligible recipients receive optimal health care.

Blue Cross—Medi-Cal's "Clearinghouse"

Medi-Cal is a vast program . . . . In support of Medi-Cal, Blue Cross acts—as does Blue Shield in its particular field—as a "clearinghouse" in behalf of the State of California to:

1. Receive bills for services rendered to eligible people, determine compliance with regulations and approve for payment those bills that meet the requirements of law and regulation, including those that apply to the appropriateness of costs and charges.

2. Maintain all necessary records and furnish the State all necessary information and reports.

3. Provide liaison and coordination with providers and groups, organizations, committees representing them, or other interested parties.

4. Apply safeguards against unnecessary utilization, abuse and fraud.

Reimbursement

Blue Cross' experience in cost-related reimbursement is unequalled. Blue Cross has a staff of accountants trained in hospital accounting fully qualified to review financial statements, determine allowable cost and apply a reimbursement formula.

Since the State initially adopted a formula similar to the one Blue Cross of Southern California uses, Blue Cross was able to provide an existing staff of experts.

Understandably, confusion could develop if a single provider, for example, was subject to audit by Blue Cross for its business; by another Medicare intermediary for Medicare claims; and by a state agency for Medi-Cal. As it is, *in most instances, a single audit suffices.* The hospital can supply its cost figures to Blue Cross, and Blue Cross can determine payment for all.

Relations with Providers

An important advantage of Blue Cross' administration of the Medi-Cal program is its long-term favorable relationship to hospitals. Actually, the hospitals, along with the general public, have a voice in the policy and operations of Blue Cross through board membership. Blue Cross is sponsored and supported by hospitals; Blue Cross works closely with recognized hospital organizations; the contractual relationship between hospitals and Blue Cross is yet another bond between the providers of institutional care and the fiscal intermediary in the Medi-Cal program. The hospitals and the general public are accustomed to working with Blue Cross.

Evidence of provider preference for Blue Cross can be found in the fact that 92% of all Medicare participating hospitals in California selected Blue Cross as intermediary under that program. So did 60% of extended care facilities and almost all home health agencies. While selection by provider is not permitted under Medi-Cal, it can be assumed that there would be essentially the same ratio of preference for Blue Cross.

This provider rapport works to the advantage of the Medi-Cal program in other ways. Blue Cross field representatives, who regularly visit hospitals and other providers, help train personnel in administrative practices involving Medi-Cal. They also serve to answer questions and solve problems that might arise, in advance.[26]

Despite their testimony to the Senate subcommittee, these agencies do not always act in the interests of health consumers. The California Medical Association sought to obtain a higher fee schedule, while Blue Shield recommended that Medicare pay fees in the 90th percentile of all claims in an area for that procedure under California Blue Shield plans. Medicare and Medi-Cal were then paying fees in the 60th percentile, and adequate numbers of physicians were available at those fees.

Notes

1. See HEW, National Center for Health Statistics, *Utilization of Short-Stay Hospitals by Characteristics of Discharged Patients, U.S. 1965,* pp. 1-6.

2. W. J. McNerney, *Hospital and Medical Economics* (1962), vol. 1, p. 158.

3. HEW, Public Health Service, *Medical Care Financing and Utilization* (1962), pp. 158-62.

4. Ibid., pp. 173, 177, 185, 186, 222.

5. P. A. Lembcke, "Is the Operation Necessary?" *New Republic*, November 9, 1963, p. 16; see H. M. Somers and A. R. Somers, *A Program for Research in Health Economics* (1967), p. 80.

6. U.S. Senate, Committee on Governmental Operations, Subcommittee on Executive Reorganization, *Hearings on Health Care in America* (April 1968), part 1, pp. 15-16, 168-69.

7. Ibid., p. 441.

8. U.S. Senate, Committee on Finance, *Staff Report: Medicare and Medicaid, Problems, Issues and Alternatives* (February 1970), p. 126.

9. Ibid., p. 128.

10. U.S. Senate, Special Committee on Aging, Subcommittee on Health of the Elderly, *Hearings on the Economics of Aging: Toward a Full Share of Abundance,* Senate Report no. 91-1 (July 1969), part 3, p. 652.

11. HEW, Social Security Administration, *Social Security Handbook* (February 1969), p. 371.

12. *Wall Street Journal,* December 6, 1973.

13. R. E. McGarrah, Jr., and L. R. Judd, *PSRO: Doctor Accountability or Consumer Disaster?*

14. Veterans' Administration, Department of Medicine and Surgery, *Report of the Committee on Measurement of the Quality of Medical Care* (April 1959).

15. Ibid., p. 18.

16. U.S. Senate, *Developments in Aging,* Senate Report no. 91-875 (1969), pp. 81-86.

17. HEW, *Report of the National Conference on Medical Costs,* Washington, D.C., June 27-28, 1967, pp. 62-64.

18. *Report of the National Advisory Committee on Health Manpower* (November 1967), vol. 1, pp. 38-39.

19. Ibid., pp. 40-42.

20. Ibid., p. 42.

21. Ibid., pp. 39-40. See also P. A. Lembcke, "Medical Auditing by Scientific Methods," *Journal of the American Medical Association,* October 13, 1956; M. A. Morehead et al., *A Study of the Quality of Hospital Care Secured by a Sample of Teamster Family Members in New York City,* Columbia University School of Public Health and Administrative Medicine, New York (1964).

22. American Medical Association, *Report of the Commission on the Cost of Medical Care* (1964), pp. 50-52.

23. School of Public Health and Administrative Medicine, Columbia University, *Prepayment for Medical and Dental Care in New York State* (October 1962), especially chap. 1.

24. Ibid.

25. U.S. Senate, Special Committee on Aging, Subcommittee on Health of the Elderly, *Hearings on Costs and Delivery of Health Services to Older Americans* (October 1968), part 3, pp. 717-18.

26. Ibid., pp. 720-21.

PART IV

Insurance

12

Medical Insurance Today

History of Health Insurance

In the early 1900s, health care was financed in a simple way: individuals paid at the time of illness. This process was gradually replaced by the regulated collection of small amounts of money from many people in the form of private health insurance.

Today in the United States two types of private health insurance exist: the "nonprofit" tax-exempt Blue Cross and Blue Shield, and the private commercial insurance companies. The biggest push for private health insurance came during the Depression. In the thirties, people did not have enough money to pay their hospital bills, thus putting the hospitals in financial trouble. As a result, hospitals organized a prepayment plan called Blue Cross. Plan enrollees would pay a monthly amount to Blue Cross, and it would pay the hospital bills.

Similarly, during the late thirties, physicians found that patients could not pay them at the time of receiving care. State medical associations (local AMAs) sponsored Blue Shield plans. Patients would pay monthly sums to Blue Shield and Blue Shield would pay the doctors for their services.

Commercial insurance companies insured people against sickness as early as the nineteenth century, but these policies became widespread only after World War II. This happened because labor unions began to demand health benefits for their workers. Employers started paying part of the employees' wages into health and welfare funds. These large funds were used to buy private health insurance at *group* rates, which were lower than individual rates.

Commercial companies captured a large share of the union market due to their practice of *experience rating*. By this mechanism, each group in the population is charged a different rate, depending on how much it uses hospitals and doctors. In this way, insurance companies give lower rates to healthy and young people, and higher rates to sick, poor, and old people, who need more medical attention.

The Blues used to charge the population one rate (*community rating*) but finally began using experience rating themselves in response to commercial insurance company pressure.

All types of health insurance have *deductibles*, that is, amounts the individual must pay for services before the insurance company will begin to pay. Insurance policies generally make patients also pay part of the cost of services (called *coinsurance*). For example, a policy will specify that the company will pay 80 percent and the individual will pay 20 percent of the cost above the deductible, or the company will pay for sixty days of care, and the individual must pay for any additional care needed. Every insurance policy leaves many medical services uncovered, such as dental care, outpatient psychiatric care, outpatient drugs, and preventive medicine.

By 1970, slightly more than 150 million persons—60 million employees and 90 million dependents—were covered by health insurance. But there are over 20 million Americans who have no insurance coverage (and neither Medicaid nor Medicare), and they have difficulty finding a doctor who will see them. These people must go to public hospitals, which are inadequately staffed, underfinanced, and in need of improvements. Of people discharged from short-stay hospitals in the 1958-60 period, 32 percent had no insurance payments; 49 percent of those aged sixty-five and over had no insurance payments.

In 1970 private insurance payments totaled $15.8 billion, or 25 percent of personal health expenditures, and 40 percent of consumer expenditures. Private insurance payments for *hospital care* constituted 36 percent of personal health expenditures and 75 percent of consumer expenditures; for *physicians' services*, private insurance payments were 36 percent of personal health care, and 48 percent of consumer expenditures.[1]

The insurance payment rates ranged from 41 percent for males in the $2,000 income group to 83 percent for those earning $7,000 and over. The number of health insurance policies in force varied greatly by occupation, ranging from 35 percent to 67 percent.

Group policies are far less costly than individual policies. Expenses for the latter run as high as 40 percent to 50 percent of premium income.

Blue Cross

The management of local Blue Cross plans is traditionally dominated by hospital representatives: 50 percent of the Blue Cross board members are hospital administrators and trustees.[2] Other Blue Cross directors are businessmen and doctors with hospital ties.

What is the effect of the hospital domination of Blue Cross boards? It has tended to channel as much money as possible to hospitals. This is done by the "cost-plus" method of reimbursement. Blue Cross negotiates with hospitals every year or two about which costs it will reimburse. Rarely will it refuse to pay for items the hospitals want reimbursed. Thus Blue Cross allows hospitals to continue to raise rates without questioning the reasons for the increases. Only one-fifth of the Blue Cross plans make audits of hospital accounts.[3]

If Blue Cross used its power, it could change the practices of hospitals. In New York City, for example, Blue Cross pays for over two-thirds of hospital costs; with this leverage, it could better control costs.

Blue Shield

Blue Shield plans are controlled by local or state medical societies. About two-thirds of Blue Shield board members are doctors. Blue Shield protects physicians' fees through its method of reimbursement. It generally pays doctors their "usual and customary" fees. These can be raised by the doctors themselves in an area. When Blue Shield makes a contract with a doctor, that doctor generally cannot charge patients above what the plan pays the doctor. However, many doctors do not participate in Blue Shield. They charge patients any fee they wish, and Blue Shield reimburses the patient for only the amount it considers a usual and customary fee for the particular service.

Commercial Insurance Companies

Unlike the Blues, which were organized to assure the payment of bills to hospitals and doctors, commercial insurance companies sell health insurance for the purpose of making a profit. About 1,000 companies offer accident and health insurance, covering 125 million people. In 1970, the commercials took in $8.7 billion in premium income. Although the total volume of commercial insurance company business is slightly greater than that of the Blues, no one commercial company is as big as Blue Cross.

Most of the top health insurance companies are also the biggest life insurance companies. Prudential and Metropolitan Life, the two largest, each have $30 billion in assets, making them substantially bigger than General Motors, Standard Oil of New Jersey, and IT&T, and the equals of Bank of America and Chase Manhattan Bank.

Commercial insurance companies have a different relationship to doctors and hospitals from that of the Blues. The commercials contract with the patient and do not deal with the providers. This means that patients often have to fight to collect money from the insurance company. On the other hand, commercials, like consumers, have become concerned with the rise in hospital charges, since they too must pay out more when hospital rates go up. In the past, commercial companies paid the patient only a stipulated sum for each service. As a result of competition, many of these plans now pay the full daily hospital rate, except for deductibles, coinsurance, and certain limitations.

Independent Group Plans

Independent group plans, such as New York's Health Insurance Plan, the Kaiser-Permanente Health Plan, and the Ross-Loos Clinics, are more progressive than the traditional insurance companies. They are more generous in providing benefits for professional services, they use capitation reimbursement, and they generally act as their own insurance companies.

The Kaiser-Permanente Health Plan—one of the largest group practices in the United States—is considered a health maintenance organization (HMO) prototype. Many health planners and government leaders believe HMOs will be America's future health delivery system. The income of HMOs is based on prepayment, and they provide relatively complete and continuous care for a subscribing clientele or population.

According to the Department of Health, Education, and Welfare, an HMO is any organization that is "fiscally responsible" and agrees to provide or arranges for other organizations to provide certain inpatient and outpatient health care services to a limited group of "enrollees."[4] Subscribers pay a set monthly fee to the HMO regardless of how little or how much service they use that month. Enrollment in an HMO covers at least part of the cost of many health services, though the enrollee may have to pay substantial deductibles and coinsurance in many cases. Except in certain emergency situations, an HMO will not pay for care given by hospitals, clinics, or doctors not associated with that HMO.

The definition of an HMO can be very misleading. HMOs do not have to be prepaid group practices in which doctors receive annual salaries. They can include solo fee-for-service practices, as exemplified by foundations for medical care, large hospitals with outpatient clinics, and university medical centers.

Among the many accomplishments of various HMOs are reductions in inpatient utilizations, improved use of manpower, and provision of more complete care at a more economical cost to subscribers than individual practice plans.

National Health Insurance

There is no doubt that America's future health care will be under some form of national health insurance. Almost every vested group— the AMA, the Nixon administration, and the private insurance companies—has a bill for such insurance before Congress.

But passage of national health insurance will take some time, because disagreements among the parties are great. Unresolved issues relate to the degree of compulsion, the site of control, the treatment of current programs, the benefits and costs of the program, the methods of finance, the acceptance of a budgetary system, and the reimbursement system for doctors and institutions.

Enrollment in Present Insurance Plans

By 1968, 87 percent of Americans under age sixty-five were covered by insurance for hospital care. By 1965 the Blues had an enrollment of 64 million for hospital care. Private commercial insurance companies enrolled 97 million, and the independent plans subscribed almost 7 million.[5]

The upward trend of enrollment (for all ages) has been uneven. From 1955 to 1970 the overall rise was from 102 million to 194 million. For the Blues, the gain was less than 100 percent. For insurance companies, enrollment doubled, with group policies gaining much more than individual ones. Independent plans rose by about three-quarters.[6]

Community versus Experience Ratings

One of the biggest changes in health insurance occurred around rate schedules. As Blue Cross rates escalated, low- and middle-income groups were increasingly excluded from the community rates (a single rate for one group) upon which Blue Cross had been built.

Competition from private commercial insurance companies forced Blue Cross to offer experience rating. Those groups who choose experience rating are the ones whose members use little hospital care and can thus obtain a reduced rate. Those who use more hospital services remain community-rated. They tend to be lower-income groups, they have riskier jobs, they work for smaller employers, they have larger families, and they are less able to afford the kind of care that would prevent hospitalization. Unfortunately, for these people, Blue Cross tends to raise its rates.

In 1970, in New York and Philadelphia, the community-rated group alone bore the rate increases. Whether experience-rated groups had their rates raised proportionately is not known. The New York Blue Cross proposed to divide the community-rated subscribers, who represented 60 percent of its membership, into three categories: direct pay subscribers, subscribers in groups of over 100 members, and those in groups of fewer than 100. Each group was experience-rated. The direct pay subscribers especially would suffer under this plan, because they include many disabled and unemployed persons. Blue Cross then asked for a raise of 36 to 57 percent for this group, and it revoked its previous contracts, which had provided full benefits for 120 days. Thus, Blue Cross concentrated its high rates on those least able to pay.[7]

Coverage

In 1966, private commercial insurance companies accounted for a substantial part of the covered population: 97 million enrolled for hospital benefits, 94 million for surgical benefits, and 58 million for in-hospital physicians' visits. Those over age sixty-five accounted for 5, 4, and 3 percent of the coverage for these three services, respectively, although roughly 10 percent of the persons hospitalized are sixty-five or older. For surgical services, 80 percent of the population under sixty-five was covered, and for in-hospital visits 66 percent. For other services coverage was much lower: 2.6 percent of the under-sixty-five age group was covered for dental care, 8.9 percent for nursing-home care, and 44.6 percent for visiting nurse service.[8]

Beginning at about age forty, coverage declines markedly with advancing age, especially for hospital and surgical benefits. Thus, whereas in 1961-63 70.3 percent of the population had hospital insurance, only 54.0 percent of those sixty-five and over were so insured. The picture is not a consistent one, however, for various types of coverage by ages (see table 12.1 and figure 12.2).[9]

Historical Trends in Coverage

From 1940 to 1960 the proportion of persons with hospital insurance who also had surgical insurance rose from 43.5 percent to 91.7 percent. Those who also had regular medical insurance rose from 24.4 percent to 66.3 percent. From 1950 to 1960, the largest relative increases in coverage were for regular medical expense, surgical expense, and hospital expense, in descending order. Early hospital coverage helps explain its small relative rise in the 1950s. From 1960 to 1965, the order of relative increases in covered expenses was major medical, regular medical, surgical, and hospital.[10] For the number of people covered by each type of insurance from 1940 to 1960, see table 12.3.

Group Health Coverage

In 1967 the Health Association of America studied the nature and scope of group health insurance for fifty-six companies. The association found that these companies accounted for 66 percent of group health insurance premiums among insurance companies. A recent survey reveals that under group insurance policies "the number of persons with major medical expense coverage is equal to about three-fourths of the total number with some hospital or surgical expense coverage."

At the end of 1966, 39 million people under age sixty-five were

TABLE 12.1 Percentage Enrolled in Private Plans by Age, Type of Plan, and Type of Care, 1970

Age and Type of Plan	Hospital Care	Surgical Services	Physicians' Services			Dental Care	Prescribed Drugs (Out-of-Hospital)	Private-Duty Nursing	Visiting Nurse Service	Nursing Home Care
			In-Hospital Visits	X-ray and Laboratory Examinations	Office and Home Visits					
All ages										
Blue Cross-Blue Shield	36.0	35.7	40.5	32.8	20.3	2.2	24.2	22.6	26.7	69.5
Insurance companies	60.1	58.9	53.4	60.3	70.2	54.8	71.2	71.5	67.1	24.0
Group policies	39.4	43.4	44.5	55.0	62.5	54.3	66.4	65.8	61.7	13.9
Individual policies	20.7	15.5	8.9	5.3	7.7	.5	4.8	5.7	5.4	10.1
Independent plans	3.9	5.4	6.1	6.9	9.5	43.0	4.6	5.9	6.2	6.5
Under sixty-five										
Blue Cross-Blue Shield	35.1	34.4	39.1	31.5	19.4	2.3	23.9	22.2	26.2	65.2
Insurance companies	61.0	60.2	54.8	61.7	71.2	54.5	71.7	72.0	67.8	28.0
Group policies	40.9	44.8	46.0	56.4	63.5	54.0	66.9	66.2	62.3	16.0
Individual policies	20.1	15.4	8.8	5.3	7.7	.5	4.8	5.8	5.5	12.0
Independent plans	3.9	5.4	6.1	6.8	9.4	43.2	4.4	5.8	6.0	6.8
Sixty-five and over										
Blue Cross-Blue Shield	49.7	58.6	62.7	58.1	42.5	1.5	34.6	33.5	41.5	93.2
Insurance companies	46.4	36.0	30.8	34.2	46.2	79.4	56.4	56.5	47.6	2.2
Group policies	15.9	18.7	20.3	30.6	39.9	79.4	52.6	51.9	43.8	2.2
Individual policies	30.5	17.3	10.5	3.6	6.3	–	3.8	4.6	3.8	–
Independent plans	3.9	5.4	6.5	7.7	11.3	19.1	9.0	10.0	10.9	4.6

FIGURE 12.2 Percentage of Aged Covered by Health Insurance, 1959

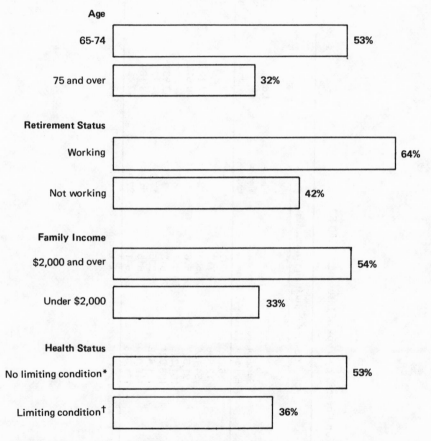

Source: HEW, *Chart Book of Basic Health Economics Data,* Health Economics Series no. 3 (February 1964), chart 19.

* No chronic condition or only those not limiting major activity.
† Chronic condition limiting or making it impossible to carry on major activity.

TABLE 12.3   Population Covered by Type of Insurance, 1940-60

| Year | Covered Population (Thousands) | | | | | Percentage of Persons with Hospital Insurance Who Also Have: | |
	Hospital Expense	Surgical Expense	Regular Medical Expense	Major Medical Expense	Loss of Income	Surgical Insurance	Regular Medical Insurance
1940	12,312	5,350	3,000	—	*	43.5	24.4
1945	32,068	12,890	4,713	—	*	40.2	14.7
1950	76,639	54,156	21,589	—	37,793	70.7	28.2
1955	107,662	91,927	55,506	5,241	39,513	85.4	51.6
1956	115,949	101,325	64,891	8,876	41,688	87.4	56.0
1957	121,432	108,931	71,813	13,262	42,939	89.7	59.1
1958	123,038	111,435	75,395	17,375	41,870	90.6	61.3
1959	127,896	116,944	82,615	21,850	43,169	91.4	64.6
1960	131,962	121,045	87,541	27,448	42,436	91.7	66.3

Source: HEW, *Medical Care Financing and Utilization*, Health Economics Series no. 1 (1962), p. 91.

* Not available.

covered by group supplemental major medical policies. Over two-thirds had maximum benefits of $10,000 or more. The vast majority (94 percent) of the policies had some kind of "corridor" or deductible amount. Approximately 70 percent of those covered (employees and dependents) had deductibles of $100; 12 percent had smaller deductibles, and 15 percent had larger. About two-thirds of the covered population had a coinsurance arrangement of 80-20 (80 percent of the costs paid by the insurer, 20 percent borne by the individual).

Nearly four-fifths of the people covered by comprehensive major medical benefits were under "all cause plans"; the remainder were under "each cause plans." More than nine-tenths of the insured were covered for maximum benefits of $10,000 or more; one-fourth were covered for $20,000 or more. About two-thirds of those covered by comprehensive major medical policies had some full-payment coverage, generally for hospital or surgical expense.

Regional Coverage

Private insurance company coverage does not vary by regions nearly as much as Blue Cross and Blue Shield do. (Of course, percentage differences from minimum to maximum are larger by states than by regions.) For hospital benefits, Blue Cross enrolled 80 percent in Rhode Island as compared to 12 percent in New Mexico.

Of the total population in 1960, 31 percent were Blue Cross members. The Northeast region was highest in the proportion of Blue Cross members to total population (49 percent), and the West and Southwest were lowest (only 13 percent). Admission rates per thousand persons and days per thousand persons were higher for Blue Cross subscribers than for the total population, but the average length of stay was approximately the same (see table 12.4).[11]

Large differences are revealed in special categories. Thus a day at a hospital for obstetrical patients under Blue Cross cost a minimum of $22.79 in 1961 in Rhode Island and a maximum of $55.92 in Los Angeles. The difference was 145 percent.[12] Differences in coverage are not tied wholly to those in per capita income. The range is greater for coverage than for differences in premium income. Table 12.5 shows numerous comparisons of minimum and maximum values.

Insurance Coverage and Income

As might be expected, insurance coverage rises with income. For example, only 34 percent of the people with family incomes of less

TABLE 12.4   Blue Cross and Total Population Hospital Use by Region, 1960

	Total	North-east	Middle West	South and Southwest	Northern Plains	West and Southwest
Percentage of population in Blue Cross	31	49	39	18	27	13
Admissions per thousand persons						
Total population	128	126	129	126	147	121
Blue Cross	139	126	141	154	164	146
Days per thousand persons						
Total population	974	1,110	1,017	832	1,129	794
Blue Cross	1,060	1,025	1,164	995	1,194	881
Average length of stay (days)						
Total population		7.61	8.83	7.87	6.62	7.66	6.56
Blue Cross		7.63	8.11	8.23	6.47	7.27	6.04

Sources: HEW, *Medical Care Financing and Utilization,* Health Economics Series no. 1 (1962), p. 118; Blue Cross Association, "Utilization Report, Second Quarter, 1961," *Statistical Bulletin no. 2F,* table 4, p. 6.

than $2,000 have hospital insurance, but 88 percent of those with incomes of $10,000 and over are covered. Enrollment is higher for whites than for nonwhites; for those employed than for the unemployed; and for white-collar workers than for laborers (for example, 84 percent of professional workers and managers are covered, while only 60 percent of farm laborers are). Attachment to the labor market is a very important source of medical coverage.

In part, the regional variations in coverage are related to regional variations in income per family or per capita. But an examination of the relationship of income and coverage does not reveal a consistent result. Many more families with incomes of less than $4,000 have coverage of hospital expenses than do families with incomes over $7,000. But those earning more than $7,000 have more comprehensive coverage. The figures for these types of coverage are given in table 12.6.

Inadequate Coverage and Benefits

Private health insurance plans do not provide complete coverage for hospital care and physicians' services that are associated with hospitalization. A major medical plan offered by Connecticut General

TABLE 12.5 Minimum and Maximum Benefits and Coverage by Region

Item	Year	Minimum		Maximum		Percentage Difference
		Amount	Region	Amount	Region	
Per capita premium income	1968	$26.76	West South Central	$49.35	Middle Atlantic	82%
Per capita personal income	1968	$15.92	East South Central	$27.77	West	74%
Percentage covered by Blue Shield hospital benefits	1968	18.3%	West South Central	54.9%	Middle Atlantic	200%
Percentage covered by Blue Shield surgical benefits	1968	16.7%	West South Central	51.3%	New England	208%
Percentage covered by Blue Cross-Blue Shield	1960	13.0%	West	49.0%	New England	277%
Per capita premium income of insurance companies	1968	$39.90	Middle Atlantic	$66.90	West South Central	66%
Hospital admissions per 1,000, Blue Cross	1960	12.6	Northeast	16.4	North Plains	30%

Sources: HEW, *Medical Care Financing and Utilization,* Health Economics Series no. 1 (1962), p. 118; *Enrollment and Finance of Blue Cross and Blue Shield* (1968), p. 3; *Health Insurance Coverage of Adults Who Died in 1964 or 1965,* Series 22, no. 10, p. 9.

TABLE 12.6 Coverage for Hospital Care and Comprehensive Care by Income and Region, 1961-63

	Percentage Covered			
	Hospital Care		Hospital, Surgical, and Physician's Visit Care	
	Family Income		Family Income	
Region	$4,000 and Less	$7,000 and More	$4,000 and Less	$7,000 and More
Northeast	15.3	5.9	11.0	18.1
North Central	10.5	6.1	8.9	11.3
South	10.7	4.6	11.5	14.9
West	7.5	3.3	36.4	45.0

Source: Adapted from HEW, *Medical Care Financing and Utilization,* Health Economics Series no. 1-A (1962), p. 55.

begins paying for covered services after the consumer has paid a $750 deductible. A similar plan by Prudential offers major medical plans with deductibles ranging from $500 to $2,000. A group Blue Cross plan requires the policy holder to pay 20 percent of the hospital bill after seventy days. Innumerable additional cases could be listed.

Many policies will not insure or will only partially insure the ill. Blue Cross states in its policy, "If at the time your application is reviewed a condition is found which excludes you from enrollment, you may be given an opportunity to join with a waiver for that condition." In other words, if a person has an illness (such as diabetes or heart trouble), medical expenses will be covered for other illnesses only.

The elderly, under experience rating, pay more for their insurance. A Prudential policy offering hospital coverage costs $318.36 per year for a twenty-six-year-old woman and $482.36 per year for a sixty-eight-year-old woman.

Every insurance policy leaves many medical services uncovered or partially covered. The services most frequently uncovered are dental care, outpatient psychiatric care, preventive medicine, and outpatient drugs. Only 2.6 percent of the people under sixty-five years old are covered for dental benefits, for example.

Insurance spokesmen claim that policy provisions for deductibles, uncovered services, and partially covered care prevent the policy holder from "overusing" health facilities, since he has to pay for part of his own care. In reality, the need to make out-of-pocket payments prevents many people from using *needed* health care services.

The enormous expenses now incurred for medical care are not getting any smaller. The average person is insured for less than 40 percent of his health care costs, and costs continue to rise. This can mean unexpected health care expenditures of $2,000 for the $15,000-to-$20,000 income group, or $300 for the $5,000 income group, which may be catastrophic.

In 1969, the daughter of two federal government employees had a sudden attack of intestinal disease with complications in the liver and lungs. She was hospitalized for forty-four days, resulting in a bill of $7,571. Even with her parents' comparatively good federal health insurance, the family had to pay $1,550 out of pocket.[13]

Tables 12.7 and 12.8 illustrate substantial noncoverage of important categories. Coverage for the items listed in table 12.7 ranges from 50 to 80 percent; for dental care it is 6 percent and for prescribed drugs and nursing care it is a little more than 50 percent. A much smaller proportion of those sixty-five and over are covered than of all ages (see table 12.8). For example, 80 percent of the population at all ages have hospital coverage, but only 51 percent of those sixty-five and over. In 1970, gross enrollment was 210 million people, but only 96 million were covered for physicians' office and home visits and only 12 million were covered for dental care. Potential gains are substantial in these areas. Possibilities are also revealed by the coverages of each type of insurance organization—e.g., hospital care with a coverage of 49 percent for Blue Cross-Blue Shield; accident and health is 46 percent, and independents 4 percent. There clearly is much room for improvement.

TABLE 12.7   Percentage of Population Covered by Private Health Insurance, 1970

Type of Coverage	Population Covered
Hospital care, civilian population	80%
Physicians' services, surgical	78%
Physicians' services, in-hospital visits	72%
X-ray and laboratory examinations	70%
Out-of-hospital care	50%

Source: M. S. Mueller, "Private Health Insurance in 1970: Population, Coverage, Enrollment and Financial Experience," *Social Security Bulletin*, February 1972, p. 4.

TABLE 12.8   Coverage of Total Population and Aged

Type of Coverage	Population Covered	
	All Ages	65 and Over
Hospital care	80%	51 %
X-ray and laboratory costs	70%	37 %
Dental care	6%	0.6%
Out-of-hospital care	50%	16 %

Insurance Organizations

Blue Cross and Blue Shield Coverage

According to a 1970 HEW study, the benefits of the most widely held Blue Cross and Blue Shield contracts are largely focused on hospital inpatient care. The plans allow a specific number of hospital days and cover all or most of the charges for special hospital services. They provide some coverage of surgery, obstetrics, and in-hospital medical visits. The coverage outside the hospital is noticeably meager, however. Fewer than half the plans provide basic coverage of X-ray and laboratory examinations for ambulatory patients. Only a few plans provide basic coverage of physicians' office and home services. There is no coverage of outpatient drugs or appliances. Nursing service benefits are rare, and preventive care and health maintenance services are not covered. Most of the plans cover care in mental hospitals and tuberculosis hospitals, but on a very restricted basis.[14]

In the late 1940s, insurance companies began to offer major medical coverage built on the principle that all types of health care expenses contributing to the costs of potentially major or catastrophic illness should be covered. Under major medical contracts, physicians' office and home visits, out-of-hospital drugs, appliances, and private duty nursing were first covered.

In recent years, change has proceeded at an accelerated rate. Coverage of hospital care for 365 days has become common. Blue Cross-Blue Shield coverage of out-of-hospital X-ray and laboratory costs has greatly increased. Coverage of treatment for mental illness has improved, although it is still far below general hospital coverage. Services that insurance spokesmen, twenty years ago, held could not be covered—such as doctors' office visits and dental care—are now included in policies.[15]

With prepayment of health expenses, the low- and middle-income families give medical care a much higher priority in their spending budgets than would otherwise be necessary.[16] Most people with major medical coverage "have some protection against practically all types of health care expenses, other than those for dental care, eyeglasses, routine health checkups and nursing home care."[17]

A problem arises in group major medical insurance plans: these policies provide reimbursement of 78 to 80 percent of the charges incurred—if customary and reasonable. As this type of insurance grows, "a point may be reached at which charges not paid or reimbursed by insurance will cease to provide a standard of usual, customary and reasonable charges."[18]

Commercial Insurers and Independent Plans

A 1970 survey reports that relative outlays for physicians' services were much larger for independent health plans than for health insurance generally.[19] Union and community plans account for the largest outlays by independent plans. Their coverage of services is wider than that of other types of insurance. Unions are especially strong in coverage of services other than hospital and physician care (see table 12.9).

There are large differences in the financial experiences of various independent health insurance plans. For example, in seven categories of plans, benefit expenditures ranged from 82.1 percent to 97.5 percent of income.[20]

An examination of premium income also points to relative gains of commercial insurance companies over Blue Cross-Blue Shield. In 1962, the Blues received 42 percent of the total premium income, whereas insurance companies obtained 51 percent. Moreover, insurance companies enrolled almost 30 percent under the expensive individual policies; the Blues apparently enrolled about half as

TABLE 12.9 Percentage Covered for Specific Services by Independent Plans

Type of Service	Percentage of Enrollees Covered	
	Community Plans	Union Plans
Surgical-obstetrical services	98.5	72.2
Physicians' home calls	98.4	33.1
Drugs out of hospital	8.2	43.4

many, proportionally, under individual contracts. In recent years, government coverage in general has tended to stabilize the relative share of private insurance companies.[21]

Insurance and the Medical Economy

Insurance has had a large impact on the market for medical services. Private insurance and, in recent years, government insurance have greatly added to the flow of cash to medical markets. The increase has been so great that a disproportionate share of the additional funds has gone into rising prices and rising incomes of the purveyors of medical services, while a disappointing share has gone to provide additional services.

In part, the erosion of new funds stems from two factors: (1) excessive use of the system of compensating purveyors on the basis of customary and reasonable charges, and (2) the tendency of third parties to function inadequately as controlling forces for economical purchasing and high quality services. Under escalating demand, the tendency is to overplay the financial problems and underplay the provision of adequate facilities and manpower. As third-party payments grow to the point where they provide 80 to 90 percent of hospital costs, price control and quality control become increasingly difficult.

Attachment to the Labor Market

Insurance companies have also improved their relative position because they find it easier to deal with large national groups than their competitors do. Undoubtedly the most important source of medical insurance comes from labor negotiations. In 1954 total contributions of employers and employees under employment benefit plans amounted to almost $7 billion. In 1964 these contributions totaled more than $17 billion, with benefits itemized as shown in table 12.10.

From 1954 to 1964 the percentage of the population covered by this type of benefit increased greatly. For example, the proportion of wage and salary workers covered for hospitalization rose from 59 percent to 73 percent. Contributions increased from 0.65 percent to 1.18 percent of wages and salaries (see table 12.11).

TABLE 12.10   Employer-Employee Benefits, 1964

	Amount (Thousands)
All wage and salary workers	
Life insurance and death benefits	$2,039
Hospitalization	3,804
Surgical and regular medical	1,846
Major medical expense	965
Workers in private industry	
Temporary disability benefits and sick leave	1,369
Retirement	6,890

Source: Adapted from HEW, *Medical Care Financing and Utilization*, Health Economics Series no. 1-A (1967), p. 45.

Financial Experience

Premiums, Claims, and Expenses

Insurance companies depend primarily on premiums for income and use this income primarily to cover losses (claims) and operating expenses. As losses rise in relation to premium income and as operating expenses decline, the policy holders obtain an increasing share of premium income. Table 12.12 gives a few statistics on the changes that occurred from 1950 to 1966. The large rise in losses (claims) was counterbalanced by the reductions in operating expenses and underwriting gains.

In 1966, commercial insurance companies received $5.4 billion in premium income from group plans, roughly 8 1/2 times the 1950 figure. In this same period, claims increased from 76.5 percent to 87.8 percent of premiums (see table 12.13). This rise in claims as a proportion of income is explained by the reduction in operating expenditures and underwriting gains. In absolute terms, claims increased $538 million. Claims against Blue Cross increased much less—4.9 percent or $175 million. Blue Cross's subscription income rose from $434,000 to $3,711,000 from 1950 to 1966, a rise 7 1/2 times. Thus, the rise of premium income was roughly equal, proportionally, for Blue Cross and the commercial insurance companies, but the latter provided a greater return (claims were a higher percentage of premiums) than Blue Cross through their reductions in operating expenses and greater decline in underwriting gains. By

TABLE 12.11 Coverage and Contributions under Employee-Benefit Plans, 1954–64

Year	Life Insurance and Death	Accidental Death and Dismemberment	Hospitalization	Surgical	Regular Medical	Major Medical Expense	Temporary Disability, Including Formal Sick Leave	Supplemental Unemployment	Retirement
			Percentage of All Workers Covered					Percentage of Workers in Private Industry Covered	
1954	48.6	26.4	58.8	52.6	32.1	1.5	50.0	–	31.0
1956	52.4	30.4	62.8	58.5	40.0	6.3	50.3	4.1	34.4
1957	54.6	32.2	64.7	61.0	43.4	9.0	50.4	3.8	36.7
1958	56.7	33.4	66.5	62.9	46.0	11.2	49.7	3.6	39.3
1959	58.0	34.2	66.4	63.6	48.7	13.6	49.4	3.8	40.3
1960	58.1	35.5	68.7	65.9	51.0	16.6	49.0	3.4	42.3
1961	60.5	36.2	71.5	68.5	54.6	19.7	49.3	3.6	44.5
1962	60.3	37.4	71.4	68.4	54.9	21.3	49.2	3.6	45.1
1963	61.5	40.1	73.1	70.0	56.8	23.8	49.5	3.6	45.9
1964	63.5	42.2	73.0	70.1	58.3	24.9	49.9	3.6	46.4
			Percentage of All Wages and Salaries Contributed					Percentage of Wages and Salaries in Private Industry Contributed	
1954	0.39	0.02	0.65	0.37		0.01	0.48	–	2.17
1956	.46	.02	.73	.41		.04	.48	0.07	2.23
1957	.47	.02	.79	.45		.07	.51	.09	2.38
1958	.51	.03	.85	.47		.12	.53	.06	2.45
1959	.52	.03	.90	.48		.14	.51	.06	2.52
1960	.54	.03	.96	.49		.18	.53	.05	2.47
1961	.58	.03	1.05	.54		.24	.53	.05	2.47
1962	.59	.03	1.10	.56		.26	.54	.07	2.45
1963	.62	.03	1.14	.55		.28	.53	.06	2.46
1964	.63	.03	1.18	.57		.30	.51	.05	2.56

Sources: "Ten Years of Employee-Benefit Plans," *Social Security Bulletin*, April 1966, table 2, p. 7; HEW, *Medical Care Financing and Utilization,* Health Economics Series no. 1-A (1967), p. 46.

TABLE 12.12 Increase in Losses and Decrease in Operating Expenses and Underwriting Gains, 1950-66

Insurance Plan	Percentage Change		
	Losses	Operating Expenses	Underwriting Gains
Commercial companies	+11.3%	−2.9%	−8.4%
Blue Cross	+ 4.9%	−3.5%	−1.6%

Sources: HEW, Office of Research and Statistics, *The Health Insurance Business of Insurance Companies, 1948-66* (1968), table 7; HEW, Office of Research and Statistics, *Enrollment and Finances of Blue Cross and Blue Shield Plans, 1968* (December 8, 1969), table 8.

1968, the Blues had accumulated reserves of almost $1.4 billion. Large reserves are needed to deal with rising costs, as premiums are increased sluggishly. Blue Shield's ratio of operating expenses to subscription income is almost twice that of Blue Cross (see table 12.14).

The subscription income of all insurance organizations is shown in table 12.15. For Blue Cross, as the percentage of subscription income represented by claim expenses rose from 88 percent to 96 percent, operating expenses dropped from 8.4 to 5.7 percent of subscription income.

Commercial health insurance claims use up most of their premium income (see table 12.16). Claims for Blue Cross-Blue Shield together were 91.9 percent of premium income in 1966. For commercial insurance company group and individual plans together, claims were 81.9 percent of premiums. Hence enrollees in the Blues got much more of their premiums back than insurance company subscribers did. This is explained largely by the great number of individual policies carried by the commercial companies, and it reflects the relative overcoverage of hospital care as against physicians' services by the Blues. Benefits from the commercial companies suffer because of the large emphasis put upon factors such as coinsurance, which force consumers to pay a large share of their medical costs themselves.

Another interesting aspect of competition among insurance organizations relates to their retentions, which are used for operating expenditures, additions to reserves, and profits. The commercial companies retain substantially higher percentages of income than the Blues. For example, in 1964 retentions by Blue Cross-Blue Shield

TABLE 12.13 Premiums, Losses, and Expenses of Commercial Group Plans, 1948-66

Year	Amount (Millions)				Ratio to Premiums Earned		
	Premiums Earned	Losses Incurred	Expenses Incurred	Net Underwriting Gain	Losses Incurred	Expenses Incurred	Underwriting Gain
1948	$ 391	$ 284	$ 64	$43	72.6	16.5	10.9
1949	476	353	76	46	74.2	16.1	9.8
1950	633	484	99	50	76.5	15.7	7.8
1951	845	732	123	-10	86.6	14.6	-1.2
1952	1,003	866	137	*	86.4	13.6	†
1953	1,235	1,058	162	16	85.6	13.1	1.3
1954	1,377	1,132	202	43	82.2	14.7	3.1
1955	1,581	1,335	221	25	84.4	14.0	1.6
1956	1,881	1,620	252	9	86.1	13.4	0.5
1957	2,179	1,924	*	*	88.3	‡	‡
1958	2,334	2,045	315	-26	87.6	13.5	-1.1
1959	2,598	2,282	349	-33	87.8	13.4	-1.2
1960	2,922	2,552	384	-14	87.4	13.1	-0.5
1961	3,191	2,794	427	-29	87.5	13.4	-0.9
1962	3,548	3,110	462	-25	87.7	13.0	-0.7
1963	3,910	3,449	512	-50	88.2	13.1	-1.3
1964	4,390	3,881	565	-56	88.4	12.9	-1.3
1965	4,914	4,352	613	-51	88.6	12.4	-1.0
1966	5,424	4,761	694	-31	87.8	12.8	-0.6

Source: HEW, Office of Research and Statistics, *The Health Insurance Business of Insurance Companies, 1948-66* (1968), table 7.

* Less than $500,000.
† Less than 0.05 percent.
‡ Data not available.

TABLE 12.14   Income, Claims, and Expenses of Blue Cross-Blue Shield, 1968

Item	Blue Cross		Blue Shield	
	Amount (Thousands)	Ratio to Subscription Income	Amount (Thousands)	Ratio to Subscription Income
Earned subscription income	$3,711,798		$1,709,548	
Total income	3,776,487		1,747,867	
Claims expense	3,571,797	96.2	1,481,070	86.6
Operating expense	211,698	5.7	180,154	10.5
Net income (underwriting gain)	−7,008	−1.9*	86,643	2.8*
Reserves	801,389		578,390	

Source: HEW, Office of Research and Statistics, *Enrollment and Finances of Blue Cross and Blue Shield Plans, 1968* (December 8, 1969), p. 8.

* Ratios to total income are: Blue Cross, −0.2; Blue Shield, 5.0.

were 5.6 percent of income; for insurance companies generally they were 19.1 percent, and for individual contracts of insurance companies they were 45.5 percent (see table 12.17).

Roughly one-third of the premium income earned in 1966 by commercial insurers came from individual policies. The major items were accident and health, noncancelable accident and health, and hospital and medical. For those three types of policies, the losses incurred ranged from 46 percent to 59 percent of premiums.[22]

From 1960 to 1966 insurance premiums increased, especially for major medical policies (see table 12.18). The large relative increase for group policies also stands out. This suggests the increasing impact

TABLE 12.15   Subscription Income of All Insurers, 1966

Organization	Amount
Total	$10,561,000
Blue Cross	3,086,000
Blue Shield	1,242,000
Commercial insurance companies	
Group plans	3,987,000
Endowment	1,608,000
Independent health plans	611,000

TABLE 12.16   Ratio of Claims and Expenses to Income, All Insurers, 1966

	Percentage of Premium Income	
Organization	Claims	Operating Expenses
Blue Cross	93.4	4.9
Blue Shield	88.0	9.7
Commercial insurance companies		
Group plans	93.1	12.8
Individual contracts	54.4	43.2
Independent health plans	90.7	6.1

Sources: HEW, *Private Health Insurance and Medical Care Conference Papers* (1968); HEW, Office of Research and Statistics, *The Health Insurance Business of Insurance Companies, 1948-66* (1968), table 7.

of large contracts.[23] From 1950 to 1965, benefits under commercial companies' group policies increased by 9 times; individual and family policy benefits increased by 2-2/3 times. This relative expansion of group benefits is indeed welcome.

The commercial companies advanced at an uneven pace. From 1945 to 1966 the number of companies increased from 145 to 1,000 (or 6 times); health care coverage rose from $89 million to $3,871 million (41 times); and wages rose from $116 million to $1,052 million (8 times). These statistics point to the increasing relative gains for health care as against programs that replace wages lost on account of illness.

The hospital benefits paid by commercial insurers rose 32 times, and surgical benefits 19 times. Marked increases also occurred in major medical supplemental policies, but this became a substantial item only in the late 1950s. In this period, the advances of commercial companies were striking, especially in hospital coverage.[24]

Effect of Group Size

As might be expected, Blue Cross benefits are a higher percentage of subscription income for larger group coverage than for individual or smaller group plans, and operating expenses tend to decline as group size increases (see table 12.19).

The twenty-five largest commercial insurance companies, which account for most premiums earned ($4.1 billion), show the possibilities of paying out more in claims by cutting expenses of operations (see table 12.20). Note the range of expense ratios—from 6.5 percent

TABLE 12.17   Benefits and Retentions as Percentages of Income, All Insurers, 1964

	Percentage of Income					
	Benefits			Retentions		
Organization	Total	Hospital Care	Physicians' Services	Total	Hospital Care	Physicians' Services
Total	87.2	88.7	84.1	12.8	11.3	15.9
Blue Cross-Blue Shield plan	94.4	96.0	90.4	5.6	4.0	9.6
Blue Cross	96.1	96.2	92.1	3.9	3.8	7.9
Blue Shield	90.3	88.9	90.4	9.7	11.1	9.6
Insurance companies	80.9	81.9	79.1	19.1	18.1	20.9
Group	91.7	95.5	86.2	8.3	4.5	13.8
Individual	54.5	54.3	55.0	45.5	45.7	45.0
Independent plans	90.2	89.8	90.3	9.8	9.9	9.7
Community	90.5	90.6	90.4	9.5	9.5	9.5
Employer-employee union	89.9	89.9	89.9	10.1	10.1	10.1
Medical society	85.7	100.0	80.0	14.3	*	20.0
Dental society	100.0	—	100.0	*	—	*
Private group clinics	84.3	84.0	84.4	15.7	16.0	15.6

Sources: HEW, *Medical Care Financing and Utilization,* Health Economics Series no. 1-A (1967), table 36; adapted from Social Security Administration, "Private Health Insurance in the United States: An Overview," *Social Security Bulletin,* December 1965, table 7, p. 19.

*Less than $100,000.

to 25.7 percent of income. Substantial cuts by the high expense companies would provide more funds for financing claims.

Unsolved Problems in Private Health Insurance

It is generally agreed that health insurance benefits are inadequate. It is certain the situation will not improve when the costs of services per capita are rising from 5 percent to 7 percent a year. In other words, annual increases in benefits are required just to maintain the status quo.

TABLE 12.18   Increases in Premiums, 1960-65

Type of Policy	Percentage Rise
All	58
Major medical	146
Group	70
Individual and family	61

TABLE 12.19   Expenses by Group Size

Group Size	Percentage of Income	
	Claims	Operating Expenses
Enrollment under 100,000	89.0	7.6
Enrollment of 1,000,000 or more	95.6	4.4

Source: HEW, *Financial Experience of Health Insurance Organizations in the United States,* Research Report no. 12 (1968), table 3.

Various approaches have been suggested to improve the benefit structure. One alternative is to introduce postpayments—that is, to finance benefits to some extent by exploiting the consumer credit market as a supplement to voluntary prepayment.

The theory behind the postpayment program would be to cover benefits that are required but not actually covered by prepayment plans. The postpayment is in fact a line of credit or a loan adequate to cover the difference between benefits financed by prepayment and benefits not covered. These benefits are estimated to total in the range of $2 billion to $20 billion. The medical expenses that might be financed by postpayment are suggested by the services now covered by private insurance.[25]

How much additional coverage will be obtained will depend on the comprehensiveness of the benefits sought, the number who participate, the recourse to corridors (deductibles) and coparticipation clauses, and the impact of postpayment on voluntary prepayment plans. In general, postpayment premiums for specific additional services would be substantially lower than premiums for equal additional coverage under prepayment programs.[26]

TABLE 12.20   Maximum and Minimum Expenses of Commercial Insurers

	Percentage of Premiums	
	Claims	Operating Expenses
All	90.1	10.8
Maximum	94.7	25.7
Minimum	76.7	6.5

Source: HEW, Office of Research and Statistics, *The Health Insurance Business of Insurance Companies, 1948-66* (1968), table 10.

Another approach to improve benefits is to contain the inflationary forces. Chapter 7 on prices deals with this to some extent. Rising costs are largely translated into higher prices. For example, increasing capital costs have an impact on prices. Representatives of hospital interests have urged that capital investments be heavily financed by government in order to reduce to a minimum their effect on charges to patients.[27]

A third possible route is the extension of coverage through employer-employee negotiations for health insurance. In a recent year it was estimated that three-quarters of the coverage for health insurance was provided through such negotiations. Since the degree of coverage and the percentage of wages thus mobilized vary greatly, maximum exploitation of this area could be fruitful. It is of some interest here that the governor of New York recently proposed a payroll tax negotiated by labor and management that would be used to finance medical insurance, as a means of relieving the government of heavy health care outlays.[28]

There are many deterrents to liberalization of benefits. One is the rate at which the cost of benefits is expanding and the general tendency of expenditures to increase more rapidly than projected. Apparently the Department of Health, Education, and Welfare was criticized during the gestation period of Medicare for underestimating the likely costs. Critics extrapolated recent increases in hospital costs, and found that the projected increases would exceed the increases in wages. Hence, hospital costs would ultimately absorb all rises in income. The HEW actuaries held that restraints would be put on the rise of hospital costs before such a situation occurred, and that projection of the most recent rises in hospital costs was unjustified. Yet the critics had a point, in the extreme: the history of welfare programs is one of costs greatly exceeding estimates made before enactment of the program.[29]

Another deterrent to liberalization of benefits is the failure of manpower and facilities to increase in response to increases in financing. The Medicare and Medicaid programs, though supportable for many reasons, probably would have been much more effective if more time had been available for adjustments to facilitate such massive programs. (Professor Eveline Burns has developed a theory about the pace at which new and complicated programs should be introduced.[30])

Insurance companies have always favored coverage of hospital services and physicians' services in hospitals. In a recent year these services accounted for 70 percent of benefits. With hospital care so costly, an obvious way of increasing the real benefits accruing from rising premiums is to cultivate substitute services that are less costly. Hence the recent stress in many plans on such services as home care and extended care facilities.

An interesting approach to saving costly hospital days is a Blue Cross proposal for preadmission testing. This would mean a substitution of outpatient laboratory and X-ray testing for inpatient testing. It would save hospital days and cut costs as well, because more testing could be scheduled for "slack times." Blue Cross claims it could finance out-of-hospital testing as it now finances in-hospital tests.[31]

Still another approach to saving hospital costs is the capitation method of reimbursing hospitals. The original Blue Cross capitation plan provided that each subscriber would pay a small amount each month to Baylor University. But the multiplicity of individual hospital-sponsored prepayment plans began to interfere with freedom of choice of physician and hospital. The patient would choose the hospital to which he was paying a premium, not the hospital recommended by the doctor. The inefficiency of separate enrollment drives also became troublesome. Hence multiple-hospital plans emerged, and Blue Cross maintained their characteristics: regular payment by subscribers, service benefits, comprehensive benefits, community rating, and hospital sponsorship. But one important change occurred: "The basis of payment to the *hospital* was changed from *per subscriber* (sick and well alike) to *per diem* for those subscribers who were patients." The hospital then had an interest in seeing enrollees stay for longer periods, because this brought more income. This resulted in unnecessary admissions, excessive stays, and duplication of facilities.

Group-Practice Health Plans

Community group-practice plans account for only about 4 percent of insurance enrollment today. They are important because of their experimentation, their comprehensive coverage of benefits, and their attempts at preventive medicine in contrast to "mainstream" medicine. Group prepaid voluntary comprehensive insurance plans provide coverage for many services that are underfinanced by the Blues. Yet, despite their great promise, their growth has been disappointing. In thirty-five years it has merely matched the growth of the population.

There are various reasons for this disappointment. One is clearly the failure of group-practice plans to enlist the cooperation of the family doctor. The plans must establish a position for the family doctor vis-á-vis the specialist that would induce cooperation among family doctor, pediatrician, and obstetrician. It is hoped that, through the leadership of teaching hospitals and medical schools, this situation will be corrected.

One of the most successful prepaid group-practice plans is the Kaiser-Permanente Medical Care Program—sometimes dubbed the model health maintenance organization. Kaiser-Permanente has been operating in California for over thirty years. Its membership exceeds 2.5 million, in California, Portland, Hawaii, Denver, and Cleveland. Other smaller groups are the Health Insurance Plan (HIP) in New York, the Ross-Loos Clinic in southern California, and the Group Health Cooperative in Puget Sound, Washington.

All of these groups provide hospital coverage. With one exception they do not provide benefits for nursing home or extended care facilities. They all provide comprehensive coverage for physicians' services, but none pays for home nursing. Partial charges are made for prescribed drugs outside the hospital and for immunizations and injections. In-hospital visits, diagnostic X-ray and laboratory work, X-ray therapy, and physical therapy are also partially covered. Outpatient psychiatric care and dental care are not covered.

Advantages

Group-practice plans have lowered hospital and surgery over-utilization and reduced costs. Kaiser-Permanente, for example, can provide a package of services at lower charges than identical services would cost in "mainstream" medicine. It reduces costs by lowering the use of services by its members. Kaiser members spend half as many days in the hospital as a similar proportion of Blue Cross-Blue Shield subscribers (compare the Blues and group practice plans in figure 12.21). Surgery for tonsillitis and gynecological problems performed by Kaiser is distinctly lower than in fee-for-service practice (see figure 12.21 and table 12.22).

Prepaid group-practice plans characteristically experience markedly

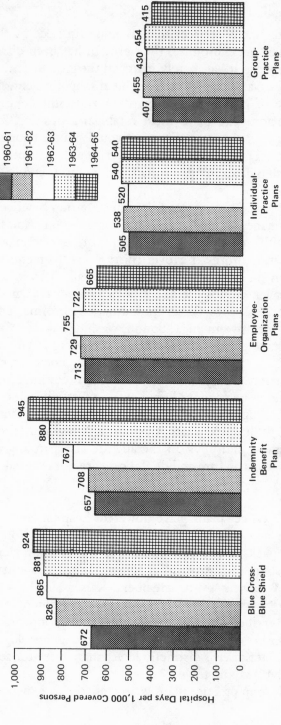

FIGURE 12.21 Hospital Utilization by Federal Employees, 1960-65

Source: G. Perrott and J. Chase, "The Federal Employees Health Benefits Program," *Group Health and Welfare News—Special Supplement,* May 1967.

TABLE 12.22   Hospital Utilization by Age Group, 1962

	Hospital Days per 1,000 Members	
Age	Group Practice	Blue Cross
19-44	345	549
35-44	464	854
45-59	756	1,237
55-64	1,247	1,880
65 and over	1,256	2,220

less utilization of inpatient services. Nonmaternity hospitalization in the contract term ending December 31, 1965, was 415 days per thousand members under the Federal Employees Health Benefits Program compared with 924 days for Blue Cross-Blue Shield subscribers and 945 days for those covered by insurance companies.

Problems of Health Maintenance Organizations

The large group prepaid practices—the health maintenance organizations—tend to lower the availability of services that are not presently in excess. At Kaiser-Permanente, for example, ambulatory care is not easily accessible. Most Kaiser subscribers complain of waiting on the phone to make an appointment, waiting until an appointment is available, and waiting at drop-in and emergency clinics. In a study conducted by the California Council for Health Plan Alternatives, 30 percent of the respondents had to wait more than one month for an appointment, and 27 percent had to wait from one to two hours to see a doctor at a drop-in clinic.[32]

Thus cost reduction goes hand in hand with a general inaccessibility of services. The reason for this is the working of the profit motive. Whether profit-making or technically nonprofit, private corporations have always committed themselves to maximizing their income, reducing their expenditures, and using the surplus for expansion. Private HMOs have an incentive to limit services by hiring an inadequate number of physicians and other personnel so that patients will be discouraged from seeking care. In this way, expenses go down, and surplus goes up.

Although HMOs claim they provide preventive measures so that medical care is less costly for the patient as well as for the physicians in the group practice, in the short run this is not true. Annual Pap smears, breast examinations, blood pressure checks, glaucoma screening, and other valuable early diagnostic procedures cost large amounts of money and require more medical personnel. The savings—in reduced numbers of seriously ill patients—come only many years later, far beyond the projections of HMO planners. Kaiser-Permanente, for example, has been able to offer multiphasic screening because of large federal grants; with cutbacks in the grants, Kaiser is reducing the screening.

Notes

1. Statistics from *Compendium of National Health Expenditures Data* (1972).

2. J. Ridgeway, "Blue Cross," *Ramparts*, May 1971.

3. Ibid.

4. Senate Bill 1182, section 1101 (1971).

5. HEW, *Private Health Insurance Medical Care Conference Papers* (1968), p. 51.

6. Ibid., p. 8 (my calculations).

7. For more information on Blue Cross, see the following: J. Ehrenreich, "The Blue Cross We Bear," *Washington Monthly*, November 1969, pp. 17-26; *New York Times*, August 12, 1969; R. Kotelchuck, "Trying to Shake the Blues," *Health/PAC Bulletin*, March 1971.

8. HEW, *The Benefit Structure of Private Health Insurance*, by L. S. Reed and W. Carr (1968), p. 105.

9. HEW, *Health Insurance Coverage of Those Who Died in 1964 and 1965*, Series 22, no. 10 (1969), p. 8.

10. HEW, *Medical Care Financing and Utilization*, Health Economics Series no. 1-A (1962), p. 50.

11. Ibid, p. 118.

12. HEW, *Maternity Care Utilization and Financing*, Health Economics Series no. 4 (1964).

13. E. Hoyt, *Your Health Insurance: A Story of Failure* (1970).

14. HEW, *Benefit Structure of Private Health Insurance* (1970), p. 43.

15. Ibid., p. 106.

16. Ibid., p. 107.

17. Ibid., p. 78.

18. Ibid., p. 79.

19. HEW, *Health Insurance Plans Other Than Blue Cross or Blue Shield Plans or Insurance Companies, 1970 Survey*.

20. Material in this section is from HEW, *Medical Care Financing and Utilization*, Health Economics Series no. 1-A (1967), p. 42, and HEW, *Independent Health Insurance Plans in the United States, 1965 Survey*, Research Report no. 17 (1966), pp. 6-17, 28-38, 42, 50.

21. HEW, *Financial Experience of Health Insurance Organizations of the United States*, Research Report no. 12 (1966), pp. 51, 55.

22. HEW, Office of Research and Statistics, *The Health Insurance Business of Insurance Companies, 1948-66* (1968), table 6.

23. See HEW, *Medical Care Financing and Utilization*, Health Economics Series no. 1-A (1967), p. 40.

24. HEW, Office of Research and Statistics, *The Health Insurance Business of Insurance Companies, 1948-66* (1966), tables 8, 9.

25. R. D. Eilers, "Post Payment Medical Expense Coverage: A Proposed Salvation for Insured and Insurer," *Medical Care*, May-June 1969, tables on pp. 194-95.

26. See discussion in chapter 1.

27. K. Williamson, "Trends in Federal Spending—and Some Predictions," *Hospitals*, October 16, 1968, pp. 67-70.

28. A. M. Somers, "Financing Medical Care in the United States," *New England Journal of Medicine*, September 29, 1966, pp. 702-9; J. M. Stone, "National Compulsory Health Insurance: Time for a Positive Program," *Hospitals*, May 1, 1969, p. 59.

29. Somers, "Financing Medical Care," p. 707.

30. E. Burns, "Health Services for All: Is Health Insurance the Answer?" *American Journal of Public Health*, supplement, January 1969, p. 13.

31. J. C. Troxel, "Pre-admission Testing—a Blue Cross Proposal," *Illinois Medical Journal*, September 1968, pp. 295, 304.

32. J. Carnoy, L. Coffee, and L. Koo, "Corporate Medicine: The Kaiser Health Plan," *Health/PAC Bulletin*, November 1973, pp. 4-18.

13

History of
National Health Insurance

Health insurance is a financing mechanism to guarantee that physicians and hospitals are paid. Health insurance answers one part of the health care crisis—the financial instability of many providers. It helps the medical user only indirectly: a patient will not be turned away simply because he cannot pay his bills. In this sense, most national health insurance proposals would subsidize the incomes of doctors, hospitals, nursing homes, and private insurance companies (except for the Kennedy proposal). Yet a national health insurance program with *broad benefits* will increase the purchasing power of consumers, and this will help reduce the financial barriers to obtaining health care.

National health insurance does not restructure the delivery of health care. It cannot guarantee that there will be doctors and hospitals to provide care for everyone who needs it. It cannot promise that care will be of high quality and offered in a humane way. It cannot pledge that the spiraling costs of health care will be controlled. Nor can national health insurance guarantee that the financial burden of providing health care to everyone who needs it will be shared equitably by the entire population.

Current national health insurance proposals do include provisions to control costs. This is done mostly through financial incentives to providers to deliver care in more "efficient" ways. Prepaid group practice is often cited as the most efficient way to organize the health delivery system, while the fee-for-service system encourages expensive and sometimes unnecessary surgical and laboratory procedures. Efficiency, however, does not ensure high quality health care, and schemes to reduce costs can eliminate necessary services. Under a prepayment arrangement, the provider might profit by discouraging his patients from seeking care or by not giving expensive treatments even when they are needed. Thus, the use of financial incentives to reorganize health care delivery turns out to be an inefficient and expensive way to achieve that goal.

Origins of National Health Insurance

About 100 years ago, European governments began paying for their people's health care. In the United States, a small group of professionals fought national health insurance in 1912.[1] In the 1930s national health insurance proposals were again raised in discussions of new Social Security legislation. At least ten congressional proposals were sponsored between 1939 and 1950. Progress was slow despite the increasing interest of Franklin D. Roosevelt. In 1939, Roosevelt had written "that a comprehensive health program was required as an essential link in our national defense." By 1945, Senators Murray and Wagner and Congressman Dingell had introduced a bill for an ambitious program that was to be financed by a 3 percent payroll tax. Dr. I. S. Falk, an authority in this field, followed with a plan.[2]

The American Medical Association fought national health insurance. Its members feared possible loss of income, especially by high-priced doctors, interference with their freedom of choice, rising government control of their professional activities, and termination of the privilege of refusing patients. The issues were largely ideological. In late 1945, the AMA journal carried an editorial saying:

The insidious strategy that has been employed in recent years, leading towards the culmination by approval of the President of the United States, is clearly apparent.... Since the time when Michael Davis and his associates engineered the formation of the Committee on the Cost of Medical Care, down to the present, a gradual enlistment has been secured in behalf of socialized medicine of every agency that could be induced to combine in a movement towards socialization of the American system of Government. Around their banner have rallied the members of the so-called Boas Physicians Forum, certain Doctors of Philosophy in the field of economics and sociology, the socialist element in the Public Health Association and those employed in governmental health agencies who thirst for increased power and expansion of the bureaus that they serve. Let the people of our country realize that the movement for the placing of American Medicine under the control of the Federal Government through a system of Federal compulsory sickness insurance is the first step towards a regimentation of utilities, of industries, of finance, and eventually of labor itself. This is the kind of regimentation that led to totalitarianism in Germany and led to the downfall of that nation.[3]

In 1949, the AMA, fearing government control over doctors' fees, hired the public relations firm of Whitaker and Baxter to wage a nationwide advertising campaign against national health insurance. The campaign equated national health insurance with socialism. Full-page ads in newspapers and magazines pictured government destroying the doctor-patient relationship. The AMA paid $5 million for advertising and lobbying. National health insurance remained a dead issue throughout most of the 1950s.[4]

In 1949, I appeared before the Senate Subcommittee on Labor and Public Welfare to support national health insurance. The following is a synopsis of my presentation:

In recent years, the pressure for health insurance has greatly increased. There are various explanations. First, this is an age when the people look increasingly to the Government for security. Protection against illness is one manifestation of the desire for security. Second, the public is becoming increasingly aware of the application of the insurance principle: the costs of serious illness are reduced for the population. ("An unlucky sixth of our people . . . pays in one year half the total sickness bills paid by everybody.") In the thirties, one expert observed that one in fifteen requires hospital care in any one year; and these expenditures account for one-half of all medical expenditures.

This leads to the third point, namely, as the Committee on the Cost of Medical Care observed, the quest for medical security stems from the uneven distribution of medical care. The poor experience more illness and receive less care. To cite examples: One survey revealed 282 illnesses per 1,000 persons for those on relief, and 233 per 1,000 for those in comfortable circumstances. Another survey revealed that families on relief or receiving $1,000 income or less received the aid of a physician for disabling illness 78 percent of the time; those with incomes of $5,000 or over, 89 percent. Those over the age of sixty-five experience four times as many days of disabling illness as the population as a whole, but spend only twice as much per capita on medical care.

Fourth, the aging of the population is a relevant consideration. In 1900 this country had but 3 million, or 4 percent of the population, aged sixty-five and over; in 1948, 11 million, or 7-8 percent; by 1975, 18 million, or 11 percent. Medical expenditures are a substantial part of all outlays by the old. As the population ages, the need for medical services will rise greatly; and particularly for those with limited resources. . . .

Fifth, the inadequacy of medical service has put pressure on the Government to do something. This inadequacy arises in part from the high level of employment in recent years, in part from the diversions of manpower to the military, in part from the improved standard of living which is reflected in a desire for more and better medical standards, in part from the failure of medical facilities to expand adequately, and in part from the uneconomical organization of medicine.

In short, many reasons can be adduced for the increased interest in health insurance. The program, I would emphasize, is one for achieving a better distribution of expenditures for medicine and an increased outlay. The country cannot afford to allow private choice to determine total outlays on medicine any more than it does in education. Surely consumers need some guidance when they spend $7.4 billion for medical care and health expenses, as compared to $2.75 billion for tobacco, $2.3 billion for personal care (largely beauty care), $15.5 billion for transportation, $9.4 billion for recreation.

1. *The Need of More Services*

Once the Government subsidizes low-income groups adequately and through insurance assures larger disbursements for medical care, then the pressure on medical facilities will rise. This will result in part because much needed medical care will now be demanded; and in part because once the expenses are pooled, there is a tendency to be wasteful of use of medical facilities. In my opinion the first factor is much more important than the second.

I shall say something presently about the need of additional services, and in this statement I emphasize the need of additional outlays on medicine. But we must italicize the following:

a. The response of trained personnel is a slow process. It has been altogether too slow in the professional medical field. Vigorous legislation is required to increase the personnel.

b. It follows that any rise of outlays in the short run will merely increase the rewards of those already entrenched in the industry or profession (as has largely happened since 1932), unless vigorous measures are taken to improve the organization and make more effective use of trained personnel and physical facilities.

c. Much better use could be made of existing personnel and facilities, thus assuring a rise in services corresponding to the suggested increase in outlays. Furthermore, the training of subsidiary personnel could be accelerated much more quickly and with more immediate results than that of the doctor or dentist. . . .

2. *Past Growth Disappointing*

It is important to provide additional doctors, dentists, and facilities. In the past the expansion of medical facilities has been disappointing. For about forty years the enrollment (around 20,000) and the output of graduates (about 5,000) in medical schools has remained roughly unchanged. Yet in this period the population has increased by more than two-thirds, the money national income by ten times, and the national income in stable dollars by about five times. Indeed, the stabilization of enrollment has partly been a process of raising standards; but there are also signs of restrictionism, of protecting the interests of the present members of the trade union.

3. *The Problem of Pricing*

My object is not to belittle the important service contributed by the medical profession. They have worked hard, put in many more hours, and carried a tremendous responsibility in the last fifteen years. According to figures released by the AMA (Bulletin 67, p. 13), the charge for physicians' services (general, surgeon, specialist) was up by but 36 percent in 1948 as compared with a rise in the consumer price index of 71 percent. This indeed shows restraint on the part of the medical profession. But undoubtedly physicians have had to reduce demand on their services by raising prices; and even these figures may understate the rise, for allowance must be made for increased collections. I make a point that is important, namely, that physicians and dentists account for but one-third of medical expenditures; and any reduction in costs and prices must extend to drugs (with the highest advertising costs in any industry), hospitals, and so on.

The real issue is one of pricing and service. An improved method of financing will make it possible to employ more doctors and dentists. What is required is more business and lower fees per visit.

4. *The Market for Doctors and the Problem of Outlets for the Educated*

At the present time (1949) the country has about 200,000 doctors. This country should be able to support 400,000 doctors at our income levels—in part through making more funds available and in part through a reduction of prices charged.

Much is made of the heavy burdens put upon the budget. But it is well to take account of the rising income and tax receipts; the gains made as recovery from depression conditions emerges; the extent to which medical outlays involve transfers rather than consumption of resources; the favorable effect on income of rising medical outlays. In the mid-1950s when medical programs were being seriously considered, the Federal unified budget rose about $70 billion; by 1971 an estimated $218 billion. In this same period GNP rose from about $350 billion to more than a trillion dollars. Total taxes in relation to GNP in 1972 were estimated at 30 percent for the United States and 43 percent for Great Britain.

What we ask is more total income for medicine; better distribution of services; a diversion of expenditures and employment into this important service area. This is partly a medical problem and particularly one of organization; but it is also part of the great economic problem of finding ways to keep our economic machine from collapsing because of its highly productive efficiency.

In the 1950s, conservative trends in Washington further dulled enthusiasm for national health insurance. President Eisenhower offered only a $25 million reinsurance program to solve a problem that required $75 billion annually by 1971. Appearing before the Senate Committee on Labor and Public Welfare in the 1950s, I again advocated national health insurance because

it is comprehensive in coverage of benefits and people; because it is a vehicle for inducing employers and trade unions in their own interest to pay part of the cost; because it emphasizes preventive medicine and encourages early diagnosis; because it excludes co-insurance; because, properly implemented, it makes available insurance for the low-income groups; because in stressing preventive medicine, it cuts the pressure on hospitals (according to one study it cuts recourse to hospitals by one-half); because it gives the buyer of the service as well as the seller some control over charges and services rendered; because it relieves the physician of the concern over collecting bills and of the association of service and capacity to pay; because, as a result of centralization of facilities and personnel, it cuts overhead and saves the patients much time and energy; because it is the economical, supermarket approach to medicine; because it provides protection for those now excluded who not only suffer thereby but, with the growth of prepayment plans, find themselves discriminated against.

The British Example

Unlike the United States, Great Britain initiated its National Health Service (NHS) operations on July 5, 1948. The legislation enacted in 1946 provided that

a comprehensive national health service will ensure for every citizen that there is available whatever medical treatment he requires, in whatever form he requires it, domiciliary or institutional, general, specialist, or consultant, and will ensure also the provision of dental, ophthalmic and surgical appliances, nursing and midwifery and rehabilitation after accidents.[5]

Financing the British System

The British raise most (about two-thirds) of their health care revenue from the central government and get additional funds from local governments. The public pays very little directly for health services (see table 13.1). Currently each person pays $1 a week to the NHS out of wages and salaries. By comparison, in the United States, public funds provided 29 percent of health expenditures in 1960, and 37 percent in 1968-69.

British welfare policies depend on high taxes and correspondingly higher prices for such items as alcohol and tobacco. These taxes largely finance the welfare programs. Hence the government encourages the public to indulge in fewer luxuries in exchange for more medical care, more education, and more housing. The Englishman who can do without alcohol and tobacco avoids the heavy taxes and still gets his social services. In general, the great achievement of the British government was to provide comprehensive medical services to all, rich and poor.

A comparison of British and American tax policies shows that the British depend much more on consumption taxes. In 1960, 41 percent of the British government's revenues came from these taxes; in the United States, only 15 percent was derived from consumption taxes. Income taxes provided 55 percent of British revenues compared to 83 percent of United States funds.

Gains in Health Care under NHS

It may well be, as Professor Jewkes and other British experts claim, that the promises of NHS to provide comprehensive services have not been fully kept. The major problem has been a failure to build new facilities. The government, pressed by other demands, did not provide

TABLE 13.1 Sources of Revenues for British National Health Service, 1960

Source	Percentage Contributed
Exchequer	68
Partly exchequer and partly local rates	8
Superannuation rates	5
Payments by persons using services (deductibles for drugs)	5
National Health Insurance	14

the hospitals and other facilities needed. Hence patients experience long queues and annoying delays for elective surgery. Yet the British government does spend about 5 percent of its gross national product on NHS.

Despite its shortcomings, gains were also evident under NHS. Medical services became available to more people, diverse services were better integrated, services that had been neglected in the past now attracted more resources, luxury medical procedures were reduced, and use of excess capacity improved. Objective observers commented on these gains, especially the availability of health care to greater numbers of people, even though the quality of services may have deteriorated.

Overall, the British experience seems to me to have been highly successful. Comprehensive medical services have become available to all, with little concern over private financing for these services. Even the medical profession is almost totally in support of the program. Doctors are pleased to be relieved of concern for collecting bills from patients. Every poll seems to show overwhelming—almost unanimous—support by the population and as much as 90 percent of the medical profession.

A 1962 report by a committee of eight medical associations, including the British Medical Association stated: "A full return to purely private general practise, when remuneration is a matter of private arrangement between the patient and his doctor, and where the patient is responsible for the whole of the doctor's fee, is today, in our judgement, neither possible nor desirable."

Rise in Costs

Costs of medical care under the National Health Service have increased much beyond expectations. Yet the increase has been less for NHS than for some other programs. The NHS has achieved economies through improved use of plant, discouragement of luxury medicine, lower expenditures for drugs (about half the United States per capita outlay), and bulk purchasing.

British high officials underestimated the rise in costs. As early as 1950, the Chancellor of the Exchequer warned: "It is clear that it is not possible under existing circumstances to permit any overall increase in the expenditures on the health services. Any expansion in one part of the services must in the future be met by economies, or, if necessary, by contraction in others."[6]

Of course, rising costs were inflated further because large outlays were required to finance heavy backlogs of needed health care services. Pharmaceutical, dental, and ophthalmic services were estimated at 30.8 million pounds in the original presentation in 1948-49 and at 109 million pounds in the revised estimates for 1949-50, indicating both backlogs and early abuses. Expenditures for general practitioner services increased only from 42 million pounds to 47 million pounds, demonstrating the ungenerous treatment of GPs.[7]

Perhaps the most troublesome problem confronting the NHS is the status of the general practitioner. He has inadequate access to the hospitals, and his remuneration is often inadequate, especially in relation to the pay of the consultant (specialist). This is in part due to slow adjustment of incomes to rising prices and wages. In the 1950s the British GP experienced a drop of 20 percent in real income while the whole population averaged a gain of 20 percent. The GP's pay of $8,000 to $10,000 a year currently is earned by assuming a heavy workload—an average total of 2,500 patients under his care and perhaps twenty-five home visits a day.

When the NHS was initiated, the medical profession wanted fees for service, while the government proposed salaries. The fee-for-service plan often leads to excessive visits and procedures, while salaries provide no incentives for high quality services and often encourage doctors to give too little care. A compromise was reached, providing for reimbursement according to the number of patients cared for (capitation). Capitation provides some incentives—for example, it may encourage competition among doctors for patients.

Medicare in the United States

The Campaign for Adoption

In the late 1950s and early 1960s, a vigorous campaign was launched to provide medical aid for the aged. Senators John F. Kennedy and Clinton Anderson and Representative Aime Forand were especially active supporters. But there were disagreements on the recourse to deductibles and coinsurance, on coverage of the medically indigent, on payments for doctors' services, on the chances of rising costs and liberalization of benefits, and on sources of support. These conflicts delayed progress despite the efforts of two congressional committees.

The Kerr-Mills Act, approved in 1960, deals especially with public medical assistance to the aged. It proved to be an obstacle to the advance of Medicare, however. By July 1961, only twelve states were operating under Medical Assistance for the Aged. Even by July 1962, only 102,000 of the 17,000,000 aged were covered, and costs were merely $264 million annually. The benefits allowed were far from generous. The average monthly payment in early 1961 for vendor payments for medical care was $9.54 or 14 percent of monthly assistance payments. State income ceilings under which individuals would qualify for assistance ranged from $100 to $1,800 per year.

Much opposition to the Kerr-Mills Act stemmed from its emphasis on charity, particularly in the "means test" used. A Commission of Public Assistance commented:

Such a Means Test (as administered by a physician) is a far cry from the procedure that any responsible public agency must follow, with its accountability to public auditors, legislative committees, and taxpayers in general. The public agency is expected or required by law to assure itself that only those who meet defined eligibility conditions, receive the benefits of the program. . . . It must require a sworn statement, with legal penalties for false representations, or conduct an investigation to verify the applicant's statement, or do both. The applicant is aware that his economic status will be measured against a standard; that the service he needs and has requested will be granted him only if that standard declares him needy or medically indigent; and that at least his economic life history will be entered upon a public record.[8]

According to the Bureau of Labor Statistics, an aged couple needed $3,000 of income in 1959 ($290 for medical care in large cities and suburban areas); a city worker had to spend $600 on medical care per year. But 31 percent of the city dwellers had incomes under $2,000.[9]

Needs of the Aged

The aged incur more illnesses than others. In the mid-1950s, they constituted 8 percent of the population, but they experienced almost 40 percent of disabling illnesses lasting three months or more, and they accounted for 25 percent of the people in mental institutions.[10]

The population sixty-five and over had six times as many chronic diseases per thousand (77.8) as the younger population (which had 12.8 per thousand). These diseases require large resources for treatment. Furthermore, the old endure many more periods of limited activity than the general population. Thus, in 1957-58, the aged, who made up 7.7 percent of the country's population, accounted for 56 percent of those with limited mobility.[11]

Health expenditure patterns vary by age. The elderly spend relatively more on drugs and hospitals. This is unfortunate, since insurance coverage of drug outlays is modest, and hospital costs are rising more than any other major component of health expenditures (see table 13.2).

With large medical requirements and small incomes, the aged are in great need of health insurance. At the end of 1959, a study showed 67 percent of the whole population covered by insurance but only 46 percent of the old. In addition, a disproportionate number of those sixty-five and over have individual policies, which cost as much as 50 percent more than group insurance. One study revealed that only about half of all aged people maintain their memberships in group plans after retirement.[12]

The old are also affected adversely by the insurers' use of experience rating. When insurance companies set premiums for various population groups according to past claim experience, the old are subjected to higher charges because they incur higher medical expenditures. Insurance companies are trying to improve their coverage of the aged.[13] Thus, those sixty-five and over suffer many deprivations: inadequate insurance, loss of coverage at retirement, limited benefits, higher premiums, and less capacity to pay.

Medicare and Medicaid as Enacted

In 1965, Congress passed legislation establishing Medicare for those over sixty-five and Medicaid for people who are unable to

TABLE 13.2 Average Annual Medical Expenditures by Age, 1958

	All Ages		65 and Over	
	Amount	Percentage	Amount	Percentage
Total	$96.00	99.9	$151	99.9
Physicians' services	36.00	37.5	52	34.4
Drugs and medicines	14.50	15.1	32	21.2
Hospital care	19.00	19.7	36	23.8
Dentist's services	14.50	15.1	6	3.9
Other	12.06	12.5	25	16.6

Source: *The Aged and Aging in the United States,* Senate Report no. 1121 (1960), p. 107.

work or whose incomes are so low that they cannot pay for their medical care.

Medicare is financed by premiums deducted from people's paychecks under Social Security, and used to pay medical bills incurred by the aged. Premiums are equal irrespective of income, and this introduces serious inequities. A premium of $50 is 1 percent of a $5,000 income but only 0.25 percent of a $20,000 income. This is not a supportable theory of taxation. Rates rising with income could be set for Medicare payments.

While Medicare combats the problem of low income and large need among the old, it still leaves substantial burdens on the beneficiary. The program pays on the average only *half* of medical bills; it ignores a sizable portion of charges for physicians' services. Thus, people over sixty-five pay an average of $400 to $500 each year in medical bills not covered by Medicare. Due to the rise in costs in recent years, that is more than the average elderly person paid in total health costs before Medicare was passed.[14]

Medicaid also falls short of meeting the needs of the 40 million poor people in the United States (the government defines "poor" as a family of four earning less than $4,300). Estimates of the number of poor covered at all vary between 20 million and 30 million people. Those who have Medicaid are covered for only certain services, and Medicaid recipients often have a difficult time finding doctors and dentists who will see them.

A 1967 survey by the Social Security Administration throws much light on the medical services available under Medicare.[15] In that year—the first full year of Medicare operations—19 million people were enrolled at some time in the medical insurance program, or about 93 percent of all persons then eligible for hospital insurance benefits under Medicare. Some 15 million people, or four-fifths of all enrollees, had some covered medical services. Charges of $2.2 billion, or $152 per person, were incurred.

The proportion of the aged population using covered services rose with advancing age, from 75 percent for persons aged sixty-five to sixty-nine to 82 percent for those aged seventy-five and older. The average charge was significantly higher for whites ($157) than for others ($86). The average number of visits per person was also higher for whites than for others.

Private health insurance covers some of the gaps in Medicare. In previous years, 37 percent of the aged had private insurance coverage for surgical services and 27 percent had coverage for physicians' visits outside the hospital.[16] Enrollment in and use of supplementary medical insurance vary greatly according to race, sex, and socioeconomic status criteria (see table 13.3). Variations in supplemental medical insurance charges are also significant from group to group (see table 13.4).

Of the persons entitled to Medicare, 81 percent of those also covered under private plans that paid for hospital and surgical services used medical services, while only 75 percent of those without private health insurance used such services. Persons with Medicare who resided in urban areas had a higher utilization rate, paid higher average charges, and used more physicians' visits than others.[17] "Persons not working, with some welfare payments or services and living in the West and in urban areas were more likely to meet the $50 deductible and their average charges were higher than those

TABLE 13.3   Use of Supplementary Medical Insurance

Population Characteristic	Percentage of Enrollees Using Services
Sex	
Men	75
Women	82
Race	
White	79
Other	8
Education	
Less than seven years	76
Nine years or more	78
Health insurance coverage	
Only when confined to bed or home	94
No limitation	74
Living arrangement	
Institutional	93
Living alone	78
Work status	
Not working	79
Working full-time	67
Family income	
Less than $3,000 per year	76
More than $5,000 per year	75
Size of community of residence	
Urban	80
Rural	73

TABLE 13.4 Range of Charges under Supplemental Medical Insurance

Population Characteristic	Minimum Charge	Maximum Charge
Age	$136	$165
Race	157	186
Education	125	156
Health insurance coverage limitations	119	338
Institutional or private living arrangements	124	343
Work status	122	198
Size of community of residence	112	158

workers who were not welfare recipients, did not live in the West, or did not reside in urban areas."[18]

Compared to Medicare, Medicaid has almost insoluble problems. It is essentially a state program, with matching payments provided by the federal government to produce an incentive for cooperation by state governments. Benefits vary greatly from state to state and some states do not have Medicaid programs. Payments per capita in the highest states are about ten times those in the lowest.

Medicaid has always had serious problems, in part because the program was introduced without adequate preparation. By 1970, Medicaid expenditures were $5.9 billion. These large payments overburdened existing markets in a short period.

The federal government has gradually retreated from its original lofty standards for participating programs, and states are making increased demands for federal funds. "As approved by the President, the 1967 Amendments to the Medicaid Program established a maximum income level for Federal financial participation in the cost of medical assistance for the medically needy. The limitation was set ultimately at 133-1/3 percent of the actual payment level under the AFDC [Aid to Families with Dependent Children] Program."[19]

Utilization Reviews

Excess utilization of medical services is one of the primary causes of rising medical care prices and expenditures. One of the great disappointments under the Medicare and Medicaid programs has been the failure of utilization reviews to accomplish their purpose. These reviews are required under the law to check on hospital admissions and lengths of stay, to make certain that the least costly alternative is used. Often, however, cheap alternatives are not available. The reviews also deal with excessive charges, frauds, and the like.

All sides—for example, both public advisory boards and government officials—agree that utilization reviews have been a dismal failure, and the history of prices and utilization since 1966 confirms this fact. After three years of the new programs, even the top administration official, Undersecretary John Veneman, admitted the failure:

In both Medicare and Medicaid we feel much more can be done with utilization controls than has been accomplished to date. Peer group review must become widespread not just in hospitals but also for other medical services. But mere peer review alone is obviously not enough to control abuses and escalating costs. We have issued regulations for Medicaid which provide that starting July 1, 1970, no state may raise fees without demonstrating to the Secretary that its utilization review is effective. . . . Too often "peer review" is simply *peer justification.*[20]

This is a problem that will confront national health insurance. In fact, with increases in the number of people covered and the benefits paid, through the use of government and private insurance funds, the temptation to overutilize medical services will grow. Failure to provide effective reviews will be increasingly costly.

Inflationary Pressures

Medicare and Medicaid have caused medical costs to jump tremendously (see figures 13.5-13.9). In the past, hospitals, doctors, and nursing homes set their fees, and Blue Cross and Blue Shield paid them, without attempting to control the charges. Yet, shockingly enough, after one year of Medicare and Medicaid, hospital costs and doctors' fees were up even more, 19 percent and 7 percent, respectively.[21] In the first six years of the two programs, medical prices increased by over 40 percent compared to an increase of 20 percent in the six years before the programs started.

The average income of physicians is now over $40,000 with many specialists making well over $100,000. Insurance intermediaries also expanded their business by $10 billion a year, including several hundred million dollars for "administrative expenses." Medical equipment firms and drug companies increased their sales and profits.

FIGURE 13.5   Estimated Daily Hospital Rates, 1967-82

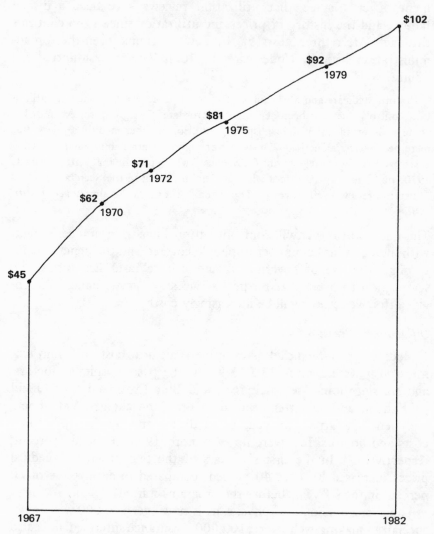

Source: U.S. Senate, Finance Committee, *Hearings on Medicare and Medicaid* (1970), chart 9.

FIGURE 13.6   Increase in Estimates of Future Hospital Insurance Benefits, 1965-69

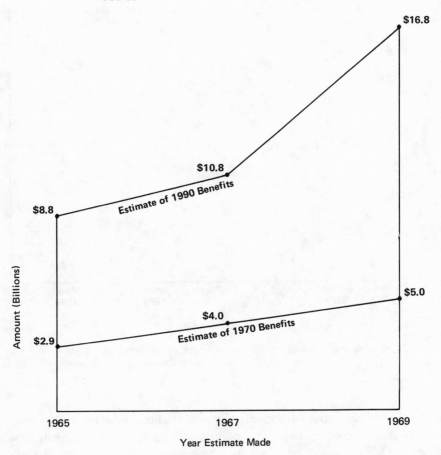

Source: U.S. Senate, Finance Committee, *Hearings on Medicare and Medicaid* (1970), chart 5.

FIGURE 13.7   Increase in Estimates of 1968-69 Federal Medicaid Costs

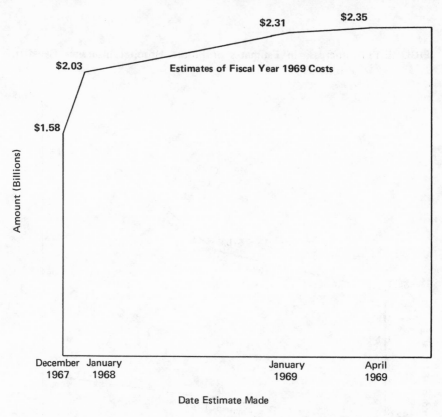

Source: U.S. Senate, Finance Committee, *Hearings on Medicare and Medicaid* (1970), chart 2.

Nursing home stocks boomed. Hospitals added new beds at a rate three times greater than the population increase. As a result, 25 percent of hospital beds are now empty, raising the rates to all patients.

National Health Insurance in the 1970s

In the years since World War II, national health insurance has been under continual consideration, but advances made by private insurance companies have delayed acceptance of NHI. Particularly

FIGURE 13.8 Increase in Vendor Payments for Medical Care, 1960-70

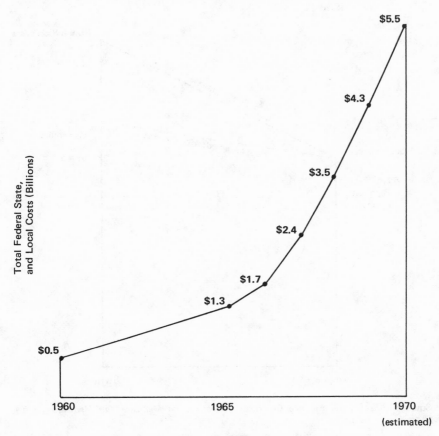

Source: U.S. Senate, Finance Committee, *Hearings on Medicare and Medicaid* (1970), chart 1.

in the 1950s, under President Eisenhower, progress toward NHI was slow.

Although the continued growth of private health insurance in the 1960s further reduced interest in NHI, it fell short of providing comprehensive benefits, covering greater proportions of the population, and financing more costs per capita. Financing was not available for programs that would meet these goals. Radical innovations were necessary to combat the burgeoning costs, the deficiencies of delivery,

FIGURE 13.9   Increases in Medicaid Costs and Numbers of People Served, 1968-70

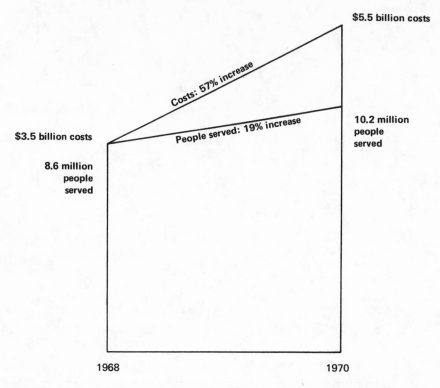

$5.5 billion costs

Costs: 57% increase

10.2 million people served

People served: 19% increase

$3.5 billion costs

8.6 million people served

1968   1970

Source: U.S. Senate, Finance Committee, *Hearings on Medicare and Medicaid* (1970), chart 3.

the shortage of funds, the slow rise of productivity, and the inadequate intervention by government.

Private insurance raised many problems: slow advances, waste in the rising contribution by third parties, failure to provide comprehensive benefits, rising costs per capita, and disappointing growth of comprehensive group prepayment insurance. These failures paved the way for introduction of a national health insurance program.

National health insurance in some form or other is likely to be enacted during the 1970s. The major contribution of NHI would be to increase the funds available for medical care and to improve the distribution of medical services. Comprehensive benefits would be provided, and financing would be facilitated through recourse to public funds and subsidies.

The problem NHI advocates face in the next couple of years is reconciliation of the various plans proposed. A number of issues need to be resolved: how much additional funding is needed and how much can be derived from cuts in current programs; the extent to which NHI financing should be public or private; the extent to which the additional burden should fall on the federal government; how much to use incentives and voluntary programs rather than compulsory ones; how much control of the program will rest with intermediaries, such as Blue Cross-Blue Shield, and how much with the government; what reimbursement methods to use; the extent to which markets for hospitals, doctors, and drugs will be controlled and how the integration and planning of these markets will be accomplished.

Numerous other problems also require attention. Through adoption of NHI, it is possible to accumulate large reserves, which may then be used to finance benefits. Actuarial deficits then rise, even as cash surpluses appear. Under NHI, it will be possible to charge low-income groups less than the cost of services and high-income groups more than the cost.

Over the years, emphasis has been put on pouring cash into NHI. But with badly provisioned medical markets, dumping $14 billion to $15 billion annually into Medicare and Medicaid within a few years has brought inflation and disorganization of these markets. Thus, one cure is first to provide improved delivery, additional personnel and facilities, and higher productivity. In the last few years, attention has been diverted from the flow of money to the increases in real resources, such as medical personnel. Several proposals for the introduction of NHI (such as the Kennedy bill) provide for cash to make the additional resources, personnel, and delivery systems available before the health program gets fully underway.

Even President Nixon, in a 1971 health message, emphasized the real, not monetary, aspects of national health care, calling for federal support for the development of health maintenance organizations "providing a comprehensive range of medical services in one location for a fixed contract fee, paid in advance by all subscribers. The Federal Government would establish a program of planning grants to aid sponsors of HMOs and a loan guarantee program providing initial working capital for new HMOs."

Financing Proposals

During the twenty to thirty years that national health financing has been under discussion, payroll taxes have generally been considered the most acceptable method of taxation. Here too the emphasis has shifted recently. There is now much more interest in financing through general revenues—as might well be expected, with costs rising from between 1 and 2 percent of payrolls to between 7 and 10 percent. The payroll tax puts a heavy burden on the poor. Opponents of this method of financing tend to support increased burdens on employers.

An interesting aspect of the financing problem is the preference of conservative groups—the American Medical Association and private insurance companies—for reliance on federal taxes or tax credits, while programs proposed by liberal groups rely relatively more on payroll taxes. The institutional groups probably seek government financing because they fear that payroll financing will bring federal control, as it has in the past. The liberal group prefers to rely heavily on transfers from private to federal financing. The Kennedy plan, for example, depends on transfers to federal financing, while Nixon's proposal favors private financing.

One of the troublesome aspects of financing is the difficulty of projecting future costs. In general, costs are greatly underestimated. In a two-year period, for example, the cost per service in extended care facilities increased by nine times.

Financing of NHI is likely to be costly even when an allowance is made for cuts in current programs. The additional costs may run as high as $50 billion. And some ambitious NHI programs appear to be underfinanced in the proposed budgets.

What can NHI contribute toward containment of inflation? While increasing resources such as hospitals and personnel, it can offset rising monetary supplies. Support of operations that improve productivity would be especially helpful. Funding from taxes would reduce the taxpayer's purchasing power and thus also work against inflation.[22]

Proposed NHI Plans

Congress has had at least ten national health insurance proposals before it. Each proposal represents the interests of one or more groups. The American Medical Association's Medicredit plan is designed for the physician; the National Healthcare bill is sponsored by the Health Insurance Association of America; the Health Care Services plan was designed by the American Hospital Association; President Nixon's 1974 bill benefits insurance companies and other large corporations hoping to move into the health care field; and the plan by Senators Kennedy and Mills is similar to Nixon's but it gives less power to the insurance companies.

The Nixon Plan

Nixon's 1974 NHI plan is a three-part insurance program under which employees and their families would be insured for standard health benefits, with the employer paying 65 percent of the premium for the first three years and 75 percent thereafter; the poor would receive federally subsidized coverage; and the aged would be covered under a revised Medicare program.

The Nixon plan is designed for families below $5,000 income; nonworking families with between $5,000 and $7,000 income; very high-risk working families earning between $5,000 and $7,500; nonworking families with unusually high medical risks (disabled and early retirees) regardless of income; and unusually high-risk employee groups. The plan is administered by private insurance companies under supervision by the Department of Health, Education, and Welfare—like the Medicare program. The program includes incentives for organizing prepaid group practices. A related bill provides grants for the education of needed health professionals. Reimbursement is made to providers on the same basis as under Medicare ("reasonable costs"). Medicare continues as is, and Medicaid would be limited to the blind, the aged, and the disabled.

Private insurance companies participating in the plan would be required to cover unlimited medical and hospital care (barring checkups for adults); outpatient drugs at low cost; limited treatment for mental health, alcoholism, and drug abuse problems; eye, ear, and dental care for children up to age thirteen; prenatal and well-baby care; family planning services; 100 days of nursing home care; home health services; blood and blood products; and other services, including X rays and laboratory tests.

For this, each family would pay a deductible of $150 per person (with a total family limit of $450) and a separate $50 deductible for outpatient drugs before benefit payments begin. Then the family would pay 25 percent of all medical costs, but—and this is a significant provision of the plan—once a family has spent $1,500 out of its own pocket, the plan would pick up all additional medical bills.

It is estimated that the federal government will need to put in $5.8 billion and the individual states $1 billion to care for the poor and aged. But President Nixon and Secretary of Health, Education, and Welfare Casper Weinberger both assert the outlay will not require new taxes—a conjecture open to doubt.

Medicredit

The plan proposed by the American Medical Association, "Medicredit," has two parts: catastrophic insurance, which is similar to Senator Long's proposal, and basic health insurance. Medicredit relies on private insurance companies but provides for government assistance to people unable to buy insurance. The program has coinsurance provisions, deductibles, and a number of services excluded from coverage. It minimizes the government's role and provides, in the AMA's words, for "free choice by every physician as to how he will conduct his practice."

National Healthcare Act

The proposed National Healthcare Act, sponsored by the Health Insurance Association of America, provides incentives for all working people to buy private insurance. Poor and "uninsurable" persons receive private insurance at government expense. The coinsurance payments are set higher for hospital care than for physicians' services, in order to discourage expensive hospitalization. The government-supported portion of the bill is administered by the states.

The Kennedy Plan

Senator Edward Kennedy's first national health insurance proposal, the Health Security Program, was a totally public system of health insurance that would have supplanted private health insurance companies almost entirely. It would have provided Americans with lifetime care, from nursery to nursing home, at an estimated cost of some $60 billion a year. Financing was proposed from a compulsory 1 percent tax on wages up to $15,000 and a 3.5 percent tax from employers, matched by an equal amount from federal general revenues. Self-employed persons would have paid a 2.5 percent tax. This money was to be placed in a Health Security Trust Fund, to be used only for health care (similar to the provisions on Social Security).

Due to political pressures from doctors and conservative politicians, Kennedy changed his proposal in April 1974, and teaming up with Representative Wilbur Mills, Chairman of the House Ways and Means Committee, introduced a measure closely resembling the Nixon Administration program.

Like the Nixon plan, the Kennedy-Mills program would cover the costs of hospitalization, major medical expenses, and catastrophic illness. It would have employers pay a large part of the premiums and retain a role for private insurance companies. It would also require the government to supply coverage for the unemployed (who would contribute 1 percent of their welfare or unemployment benefits) and self-employed (who would pay 2.5 percent of their income up to $20,000). Under the Kennedy-Mills plan, the government, rather than insurance companies, would collect the premiums, enabling it to control private profits. While the Nixon plan sets a $1,500 limit on the amount that any family would have to pay for medical care in any given year, the Kennedy-Mills bill lowers the limit to $1,000.

Notes

1. E. Feingold, *Medicare: Policy and Politics* (1966), pp. 86-101.

2. U.S. House of Representatives, *President of the United States Transmitting the Annual Message on Health and Security*, House Document no. 120 (1939), pp. 20-21; *National Health Act of 1945*, Report to the Senate Committee on Education and Labor (1945), p. 305.

3. *National Health Insurance*, Report to the Senate Education and Labor Committee (1945), p. 5.

4. *Who Will Pay Your Bills?* Health/PAC Special Report on National Health Insurance, December 1973.

5. For detailed study and source material, see S. E. Harris, *Economics of American Medicine* (1964), chaps. 16 and 17; also see A. M. Robson, "The British National Health Service and Some Lessons to Be Learned from it," *New England Journal of Medicine*, April 3, 1969, pp. 754-61.

6. *Parliamentary Debates* 9, no. 28, April 18, 1950, p. 39.

7. *British Medical Journal*, March 18, 1950, pp. 664-66; and see "The National Health Service Act in Great Britain," *The Practitioner* (1950).

8. U.S. House of Representatives, Ways and Means Committee, *Hearings on Health Services for the Aged* (1961), vol. 3, p. 1639.

9. Ibid., vol. 2, p. 925; *Social Security Bulletin*, January 1962, p. 16.

10. *Illness and Health Services in an Aging Population* (1957), pp. 1-19.

11. U.S. House of Representatives, Ways and Means Committee, *Hearings on Health Services for the Aged* (1961), vol. 1, p. 77; Public Health Service, *Health Statistics, Duration of Limitation of Activity Due to Chronic Conditions, United States, July, 1959-June, 1960*, p. 6; Ibid., *Limitation of Activity and Mobility Due to Chronic Conditions, United States, July, 1957-June, 1958*, p. 6; and *The Aged and Aging in the United States*, Senate Report no. 1121 (1960), p. 87.

12. U.S. Senate, Subcommittee on Problems of the Aged and Aging, *Hearings* (1960), p. 263.

13. Ibid.

14. *Who Will Pay Your Bills?* Health/PAC Special Report on National Health Insurance, December 1973, p. 3.

15. J. Green and J. Scharff, "Use of Medical Services under Medicare," *Social Security Bulletin*, March 1971, pp. 3-16.

16. Ibid., p. 7.

17. Ibid.

18. Ibid., pp. 8-9.

19. *Report of the Advisory Commission on Intergovernmental Problems in Medicaid* (1968), p. 9.

20. U.S. Senate, Subcommittee on Health of the Elderly, *Hearings on the Economics of Aging* (1970), p. 652.

21. HEW, *Medical Care Costs and Prices: Background Book* (January 1972), pp. 23, 41.

22. See especially HEW, Office of Research and Statistics, *National Health Insurance: A Comparison of Five Proposals*, by S. Waldman and E. Peel (July 23, 1970); HEW, *A Study of National Health Insurance Proposals Introduced in the 92nd Congress* (July 1971); *HEW Press Release*, August 5, 1971; "Estimated Costs of 12 National Health Insurance Proposals Now Awaiting Either House or Senate Action," *Congressional Record*, February 18, 1971, pp. 1-11.

14

Finances of
National Health Insurance

Goals

Proponents of national health insurance consider it a technique for increasing cash flow, improving the distribution and delivery of medical care, and controlling charges. It would modify methods for reimbursing providers not only by directly discouraging the costly fee-for-service approach but also by favoring capitation and salary reimbursement indirectly through the allocation of its medical funds. By using prospective budgeting, the supporters of national health insurance hope to operate more efficiently.

Above all, proponents emphasize either increasing supplies or containing demand in badly provisioned medical markets. Two of the major plans propose structural changes that would expedite improved provisioning of markets by introducing resource development funds. A crucial question is whether the funds should be poured into a national health system now, or should be delayed until the personnel and facilities are more nearly adequate to meet needs. Excess demand brings inflation; hence an increased flow of medical assets is needed unless measures are taken to contain demand. Increased productivity and a reimbursement method that yields incentives to keep costs down would also be helpful.

A common objective of all the NHI proposals is to provide more comprehensive benefits. Under the more liberal plans, sharing of costs with beneficiaries is discouraged; these plans call for more facilities and personnel and for postponement of benefits until the shortage of capacity, which seriously cuts output of services, is alleviated.

Distribution of health care would be greatly improved if the entire population were covered by national health insurance. The maldistribution of medical care services is a most troublesome problem. All the national health insurance plans discussed here emphasize the need to equalize distribution. Even the program proposed by private insurance interests presents three alternative plans for matching finances to needs. This plan does not estimate the costs, however.

Costs

A study by the Social Security Administration in early August 1971 revealed that the average American family may expect to pay $200 a year by 1974 to cover out-of-pocket medical expenditures. Secretary Veneman of the Department of Health, Education, and Welfare estimated family health care costs at more than $1,000 in 1973-74, with out-of-pocket payments accounting for a large part. A study by the department staff put the per capita health bill at $324 in 1969-70. On the basis of five members to a family, this estimate of costs would be $1,620 per family. The median family income in 1969 was $9,433, or only about six times the estimated health bill for 1969-70. The financial squeeze is serious for the 14.7 percent of families with incomes under $3,000 and the 28 percent with incomes of less than $5,000.[1]

It is agreed that, if medical care is financed primarily by national health insurance, the average American will be spared large expenditures. In the absence of a national program, family expenditures of some $1,000 to $1,500 a year would raise serious problems for the average family and almost insuperable problems for the 30 percent or so with incomes of $5,000 or less. Government intervention will save a large part of the average family's medical bill. Surely one important effect will be that low-income families will attract an increasing share of medical services. Many who are now excluded by lack of finances will become much stronger bidders for services. Those who have high incomes or comprehensive insurance coverage now will experience a relative loss of competitive position.

Insofar as national health insurance provides additional finances, the poor in particular gain. However, there are some offsetting factors. For example, the increase in taxes to finance the program would place an especially large burden on the poor, insofar as financing is done through payroll taxes. Another factor relates to the impact of pouring some $50 billion into badly provisioned manpower and facilities markets. The $17 billion or so in Medicare and Medicaid expenditures brought serious disturbances and inflation to medical markets. Price pressures from an even larger input of funds would force increases even though promises are made to control fees charged, to budget on a prospective basis, to provide incentives for redistributing doctors, and to mobilize efforts to facilitate the growth of manpower and facilities.

Controlling Costs

Various national health insurance proposals attempt to counter inflation. One way is to modify the method of reimbursing hospitals and doctors. Coverage of all costs of hospitals destroys the institution's incentives to keep its costs down. There is much to be said for basing reimbursement on average costs, allowing each hospital with costs below average to capture the difference. It is hard to justify reimbursement to a hospital irrespective of its performance in comparison to hospitals of similar type, size, and location.

Under public programs and Blue Cross-Blue Shield plans, physicians are generally paid on the basis of reasonable and customary charges. This is unfortunate, since neither the doctor nor the government knows what reasonable and customary charges are. Most physicians now subscribe to the fee-for-service method of compensation. That system is costly, because it creates a temptation to multiply visits and procedures. Yet this method of compensation has strong appeal for physicians and is a source of the doctor's interest in his patients. The payment of a fee also discourages patient recourse to the doctor. This has the advantage of reducing demand but the disadvantage of fostering neglect of needed care.

Some of the best known national health insurance proposals urge reimbursement on a capitation or salary basis. This method cuts costs, but it may also reduce incentives to some extent. While too many services are offered under fee-for-service methods, too few may be forthcoming under the capitation system. Some national health insurance plans shift funds with a view to discriminating against fee-for-service reimbursement systems.

Improvements in productivity are helpful in controlling costs, since price rises stem in part from the failure of productivity increases to offset the increasing labor costs of numerous services. The more liberal national health insurance plans stress the need to provide additional resources in order to lower prices, at least relatively. The original Kennedy bill in particular presented an ingenious proposal designed to yield advantages on the pricing front. It would have entrusted at least 2 percent of the receipts of the program—about $800 million a year—to a Resources Development Fund, so that an increase in resources—manpower, facilities, and so forth—could be obtained much more expeditiously than in the past. As more money came into the national health program, a prompt response of additional resources would develop to offset inflationary pressures.

Any factor contributing to rising productivity should also have a stabilizing impact. The various national health insurance plans offer numerous possibilities for gains here. For example, it is proposed that the budgeting process clearly define the number of people and the benefits that are covered. Such definitions reduce the payments to be made, yielding larger outputs in relation to the input of factors, which gives a gain in productivity. In contrast, now such budgeting checks are generally not available, with deleterious effects on outlays and prices. Failure to exploit the low-cost alternatives—nursing homes as opposed to hospitals, paramedical personnel as opposed to trade name drugs—also cuts down on productivity. Duplication of equipment and facilities, poor scheduling in hospitals, failure to integrate and plan the cooperative functioning of various services, excessive use of resources by insurance interests, and failure to exploit the economies in group prepayment programs are all signs of the need for better efficiency. A comparison of health care expenditures in relation to gross national product in the United States and in other countries, together with a comparison of measures of health, makes it evident that we are making inefficient use of large outlays for health care.

Financing of Specific Plans

In 1971 there were more than a dozen proposals for national health insurance before Congress, varying from the conservative catastrophic insurance bill by Senator Russell Long to the comprehensive health care bill by Senator Edward Kennedy. Costs of different proposals varied considerably. For example, the Long bill was estimated to require $35.1 billion of federal tax revenues, while the Kennedy plan would have required $91.4 billion in federal funds. The Nixon administration submitted a proposal that relied heavily on private rather than government financing.

Philosophic differences among plans created severe disagreement among the factions supporting one or another proposal, and, despite general recognition of the need for a national health insurance program, no bill was able to muster majority support in Congress in 1973. Early in 1974, President Nixon proposed a somewhat liberalized version of his program, now entitled the Comprehensive Insurance Plan, designed to reduce the most sharply criticized inequities of his earlier program. Shortly afterward, Senator Kennedy joined Congressman Wilbur Mills in submitting a compromise bill substantially similar to the Nixon plan but with somewhat better benefits. This bill represented a drastic curtailment of Kennedy's original comprehensive program, and it was now titled the National Health Insurance Program.

A third major bill before Congress in 1974 was the more conservative Long-Ribicoff bill, a modification of Senator Long's earlier catastrophic insurance bill. Financial aspects of these three proposals are detailed below.

The Nixon CHIP Bill

The Nixon administration claimed its Comprehensive Health Insurance Plan (CHIP) would cost $5.9 billion in new federal expenditures in the first full year of operation, projected as 1976-77. Most of the financing would come from the business sector.

The CHIP has two major components, an Employee Health Insurance Plan and an Assisted Health Insurance Plan. Under the first, employers would offer a minimum package of benefits to all full-time employees under age sixty-five and their dependents. This plan would also be available to self-employed and unemployed individuals and labor unions. Insurance would be offered through private carriers certified by the individual states.

The Commerce Department estimates that employers currently pay $15.4 billion a year in health insurance premiums for their employees. Under CHIP an estimated $5.9 billion would be added to the employers' total bill. Industry sectors hardest hit financially by CHIP, according to the Commerce Department would be agriculture, retail and wholesale trade, finance, real estate, and insurance.

The Department of Health, Education, and Welfare estimated that the cost of the CHIP would be about $415 per employee. The annual premium for a married worker would run about $600 and a single person's fee would be $240. Employers would contribute 65 percent of premium costs during the first three years of the CHIP and 75 percent thereafter. The government would offer a subsidy to any employer whose payroll expenses rose by more than 3 percent as a result of his required contribution to the cost of the insurance premiums.

Employees must pay a deductible of $150 per person under the plan, with a maximum of three deductibles per family, before reimbursements begin. A separate deductible of $50 per person would also be required for outpatient drugs. After paying the deductibles, the enrollee must pay 25 percent of all bills (coinsurance). However, a maximum liability of $1,500 a year per family is established. This means that all cost-sharing would stop after a family incurred $1,500 in out-of-pocket expenses (for both deductibles and coinsurance payments) in a single year.

The second component of the CHIP provides assistance to the poor in purchasing health insurance. Families with incomes above $7,500 and individuals with incomes above $5,250 would not be eligible for the government aid, unless they qualified as special high-risk exceptions. All persons eligible for the government-assisted plan would have the option of obtaining coverage through a health maintenance organization.

The CHIP would expand the benefits of the Medicare program. Medicare benefits would be offered on an income-related basis, with the government providing subsidies for the poor. Relatively high-income Medicare enrollees would have to pay up to $750 a year, while lower-income recipients would have a lower ceiling on their payments.

Under the CHIP, state governments would play a larger role in administering and regulating federal health programs. All state legislatures would have to enact new laws to be eligible to receive the 75 percent federal matching share in the program for poor people. A major new role is also assigned to the insurance industry. The amount of privately underwritten insurance would expand by 15 percent as a result of the CHIP requirement that all employers offer health insurance protection to their employees.

The administration's proposal is not really *national* health insurance, but rather *private* health insurance. Congress would require the purchase of private insurance policies by federal law but with no federal regulation whatsoever. Moreover, the program would legally sanction experience rating, despite sharp criticism of this practice on social grounds. It would not guarantee health care for all; health care would be the responsibility of no one. It features regressive financing and is based on patching up the present system, while providing no new cost or quality controls.

The Kennedy-Mills NHIP Bill

Like the Nixon bill, the Kennedy-Mills National Health Insurance Program (NHIP) requires private health insurance coverage with deductibles and coinsurance for families with incomes over $4,800, based on a means test. Those earning over $8,800 would be required to satisfy deductibles and pay coinsurance of 25 percent on all services up to a maximum liability for deductibles and coinsurance of $1,000 per family per year.

The Kennedy-Mills bill will be financed primarily by a 4 percent payroll tax—1 percent to be paid by employees on wages up to $20,000 and 3 percent to be paid by employers. Self-employment income is taxed at 1 percent. Health care for the poor is partially financed by general revenues and state contributions. Insurance companies remain the fiscal intermediaries, despite their pronounced failure to create an efficient system in Medicare.

The Kennedy-Mills bill has some excellent features, such as Social Security financing under a nationally coordinated health care system, and extension of covered care in long-term facilities. But it places a heavy burden on patients and consumers by its high deductibles and substantial cost-sharing in order to reduce program costs.

The Long-Ribicoff Bill

The employee insurance component of the Long-Ribicoff bill is financed by a regressive 0.3 percent tax on wages up to $9,000 paid by both employers and employees. The medical assistance component is financed 75 percent by the federal government through general revenues and 25 percent by the states. Both would be administered through the Social Security Administration, with private health insurance companies acting as financial intermediaries as they do now under Medicare.

Notes

1. Statistics from *Economic Report of the President* (1971), *Statistical Abstract of the United States* (1968), and *National Health Expenditures, Fiscal Year 1969-70 and Calendar Years 1929-69.*

PART V

Delivery

15

Issues in Delivery

Delivery in the United States needs to be greatly improved. Despite vast health expenditures (the highest in the world), this country is thirteenth among industrial countries in deaths of infants during the the first year of life, seventh among industrial countries in the percentage of mothers who die in childbirth; eighteenth in life expectancies of males, and sixteenth in the death rate for males in their middle years. In all instances, the United States ranked better twenty years ago than it does today.[1]

Experts' Views of the Problem

Mrs. Leona Baumgartner, former Health Commissioner of New York City, has summarized the problems of delivery well:

There is much talk of the health crisis—rapidly rising costs, personnel shortages, long waits to get into hospitals, nursing homes, doctors' offices, Medicare, and Medicaid. There is less talk of the disorganized, inefficient, fragmented no-system through which the Americans, rich and poor, get their medical care. . . .

Hospitals are often built where they are not needed. Patients stay in them longer than their medical status demands, sometimes because space in nursing homes is not available. Clinics operate at the convenience of staff, not customers. Some physicians spend all day in or near one hospital; others are "on the road" much of the day from one hospital to another between home calls. . . .

Every hospital feels it must provide all the latest, most sophisticated treatments, despite cost or need. Take a New England city of 175,000 with four hospitals. One already has the radiation therapy and staff necessary to treat all the patients with cancer in the city and surrounding area. There is no evidence that there are any patients who go without treatment when needed. But the other three hospitals are struggling to find personnel, space, and equipment so they, too, will have similar services. One hospital in the same town has an excellent cardiac service and is able to do all the simple heart operations the area needs—but another is searching for a cardiac surgeon. The city is less than two hours by car away from one of the nation's great medical centers where cardiac surgery, seldom an emergency, is superbly done. . . .

What is needed? A deliberate, well-financed program of remodeling the health system—aggressive planning for better use of scarce resources, merging of small inefficient hospitals, firm links of smaller community hospitals to larger regional medical centers, wider use of telecommunications to bring expertise to larger numbers, more ambulatory care, more group practice, more emphasis on early and preventive care, more "allied" health workers—all these and more.[2]

Dr. K. Kerr White describes eight alleged defects in our provision of medical care:

Defect No. 1. Personal health services frequently are not continuously available to all segments of the population except at emergency rooms of hospitals, or through telephone-answering services. General care available at the former, except for immediately life-threatening conditions, frequently is regarded by both the consumers and the profession as inappropriate and inadequate. A telephone-answering service is part of a communication system and not a personal health service. . . .

Defect No. 2. Generalists are decreasing in number and superspecialists are increasing. The rate per 100,000 population for all physicians is said to be too low, and the ratio between the two kinds of physicians inappropriate. The competence of the generalists to manage many problems that require a thorough knowledge of contemporary scientific medicine and the interest of superspecialists in early, nonspecific, and undifferentiated "complaints" on the one hand, and in chronic, terminal medical care on the other, are called into question. The American "specialist" is virtually unknown in other countries; he frequently confuses himself both with the "consultant" and the "generalist." He is perhaps best described as a "consultoid" since he is apt to have the training and aspiration of the former but does the work of the latter.

There is a serious imbalance in the distribution of medical scientists, medical practitioners, and medical administrators. In the long haul, the basic capacity of the health services system to provide "medical cure" will come from the medical scientists. In the long haul, however, everyone is dead and, in the short haul, the capacity of the health services system to provide "medical care" will come from the medical practitioners and medical administrators.

Defect No. 3. Health professionals employ their talents inappropriately, and scarce human resources are wasted. The medical care establishment tends to distribute its skill and knowledge more in accordance with selective individual utilization of services than with the collectively perceived needs and expressed demands of the community. For example, pediatricians are trained to manage complex problems but spend much of their time providing "well-child" care to "private" patients in their offices and "sick-child" care to "public" patients in health department clinics. Responsibility for coordinating the care of patients seen in the latter setting is often the responsibility of the public health nurse; the itinerant or rotating physician advises on medical problems only. The same physician in the former setting may spend his professional time coordinating the care of his patients in the absence of skilled public health nursing services. Nurses could undertake many tasks currently performed by doctors; preliminary history questionnaires and screening tests, clinical triage, instruction, counseling, health education, certain treatments and domiciliary visiting and care are examples.

Defect No. 4. Communication between different sources and levels of personal health services is inadequate. The recording, storage, retrieval, and transmission of medical information is outmoded compared to developments in other service systems of contemporary society. Information about patients' prior and present health problems and their treatment, or the reasons for referrals or consultations and their outcome, frequently are not transmitted between and within health professions and institutions responsibly, rapidly, and reliably. The technological capacity to accomplish this is available.

Defect No. 5. Inappropriate institutionalization of patients not only increases the cost of the whole health services system but may be harmful and even life-threatening. . . . There is evidence that patients removed from their natural habitats to nursing homes experience substantially higher age-specific mortality rates than do others who are not so institutionalized. The benefits of appropriate institutionalization must be balanced against the risks of inappropriate institutionalization. Conversely, many generalists in the centers of large cities are said to be without hospital privileges; they must of necessity refer or transfer their patients who need hospitalization.

Defect No. 6. Emphasis on the categorical organization of personal health services, e.g., by diseases (heart disease, cancer, and stroke), by ages (comprehensive child care centers), by geography (neighborhood health centers), by methods of financing (Titles 18 and 19), or by traditional emphasis (public health programs, clinical practice), is inimical to the development of health services organized on the basis of levels of patient care and sophistication of medical knowledge and facilities. Previous experience with regionalization, although not an argument against trying new approaches, suggests that the categorical approach, if not illogical and unworkable, is at least undesirable.

Defect No. 7. The notion that there is only one diagnostic system used in medicine, i.e., the one taught as the conventional wisdom in medical schools, appears to be at variance with the available facts. . . .

Defect No. 8. There is growing skepticism that academic medicine, community medicine (the new public health), and private medicine (the "organized" profession) always act either alone or collectively in the public interest. This tripartite division of responsibility and accountability can be confusing both to members of the health professions and to the public. There is uncertainty about who is "in charge" of seeing that society has the personal health services it can collectively command from the resources it provides.[3]

A 1970 congressional report noted:

The need for improvements in medical care delivery is indicated by the acute shortage of physicians and allied manpower, the even more acute lack of such manpower in rural and ghetto areas; the rising cost of medical care, particularly for hospitalization and related services; the uneven availability and accessibility of health services, again most scarce in rural and ghetto areas; and the development of over-specialization in medicine, due in part to the rapidity of medical science advances.

The impact of the delivery system is affected by recourse to preventive medicine; allocation of resources on the basis of age; the special treatment given to certain health needs areas such as heart disease, cancer, and stroke; and the extent to which emphasis is shifted to broad delivery programs and away from concentration on disease and episodic medicine generally.

Recently numerous attempts have been made to find the causes of the crisis in delivery. A leading expert on medical care, Dr. I. S. Falk, emphasized the inadequacies and maldistribution of personnel and facilities, deterioration of quality, and cost escalation. He is particularly critical of reimbursement policies, referring to "the idiocy of signed blank check reimbursement of practitioners and full cost reimbursement of practitioners and full cost reimbursement of institutions guaranteed under recently enacted public programs without feasible and substantial controls." Falk feels the state governments need to assume greater responsibilities for providing personal health care. A national program for personal health care and supplemental needs should be developed, and the federal and state governments should share responsibility.

In commenting on Falk's paper, Dr. W. J. McNerney, president of

Blue Cross, also favored increasing the responsibilities of state governments. He found Falk less pessimistic than other observers about
rising costs. The proponents of strong, comprehensive, and efficient
systems tend to underestimate costs. Past experience suggests that
costs will continue to rise, generally way beyond anticipated amounts.
New approaches to control of costs are badly needed. McNerney
recognized "that access to services is inadequate for a significant
minority of the population and that productivity of the delivery
system falls short of the mark." Like Falk, McNerney seeks a bold
intervention. These outstanding experts are fearful of the halfway
measures that have characterized the last forty years. McNerney also
seeks federal leadership, but would not put states in a totally sub-
servient relationship to the federal government. The states, in his
view, could contribute greatly to improving long-term medical care
and treatment of mental illness.

Goals of Good Delivery

Continuity of Patient Care

An adequate delivery system needs to provide continuity of treatment to the patient. When reimbursement is based on a fee-for-service approach, fragmentation of treatment thrives. Continuity of
treatment must be found.

Above all, patients need a primary doctor. Primary care is care
aimed at preventing the onset of illness, maintaining of good health,
and providing continuous scrutiny for early symptoms and intract-
able aspects of disease.[4] One national survey revealed that only
55 percent of the population was under the care of a general practitioner. Another survey put the figure for use of a family doctor at
64 percent for the population as a whole but only 32 percent for the
lower economic classes.

In most cases the patient moves from primary doctor to secondary
(referral) doctor and then to specialist. Specialists increasingly are
taking on the tasks of primary doctors. Dr. Sloss found that 44 percent of the time adults chose to seek care from specialists without
referral. In big cities, patients often use the outpatient services of a
hospital for primary care.[5] The poor commonly obtain treatment
through the use of emergency rooms. This excessive use of hospitals
keeps costs high and reduces the output of the hospital. Overuse
occurs because insurance often fails to cover outpatient services,

because doctors and patients find hospitalization more convenient than outpatient treatment, because doctors in solo practice do not have adequate facilities for diagnostic testing, because outpatient and extended care facilities are inadequate, and because there are not financial incentives to use less costly services.[6]

The patient wants medical care, not fragmented treatments from a coterie of specialists. The whole person is neglected as the patient is shunted from one specialist to another. The emphasis of health insurance plans in the past has been on financing serious illnesses and injuries incurring major expenditures. A report by the Southern California Research Council noted that the effect of current practices is "to concentrate demand and consumption upon the more expensive forms of treatment. In this way health care has become a discontinuous set of high cost services rather than a continuous stream of varied care."[7]

Continuity of Coverage

Delivery of medical care is now primarily a function of attachment to the labor market. Hence a recession and accompanying layoffs are likely to bring cancellation of health insurance. Blue Cross and Blue Shield try to deal with this problem by offering temporary continuance and conversion provisions. It would be helpful if unemployment insurance covered these contingencies.

In the 1958 recession, for example, a study in Michigan revealed that 33 percent of the study sample had their health coverage cancelled by May and another 24 percent at a later date. However, 38 percent covered themselves on a self-paying basis until they could return to work-related coverage. Of the 57 percent of the sample who were laid off, approximately 58 percent returned to their original groups within one year of their layoff dates. But 24 percent of the sample who were laid off in February 1958 had not returned to work a year later. Health care utilization rates are heavy during layoff periods—varying from 1.5 to 7.9 times the rates for comparable months in previous years.[8]

Preventive Health Care

Greater emphasis on preventive medicine contributes to improved delivery of medical care. It is widely held that a larger relative investment in preventive medicine would pay off in reduced financial burdens for health care. Group prepayment insurance with its emphasis on recourse to services outside the hospital encourages preventive medicine. General physical checkups are underutilized, and even when sought, they are not as effective as they might be. Medical programs neglect or underinvest in fluoridated water, although the returns greatly exceed the costs. Tests for cervical cancer are not exploited adequately and measures to cope with problems such as smoking and automobile accidents are not sufficient. Multiphasic programs also require more attention.

The Role of Hospitals

"Medicine has two Establishments, both of which contribute to our troubles. The second Establishment, hostile to the first, is based on urban hospitals. It is research and technology oriented, often salaried and provides the world's best treatment for complex illnesses. The result is that though this is the best country in the world in which to have a serious illness, it is one of the worst countries in the world to have a nonserious illness."[9] The strength of the hospital-based establishment is its domination of the medical schools.

The Advisory Committee on Health Facilities to the Secretary of Health, Education, and Welfare sees the hospital "as the principal organizing focus of a new and more effective system of delivery of health care in each community." Hospitals have been increasing their services for many years. As output is increased, the cost of a service is reduced and overhead unit costs decline. The gains may accrue to either the purveyor or the patient, depending in part on the size of the market. Gains may be manifested in reduced charges or in extended services or both.[10] But inflation and bottlenecks have brought rising costs despite gains from a rising level of output. Expansion of knowledge, provision of a variety of services, and changes of diagnoses and treatments bring increasing costs.[11]

In the ten years from 1958 to 1967, the consumer price index rose 16.3 percent, physicians' fees 37.6 percent, and hospital daily service charges 100 percent. These rising costs have reduced the net contribution of hospitals and similar institutions to the equitable distribution of health care. Gains in technology have added to costs and thus moderated the net effect of scientific advances. The cost of a day of general hospital care in the United States today includes wages for three or more workers; fifty years ago it included wages for one.

The explosion of medical knowledge has brought more patients to the hospital as well as more services and rising costs. But the rise of costs has been offset, to some extent, by the reduction in the length of the average stay. A study by W. J. McNerney found:

In five of the six selected diagnoses there was a substantial drop in average length of stay from 1938 to 1958; the greatest decreases occurred between 1938 and 1948. . . . In the sixth diagnosis, acute myocardial infarction, the picture was drastically different; the length of stay increased sharply. The percentage changes between 1938 and 1958 were as follows:

Cholecystitis and cholelithiasis	−13.8
Appendicitis	−22.7
Urinary tract infection	−22.8
Bronchopneumonia	−37.5
Delivery	−42.9
Acute myocardial infarction	+72.2

The stay for the surgical diagnoses changed least. The reduction in stay in urinary tract infection and in bronchopneumonia apparently reflects the use of antibiotics. In delivery, which showed the greatest reduction, the drop seems to reflect the effects both of early ambulation and of a change in medical philosophy regarding maternity cases. The great increase in the proportion of all deliveries that occur in hospitals may also have affected length of stay in some way. In 1939 only 51 percent of all births took place in hospitals. In 1949 the figure was nearly 87 percent. Today about 98 percent of births take place in hospitals. This great change in proportion of deliveries may also have resulted in a change of some kind in the distribution of the characteristics of the patients, which in turn may have affected length of stay.[12]

The Role of Health Maintenance Organizations

The Nixon HMO Proposals

In the late 1960s and early 1970s numerous plans were presented to improve delivery of medical services. President Nixon in 1970 was attracted to the concept of health maintenance organizations (HMOs), and at one point he envisioned HMO coverage for 80 percent of the population. But Congress at first was not enthusiastic about HMOs. Then in December 1973, Congress passed and President Nixon signed the Health Maintenance Organization bill, which authorized $375 million for the development and marketing of prepaid medical plans in every state for the next four years. The new law will override state restrictions that now prohibit or severely limit the growth of HMOs.

HMOs are characterized as voluntary groups of doctors who contract with groups of people for a wide program of health care paid for by fixed annual fees. The member groups vary in size from the Kaiser-Permanente program, with 2.5 million subscribers, over twenty hospitals, and 2,000 salaried doctors, to the East Baltimore Medical Plan, with 7,000 members and one clinic.

HMOs operate within a fixed budget that pays bonuses to physicians for efficient management. Unfortunately, these groups can dictate the type of care a patient will get: if a physician says a patient does not need hospitalization, he will not get it under prepaid benefits.

The proponents of HMOs have stressed the importance of keeping available patient options to obtain services through traditional procedures as well as through prepaid HMO systems. The Nixon HMO proposals include provision for an organized system of health care that accepts responsibility for providing "a set of comprehensive health maintenance and treatment services for a voluntarily enrolled group of persons in a geographic area" and "is reimbursed through pre-negotiated and fixed periodic payment made by or on behalf of each person or family unit enrolled in the plan."[13]

Nixon is concerned with the inefficiencies of the medical care program. To him the toughest question is not how much should be spent but rather how it should be spent. He has expressed his ideology as follows:

I believe the public will always be better served by a pluralistic system than by a monolithic one, by a system which creates many effective centers of responsibility—both public and private—rather than one that concentrates authority in a single governmental source. . . . We must encourage greater cooperation and build better coordination—but not by fostering uniformity and eliminating choice.

Nixon seemed disposed to push for HMO legislation, but he did not indicate how his HMO program would correct the maldistribution of medical care and other delivery problems that exist today: inadequate coverage of the old and the poor, neglect of long-time illnesses and of preventive medicine, lack of continuity of service, deterioration of quality, poor integration of services, inadequacy of financing methods, massive and rising costs, gaps in benefits, and failure to provide personal care. Quality control and underutilization receive little attention in Nixon's plan. (Indeed, as the government intervenes increasingly, health care coverage under fee-for-service insurance plans will be reduced.) Nixon certainly fails to deal with the problem of lack of cooperation on the part of physicians in efforts to supervise the quality and necessity of the treatments and procedures they perform. If physicians lose income because review boards deem surgery unnecessary, they will demand other financial compensation or more leisure time.

HMOs under Nixon's plan would cover only a small minority. The recourse to fixed budgets with cost-control provisions and incentives for efficiency, use of capitation reimbursement, and a frontal attack on fee-for-service will all help in controlling expenditures. But correction of inefficiencies, maldistribution, planning deficiencies, and benefit gaps will require strong central leadership.

AMA Opposition

One reason why legislation encouraging HMOs did not pass sooner was the opposition of the American Medical Association. Dr. J. R. Kernodle, chairman of the AMA board of trustees, saw dangers in "the idea that private plans serving selected, carefully controlled memberships can be publicly adapted to the needs and capability of an envisioned 90 percent of the people."[14] Private prepaid groups have been solvent in serving middle-class subscribers, but, in serving rural areas and the vast urban populations, health maintenance organizations have been much less than adequate, in the AMA's opinion. If HMOs fail to achieve large coverage, according to the AMA, the nation would have to resort to either permanent federal subsidies or a reduction in the scope and quality of medical care or increased charges. The AMA recognizes that a capitation charge would be insurance against overtreatment of patients by doctors and hospitals, as the proponents of HMOs claim. But another factor that concerns patients is undertreatment by HMOs in periods of financial stress.

Concerned over high health care costs, the AMA noted that HMOs would have per capita costs of $256 per year under the Nixon administration bill, whereas actual overall costs, public and private, amounted to $365 in 1971-72. On the whole, the AMA was skeptical of the cost reductions promised by HMO supporters. Dr. Kernodle also questioned what impact HMOs would have on the death rate, since 75 percent of the deaths in the United States are due to heart disease, stroke, and accidents.

Perhaps the greatest objection by AMA members to health maintenance organizations was expressed as follows: "Most physicians still
feel that they function best in traditional patterns of practice, and
their preferences—for their patients' sakes as well as their own—
should be respected." This is scarcely an adequate reason for pre-
serving the fee-for-service practice, which contributes so much to
higher health care costs.

The Kaiser Example

The twenty-year-old Kaiser Foundation medical care program is
one of the most successful examples of a health maintenance organization in the country. Consumer acceptance of Kaiser has been overwhelming, and among medical care programs it is considered outstanding.

The principal characteristic of Kaiser is its direct assumption of
responsibility for the organization and delivery of health services on
a prepaid basis to a defined population. The plan provides direct
health care services. It is not an insurance program that returns dollar
benefits for premiums. The basic principles behind the program are:

1. Prepayment, using a community rating approach, which distrib-
utes medical care costs among the covered population and provides
stable revenues for organizing services.

2. Practice by autonomous, self-governing, full-time medical groups,
paid on a capitation, not a fee-for-service, basis.

3. Practice in a medical center by a hospital-based group.

4. Voluntary enrollment.

5. Comprehensive benefits, including preventive care.

In the general market both hospitals and physicians are paid on a
piecework basis for illness, but Kaiser charges on a capitation basis
for all services it contracts to give. When a patient is insured only for
hospitalization, his prospect of being hospitalized is increased. When
insurance coverage is comprehensive and not on a fee-for-service payment method, the least expensive and most effective service can and
usually will be used.

An analysis by the California State Employees Retirement System
found that the total cost of health care for families in the Kaiser
Foundation plans was only 70 percent to 80 percent of the cost for
families covered by other types of insurance. "The economies of prepaid group practice appear to be of two types: primary economies

of scale and rationalization within the organized clinic, and secondary economies due to the more judicious use of hospitals, low cost drugs and other services outside the clinic."[15]

Costs per hospital day under Kaiser have increased, but they rose only about half as much as costs of community hospitals for similar services. The explanation lies in the reduced utilization under Kaiser: with hospital utilization cut by 40 percent, manpower is proportionately reduced.

Kaiser enrollment has risen at a geometric rate, with lack of personnel and facilities restraining further growth. For each 100,000 members, the Kaiser plan requires the availability of 180 hospital beds, 90 physicians organized in a full-time group, 800 ancillary personnel, and a capital investment of about $12 million.[16]

The Kaiser record is so good in part because of its espousal of group-practice plans. The yield of services to patients is much greater under group practice, according to Perroth and Chase, than under insurance benefit plans. Thus, more than 80 percent of the members received at least one covered service from group practice, while fewer than 30 percent of the insured received at least one service under insurance plans.[17]

Under the Kaiser program, charges for visits to doctors are minimal and members are urged to have physical checkups, Pap smears, electrocardiograms, and other preventive or early diagnostic tests. Fewer members suffer persistent symptoms under these conditions, and the encouragement of preventive medicine is reflected in fewer days spent in the hospital. In a recent year, the average number of hospital beds per thousand people nationwide was 3.9, but Kaiser gets along with only 1.7 beds per thousand—less than half.[18]

Notes

1. U.S. Senate, Committee on Labor and Public Welfare, *Hearings on National Health Insurance*, p. 538.

2. L. Baumgartner, *New York Times*, December 20, 1969.

3. K. K. White, "Social Policy for Health Care," paper reprinted from the *Bulletin of the New York Academy of Medicine*, pp. 198-201.

4. Southern California Research Council, *Sustaining Life in Southern California: A Proposal for Health Care Delivery* (1971), p. 55.

5. See especially T. S. Bodenheimer, "Patterns of American Ambulatory Care," *Inquiry*, September 1970, pp. 26-32.

6. Comments of Dr. M. Roemer in U.S. Senate, Committee on Labor and Public Welfare, *Hearings on National Health Insurance*, pp. 286, 742-43.

7. See Southern California Research Council, *Sustaining Life in Southern California: A Proposal for Health Care Delivery* (1971), especially chaps. 1, 2, and 5. This very helpful document facilitated my discussion.

8. W. J. McNerney, *Hospital and Medical Economics* (1962), vol. 2, pp. 1119-29.

9. F. Anderson, *New Republic*, January and February 1970; quoted in U.S. Senate, Committee on Labor and Public Welfare, *Hearings on National Health Insurance*, pp. 716-17.

10. R. M. Bailey, "Philosophy, Faith. . . ., Medical Services," *Inquiry*, March 1970, pp. 38-46.

11. W. J. McNerney, *Hospital and Medical Economics* (1962), vol. 1, especially pp. 595-96, 603, 609, 620-22.

12. Ibid., p. 603.

13. Southern California Research Council, *Sustaining Life in Southern California: A Proposal for Health Care Delivery* (1971), p. 55.

14. J. R. Kernodle, "HMOs: Can They Maintain Health?" *Wall Street Journal*, August 8, 1973.

15. U.S. Senate, Committee on Labor and Public Welfare, *Hearings on National Health Insurance*.

16. Ibid., pp. 350-55.

17. Ibid., p. 357.

18. Ibid., pp. 734-36.

16

Medical Care for the Poor

It is not possible to neglect the problems of the poor in discussing physicians, hospitals, and manpower. Such issues as the shortage of personnel, the remuneration of physicians and allied health workers, the growth of extended care facilities, rate making in hospitals, and the manner of financing hospitals are all germane. The rising cost of hospital care is a crucial issue for the masses. In short, the problems of the poor touch many chapters. These problems, in turn, cannot be discussed fruitfully without tying them to the analysis of national health insurance.

This chapter takes up a number of issues, including the relationships among health, education, and poverty; the special disabilities of the poor in terms of extent of illness and days of disability; medical care in the ghettos; the proportion of those covered under Medicare who fall in the low-income category; the new institutions such as neighborhood centers, that provide health services to low-income people, and the quality of their services; the maldistribution of physicians that results because doctors increasingly live near their practices and do not practice among the poor; the loss of benefits by the poor because of lack of communication, ignorance of rights, disagreements on ideology, problems of transportation, complexities of legislation, and poor administration; and differential treatment and ways of reducing differences.

The "Medically Indigent"

The term *medically indigent* refers to persons who cannot afford medical care even though they may not be indigent with respect to food, clothing, or shelter. These people do not have third-party coverage under Medicare, Medicaid, other governmental programs, or private health insurance. The vast majority have low incomes.

According to various estimates, there are between 20 million and 30 million Americans who have no third-party coverage. Two million of these live in California. A low estimate places medically indigent people at 10 percent of the population.

The number of people unable to afford care is growing. As medical care costs rise faster than personal income, more people will be unable to afford private care.[1]

Major Deficiencies in Care

Maldistribution of medical services is one of the most troublesome problems in the delivery of medical care. The affluent and the well educated receive more and better services than the rest of the population.

Recently, Dr. Alonzo Yerby, former Commissioner of Hospitals for the City of New York, told a White House conference:

The pervasive stigma of charity permeates our arrangements for health care for the disadvantaged, and whether the program is based upon the private practice of medicine or upon public or nonprofit clinics and hospitals, it tends to be piecemeal, poorly supervised and uncoordinated. In most of our large cities, the hospital out-patient department, together with the emergency room, provide the basic sources of care for the poor. [The out-patient departments] are crowded, uncomfortable, lacking in concern for human dignity, and to make it worse, no longer free.

This view may be a little too pessimistic. Local comprehensive health centers together with the emergency rooms of hospitals are today increasing their contribution to health care for the poor. By the late 1960s the federal government was spending about $10 billion on medical care with state and local contributions roughly equal. State and local governments spend 90 percent of their outlays on the poor and the federal government 40 percent. At an estimate of $200 per year per capita, the $10 billion might be adequate for the 50 million people in the low-income class. But the per capita cost now is in excess of $300 per year.

The poor receive inadequate services partly because they are not accustomed to planning, partly because of financial barriers, partly because they do not communicate well with medical personnel, and partly because of lack of education.

American medicine has many weaknesses—lack of planning and coordination, neglect of preventive medicine, excessive dependence on high-cost services, recourse to nonincentive methods of reimbursement, overutilization in some areas and underutilization in others. These and other weaknesses hurt the poor along with the well-to-do. But because of their inadequate participation in the flow of services, the poor feel these defects especially severely.

Shortages of medical personnel are especially troublesome for the poor. In various ways the shortages may be overcome. Improved personnel structures and reduced unit costs would be helpful. Greater use of group practice can bring economies of manpower. Substitution of ambulatory and home services for hospital care is another way to conserve manpower. Increased income among the population as a whole should bring a saving in manpower, since days of disability vary inversely with income. Where serious manpower gaps prevail—for instance, among primary physicians and pediatricians—special care should be exercised to conserve the physician's time for high-level tasks.

Comparison of Ward Patients and Others

A person's economic status influences his entry into a hospital and the treatment accorded to him. One doctor has identified three classes of patients: the unwashed, the washed, and the washed and perfumed. Ward patients and the poor receive inferior treatment, in part because physicians and nurses generally favor the more affluent. Poor patients suffer also as house physicians become increasingly interested in research and university operations.

Ward accommodations for patients generally exhibit narrow halls and dark rooms, no private toilets or bathrooms and no clothes closets, numerous well-worn beds, and a pervasive atmosphere of sickness and distress. To get elective surgery, a patient must put up the money; to get emergency service, he must be deadly ill. The intensive care unit costs $75 a day. It is not available for ward patients.

There are variations in the amount of time nurses spend with patients in the different kinds of hospital accommodations (see table 16.1). But the nurses have little time for genuine nursing. The registered nurse is often caught between conflicting orders from the house doctor and the private physician.

The decision to enter a hospital is made by the patient (rather than the doctor) more often in ward cases than among private-room patients (see table 16.2).

Conflicts may arise between the private physician and the house staff, when the patient seeks attention from a private physician. The doctors want good service for their patients. But they fear that the hospital administration will be more interested in scientific advances and intellectually prestigious teaching activities. "This diversity of interests and objectives profoundly influences the relationship of physicians with the hospital administration, the administration with physicians, and both the administration and physicians with patients."

Semiprivate and private accommodations are reserved for patients who are likely to pay their hospital and medical bills. The hospital staff is concerned if a private doctor cuts into this family income by charging fees.

No social stigma is attached to semiprivate accommodations by most people. The wards, however, bear an aura of dishonor among self-respecting persons: a ward patient presumably cannot pay his way. The medically indigent know they will be investigated and will have no choice of who takes care of them. The vast majority of the poor who have to accept ward accommodations resent the stigma attached to ward occupancy. About 90 percent of physicians have a good working knowledge of the economic status of the patients they sponsor at hospitals. The doctors are interested in the diseases of the ward patient, not in the patient himself. Private patients enjoy

TABLE 16.1   Hours of Nursing by Type of Accommodation

Type of Accommodation	Mean Hours of Nursing
Private	8.7
Semiprivate	3.6
Ward	4.9

TABLE 16.2   Principle Decision-Maker in Hospital Entrance

Decision-Maker	Type of Accommodation		
	Private	Semiprivate	Ward
Patient	8%	6%	19%
Private physician	85%	90%	10%

committeed sponsorship "while the ward patients endured the most discontinuous and disorganized sponsorship."

In their classic volume, *Sickness and Society*, Drs. R. S. Duff and A. B. Hollingshead deal with the socioeconomic aspects of medicine.[2] They are especially interested in the psychological problems of illness generally, the effects on and interactions with the family of the sick, the treatment of and attitude of medical personnel toward ward patients versus the more affluent, the impact of hospitalization on patients in different types of accommodations, the criteria used for admission of patients to hospitals and for appointments of staff, the quality of service provided, and similar problems.

In examining the quality of service, Duff and Hollingshead estimated that the correct diagnosis was made in 62 percent of the cases. The proportion of correct diagnoses was lower in medical cases (46 percent) than in surgical cases (75 percent).

The authors found that "the emotional status of a private patient was more likely to be perceived accurately than that of a semi or ward patient; the emotional status of a moderately disturbed patient was hardly ever perceived by his physician." Mental health also varied by type of accommodation (see table 16.3). Ward patients were most likely to be apprehensive and anxious about being hospitalized, while semiprivate-room patients experienced the most fear of hospitalization.

TABLE 16.3   Mental Health of Patients by Type of Accommodation

Mental Status Prior to Illness	Type of Accommodation		
	Private	Semiprivate	Ward
Healthy	8%	17%	2%
Psychotic	6%	13%	26%

Source: R. S. Duff and A. B. Hollingshead, *Sickness and Society* (1968).

Although 47 percent of illnesses were linked to family relationships, in two out of three cases, the physician had no awareness of family problems that were emerging with the illness. Patient satisfaction with care varied directly with cost of accommodations (see table 16.4). Mortality, however, was lower among semiprivate-room patients (15 percent) than among private-room patients (26 percent) or ward patients (37 percent). In cases of terminal illness, "evasions, silences, half-truths and deliberate lies then become elements in the social realities," Duff and Hollingshead noted.

The mean charge was surprisingly high for ward patients—$318, compared to $365 for private patients and $284 for semiprivate. About 20 percent of hospital bills were paid for by patients and their families, 48 percent by Blue Cross, 23 percent by other insurance plans, and 9 percent by other sources of funds.

The impact of illness is greater on ward patients, as table 16.5 indicates. This is also evident in appraisals of the conditions of patients and number of deaths by type of accommodation.

Poverty Area Case Studies

Chicago

Blacks especially suffer in the allocation of resources, as a brief discussion of the Chicago ghetto situation bears witness. In Chicago, the Cook County Hospital serves half of all the city's black patients. Blacks must travel eight times farther for hospital care than they would have to go if the nearest facilities were available to them.

By law and statutes, the poor of Chicago may choose any physicians and hospitals for medical care, and private vendors are reimbursed by the state for services rendered to the poor. But in practice, the Cook County Hospital—the one public charity hospital—is the primary hospital for blacks, and it thus serves 5 million people living

TABLE 16.4   Satisfaction with Medical Care by Type of Accommodation

Type of Accommodation	Percentage Fully Satisfied with Care	
	Medicine	Surgery
Private room	37%	56%
Semiprivate room	27%	46%
Ward	24%	28%

Source: R. S. Duff and A. B. Hollingshead, *Sickness and Society* (1968).

TABLE 16.5   Impact of Illness on Patient, by Type of Accommodation

	Type of Accommodation		
Effect of Illness	Private	Semiprivate	Ward
Minor change	57%	35%	21%
Severe hardship	8%	28%	29%

Source: R. S. Duff and A. B. Hollingshead, *Sickness and Society* (1968).

in a 1,000 square mile area. This hospital provides care to half of the black patients residing in the poverty zone, while it serves less than 1 percent of the patient population in the rest of Chicago.

Blacks receive less favorable treatment than others. Only one-fifth of black poor patients were admitted to hospitals by a private physician compared to four-fifths of other patients; 20 percent of the black poor had their hospital bills reimbursed out of public aid, while only 1 percent of other patients did; hospitals received no payment from 90 percent of the black poor and from only 2 percent of others.

Blacks need more hospitalization than others but they get less. Only 12.5 of the 6,000 physicians affiliated with white hospitals in Chicago are black. The proportion of blacks among Chicago's hospital patients is 30 percent, while the percentage of physicians available to serve them is 2 percent.

Physicians increasingly practice in higher income areas. Shortages prevail in rich suburban areas and in ghetto areas. The West Side community of West Garfield Park had 212 physicians in 1930 when its population was all white. Now there are only 13 physicians serving 63,000 black residents. A single North Shore medical building has more doctors than the entire West Side ghetto of 300,000 poor blacks.

Medicaid payments are currently 150 percent of medical payments to categorical public aid recipients. Although medical services are more expensive in Cook County than they are downstate, medical expenses per recipient in Cook County are about half those for downstate recipients.

Medicaid in Cook County has met with substantial obstacles: there are delays in certification and uncertainty about payments; the majority of claims put in by hospitals have been ignored; claim payments often take months because of red tape; the vast majority of physicians do not participate in Medicaid; the income eligibility ceilings are low; the eligible needy are ignorant of available programs; and the program is incomprehensible to vendors.

Of the 20 percent of patients who cannot afford any medical care, a majority seek help from hospitals. But hospitals cannot afford to provide much free help. A 1969 study found that "while the quality of physicians may be fairly high at the County Hospital, there is a high turnover rate, inadequate ancillary staff, much obsolescence in buildings and facilities, intolerable waiting at times, excessive length of stay, and an overriding feeling of being treated as inferior for being poor."[3]

So-called medically poor families, earning between $1,800 and $3,600 a year, are not eligible for public assistance payments for physicians' services in Cook County. If they qualify for categorically related payments (such as assistance to the blind or the aged), they are normally entitled to some benefits for physicians' services. But incredible red tape, confusion, and delays in reimbursement keep most Cook County physicians from participating in the programs.

Lack of rapport between black residents and health vendors leads the vendors to write off these patients as illiterates. Only one-third of the Negro poor have access to a physician. These few doctors, who are too weak or old to move to a higher income neighborhood, can do little more than give shots and prescribe pills.

One doctor operating in the slums performs a high volume of services and achieves a substantial income. He operates a clinic that grosses $250,000 a year, giving him a net income of $100,000 annually. The clinic has six examining rooms and is open seven days a week. The doctor handles 100 patients a day, and he is assisted by four part-time specialists and five women assistants. At that volume per day a patient gets five minutes per visit. This allows for "a quick recital of complaints, a symptomatic (instantaneous) diagnosis, a shot or prescription, and brief instruction. The doctor does not even gown his patients or wash his hands between examinations. The standard of care is symptomatic."[4]

The clinic justifies its high patient load and resultant brief visits by citing the low fees allowed by the Department of Public Aid. The physician-population ratio for welfare patients is one-tenth the rate for private patients (1:7,000 for welfare patients).[5]

"The only way this low-cost idea can work is with large volume," the doctor maintains. "Each patient is considered individually. But it is much like being a battlefield medic, since I see about 100 patients a day. . . . I have to make quick evaluations of which patients require consultations, which I can help immediately, which need surgery or hospitalization, etc."[6]

One doctor at the clinic gave injections to seventy-six patients in one day. It is often the only treatment: injections of vitamins, tranquilizers, and antibiotics are liberally dispensed.

A study showed that 19 percent of Chicago's total population—those living in areas designated as poverty areas—accounted for 61 percent of all poor families in the city, 89 percent of all public assistance recipients, 44 percent of adults with low education, 79 percent of those living in substandard housing, 67 percent of all male juvenile delinquents, and 62 percent of the unemployed. The birth rate of this population segment was 50 percent higher than that of the rest of the city, and there were four times as many nonhospital births as in the rest of the city. The proportion of mothers under age twenty was double that in the rest of the city. Illegitimate births were recorded 4½ times more often than in the remainder of the city. Infant mortality was 60 percent higher, cases of tuberculosis were double, and venereal disease occurred 5½ times as frequently as in the rest of the city. This mile square area had half the number of doctors per capita and only one-third the number of certified specialists per capita that the remainder of the city had.[7]

This socioeconomic survey of the poverty area of Chicago underlines the interrelationship of such items as income, housing, education, crime, welfare needs, medical care, and disease. The Chicago situation is illustrative of the distribution of resources, incomes, and medical care in low-income areas of other major cities.

Watts

The shortage of physicians is especially disturbing in the Watts area of Los Angeles. In the southeast district, the physician-population ratio is 38:100,000. For the whole of Los Angeles County, the ratio is 127:100,000. Of 106 practitioners in the south and southeast districts, only 17, or 16 percent, are specialists, whereas 55 percent of the nation's doctors are specialists. The Watts population therefore requires services from outside the Watts area. To get to the county general hospital by bus takes an hour's trip and sixty-eight cents.

J. T. English provides the following description of the Watts experience:

I think that those of you who are familiar with that community know it to be an "island," surrounded by super highways, in which 350,000 people live in an area that is the size of San Francisco. In that land area there is not a single hospital, not a single motion picture theater, not a single community center—except for a little coffee shop supported by Community Action funds. After the riot in Watts, even this was closed down because it could not meet the fire regulations. . . .

Today, the OEO health center is operating in Watts, and the University of Southern California School of Medicine, which really is a rather conservative medical institution, is working in that community. There are 30 full-time physicians from the faculty of this medical school practicing in the new building. They are organized in family health teams—not only the lines of categorical disease entities—so that the whole family can come for help. There is an internist to care for the adults, a pediatrician for the children, a public health nurse, a social worker, and people from the neighborhood are involved in the health team. The same family sees the same health team each time they come. In the event of need for more specialized diagnostic workup, arrangements are made to send patients, by appointment, to the University of Southern California Medical Center or to a hospital bed—not to a long waiting room line—in the Los Angeles County Hospital. The same physicians who are in the neighborhood health center follow them in the hospital or the outpatient clinic. . . .

As part of its program, the neighborhood health center has its own mini-buses to shuttle people back and forth between the hospital and the center. If it were not for these, the doctor could not be sure that his patients would get to the hospital when they need to go. The local physicians in the neighborhood are cooperating. They will participate, full time or part time, in the work of the center, and in that way they will have a chance to reduce their own alienation. Also, these physicians now have, for the first time, the opportunity for clinical appointments at the University of Southern California School of Medicine's medical faculty. *Time* magazine recently called the center "The Miracle of Charcoal Alley."[8]

OEO Findings

An Office of Economic Opportunity program reveals that an infant from a poor family has twice the chance of dying in the first year that an infant from a middle-income family has, and four times the chance of dying before age thirty-five.

A survey of 140,000 boys and girls sent to a training institution—largely dropouts from school, aged sixteen to twenty-one—revealed that 90 percent had never seen a dentist, 70 percent had not seen a doctor in three or four years, and one-third had visual defects. They averaged twenty-seven visits to the medical center in the first year. Similar revelations are found among the 1.3 million preschool youngsters in the Head Start program. Their medical costs of $40 million consumed 10 percent of the $400 million budget of Head Start.[9]

Public Medical Aid to the Poor

Many persons receiving benefits from public income transfer programs are aided by more than one such program in the form of cash, medical care, subsidized housing, and free or reduced-price food.[10] In fact, it is estimated that 26 percent of the largest federally funded income transfer programs and the major nonfederal programs, which were expected to have a gross total of 119 million beneficiaries in 1961-62, actually aided no more than 60 million different individuals. The gross number of 64 million recipients in the ten federal and nonfederal programs basing assistance on need criteria probably involves 25 million to 30 million different individuals. This figure reflects the true size of the "welfare rolls."[11]

Disparities in the income support available from government sources offer an incentive for low-income fathers to desert their families (see table 16.6). Medical benefits are between two and three times as large in New York City as in Atlanta. Substantial differences are also found in Medicare and Medicaid payments (see table 16.7). The tables indicate that an adequate income for poor people is mainly a function of where they live, how old they are, whether husband and wife live together, and how many children they have. "The unemployed mother of three in New York would receive benefits about $250 in excess of the poverty standard of about $4,000, or $1,300 above the line if medical benefits are included."

Some 38 percent of all families who were poor before receiving transfers were removed from poverty with the transfer payments.

TABLE 16.6 Medical Benefits by Type of Family and City

Family Type	City	
	Atlanta	New York
Aged couple	$986	$2,524
Mother and three children	448	1,070

TABLE 16.7   Medicare and Medicaid Payments by City

Type of Payment	City	
	Atlanta	New York
Medicare		
Hospital insurance	$162	$ 290
Supplementary medical		
insurance	70	108
Medicaid		
Old age assistance	261	864
Aid to Families with		
Dependent Children	498	1,070

Source: Adapted from J. R. Storey, "Public Income Transfer Programs," A Study for the Subcommittee on Fiscal Policy of the Joint Economic Committee of Congress, *Studies in Public Welfare*, Paper no. 1, pp. 16-17.

Cash transfer payments were most effective in providing adequate incomes for small families, whites, male-headed families, the aged, the unemployed, and urban residents. Medical benefits should be considered in analyzing the adequacy of benefits, but they are not.[12]

The proportion of income transfer recipients who receive benefits from other programs is revealed in table 16.8. The programs with the most recipients are Old Age and Survivors Insurance, Medicaid, and Medicare.[13]

From 1965 to 1975, it is estimated that public and private expenditures for coping with poverty will rise from $28.8 billion to $74.6 billion, a jump of 159 percent. The largest absolute rise is expected in social welfare spending ($19 billion). Public assistance medical payments and private health insurance benefits are estimated to experience the largest proportional increases—289 percent and 291 percent, respectively. Health expenditures are expected to rise by $13.3 billion or 206 percent.[14] With such large outlays to treat poverty, the resources that might be available for medicine are substantially consumed.

The financial and other barriers to getting medical services to the poor include fragmentation of care; the loss of work and money and the inconvenience associated with travel to and waiting for care; lack of communication and understanding between poor patients and members of medical teams; the failure of patients to plan and take preventive measures, because of ignorance, habit, or inability; racial

TABLE 16.8   Income Transfer Recipients Receiving Other Benefits, 1971-72

Programs	Number of Recipients (Thousands)	Percentage of Recipients Who Receive Other Benefits	
		Cash Benefits	Benefits Including Aid in Kind
Aid to Families with Dependent Children	11,073	12	99
Old Age Assistance	2,241	64	99
Aid to the Blind	83	34	99
Aid to the Permanently and Totally Disabled	1,103	31	99
General assistance	969	*	*
Old Age and Survivors Insurance	24,355	22-25	93-95
Disability insurance	2,925	16-20	*
Railroad retirement	994	50	85-92
Civil service retirement	1,058	*	*
Other federal employee retirement	889	*	*
State and local retirement	1,272	*	*
Unemployment insurance	1,564	9	*
Workmen's compensation	1,500	*	*
Veterans' pensions	2,297	82	91-93
Veterans' compensation	2,549	*	*
National School Lunch Program (free or reduced-price lunches)	7,900	*	*
Food stamps	11,000	*	*
Food distribution	3,513	*	*
Public housing	3,453	61	*
Veterans' medical care	89	*	*
Medicare	17,300	92-95	*
Medicaid	20,600	*	*

Source: J. R. Storey, "Public Income Transfer Programs," A Study for the Subcommittee on Fiscal Policy of the Joint Economic Committee of Congress, *Studies in Public Welfare*, Paper no. 1, p. 24.

*Not available.

discrimination; and lack of manpower and facilities, in part resulting from large expansion of government and private insurance programs. These obstacles are brilliantly detailed in the HEW study, *Delivery of Health Services for the Poor* (December 1967):

1. *Inability to pay:* The most obvious barrier to the poor's quest to obtain the whole spectrum of medical services is their lack of ability to pay for services. The provision of services by welfare systems employing "means tests" is an attempt to overcome the financial barrier, but is not entirely successful because

other barriers are erected in this effort. For example, the mere establishment of "medical indigency" can be a humiliating experience to some patients which does not encourage repetition of the attempt to secure such services.

2. *Fragmentation of care:* Outpatient clinics serving indigent patients have been described as "medical medievalism," usually dispensing depersonalized care with no one person or group concerned with the patients' needs being met over time. The system of frequent referrals to specialty clinics results in fragmented care not easily understood by the average consumer or the low-income person. To illustrate the fragmentation of medical care, Dr. George James has cited the example of the elderly indigent man who lived near one of the largest medical centers in the world. This man, picked up on a survey, had been labeled as an "uncooperative" patient by the hospital because he had stopped attending the clinics. He had 12 major pathological diagnoses at the time the survey had found him. He had been told to attend no less than 10 specialty clinics; but he was too sick to do this so he stopped attending any.

3. *Operational features of providing the services:* Physical and operational features of medical services located among the poor discourage utilization by causing excessive time lost from work; involved travel to health care facilities; long hours of waiting; lack of seats; unattractive buildings and furniture; and inconvenient hours of operation.

Lack of communication, trust, and understanding on both the part of poor patients and the doctors, nurses, and other medical personnel serving them, have raised barriers which prevent the doctor and other health team members from really getting to know and coming to grips with the patient's medical-social problems. Additionally, staffing inadequacies further frustrate the physician in his attempt to spend adequate time caring for low-income patients. Hostility and isolation may develop from this inability of the patient to relate to the doctor and his institution, and vice versa.

4. *"Low-income" attitudes toward general health care:* Part of the difficulty that the poor have with the established medical care system stems from the way in which they view the world, which may conflict with the behavior and expectations of the health personnel with whom they come into contact. People who grow up in poverty must learn to deal with the frequent immediate crises they face (i.e., making ends meet, etc.) and therefore may have difficulty in planning for the future and thinking in terms of disease prevention. Certain diseases, such as arthritis or loss of teeth may be accepted as necessary concomitants of aging. In studies of the attitudes of "blue collar" workers toward health and illness, it has been found that they tend to be less informed about illness as contrasted to "white collar" workers. In addition, they may be more skeptical about the value of prevention, early sickness consultation, and treatment, and subsequently will seek treatment at a relatively late stage of a disease. These attitudes may lead to under-utilization of services and interfere with the receipt of timely care.

5. *Racial discrimination in provision of services:* While it is difficult to get reliable statistics on subtle discriminatory practices, it is clear that racial discrimination interferes with the delivery of adequate medical care, particularly in the South, but also in the North. The situation improved somewhat with the requirement that providers of service under Medicare comply with civil rights regulations. The result has been that many younger Negroes, as well as the old, are being served in facilities previously closed to them. However, in areas where a dual hospital system existed, many facilities have been unable to change their "white only" image and subsequently are underutilized by Negroes. Three hundred hospitals in the South are still not in compliance with civil rights regulations. In addition, Negro physicians are often denied staff privileges in the better hospitals.

6. *Lack of facilities and manpower:* Lack of facilities and manpower create additional barriers in poverty areas. The urban slums and ghettos in which the poor live, as well as remote rural areas such as parts of Appalachia, have, according to many studies, a paucity of medical facilities and manpower. Since these areas are often unattractive places for physicians and their families to settle in, it is not surprising that they choose to practice in the middle and upper-class areas. The central core hospitals of most large American cities often migrate to the suburbs with a new building program after the deterioration of the central core area; those who can escape to the suburbs take their doctors and hospitals with them. In rural areas, the sparse population, long distance between settlements, general poverty, and social isolation make it difficult to attract doctors. The nature of political subdivisions and local politics often prevent the establishment of area-wide centralized medical facilities.[15]

It is clear that treating poverty is a costly matter. One important factor in the antipoverty programs is the high cost of financing and delivering health services for the aged. The most important programs now in operation are described below.[16]

Medicaid

Medicaid, sometimes referred to as Title XIX (of the Social Security Act), is a medical assistance program intended

to assist states in furnishing medical assistance to families with dependent children, and to aged, blind, or permanently and totally disabled individuals whose incomes and resources are insufficient to meet the costs of necessary services and rehabilitation and other services to help such families and individuals attain or retain capability for self-care. . . . The goal by 1975, is to cover payment for comprehensive health care services for all persons who need help in meeting their medical obligations.

By January 1968, there were thirty-eight approved state plans covering between 6 million and 8 million persons.

At the present time, under Title XIX, and until 1975 when comprehensive health services must be covered, programs must provide for in- and out-patient hospital services, physicians' services, laboratory, x-ray, and skilled nursing home services for adults. The 1967 Amendments allow as alternatives any 7 of the 14 specified services. However, the States may, and often do, set limitations on the extent of coverage provided within any one of these or other services. It is not presently known what percent of the total medical costs incurred by persons covered under Title XIX are borne by the program, nor is it known with any degree of certainty what percent of the medically indigent are covered by or make use of the various medical assistance programs. The Social and Rehabilitation Service has initiated studies which will provide this information.

Title XIX, along with other major health care programs, is straining already scarce traditional medical resources. The quality of services rendered under the program is not known, but preliminary evidence suggests that the pattern of receipt of care (as with previous welfare programs) may often be that patients are receiving care from the small percentage of practitioners (not infrequently without hospital privileges) who reside in low-income neighborhoods and must provide a large volume of service. There is also evidence, in some localities, of decreased use of county hospitals, some of which are considering an organizational shift to community hospital status.[17]

The Human Investment Program in the Department of Health, Education, and Welfare, has outlined the goals and objectives of Medicaid:

With the enactment of major health legislation in the past several years, Congress and the Administration have asserted that access to health care is the right of every citizen, not the privilege of a few. However, those among the poor who are eligible for the Medical Assistance Program (Title XIX) find that their health care ticket must compete for already scarce resources in a health care system which will be unable to fulfill their expectations for services. Nonetheless, if Title XIX receives fuller financing than it now enjoys, if there are improvements in the income limits set for determining medical indigency, if there are built-in incentives to encourage the participation of group practices, then it can form the financial underpinning for more efficient and effective organization of services. In this way, the potential benefits of recent health legislation can be realized.[18]

The objectives related to the program's intermediate health services goal (by 1973) were:

a. To reduce the social and cultural barriers to the receipt of comprehensive health services.
b. To eliminate the utilization gap between poor and non-poor in outpatient physicians' and dentists' services.
c. To assure the accessibility of preventive services and family planning to all poor persons.
d. Through more accessible ambulatory care, to reduce the utilization of in-patient hospital and emergency room services.
e. To assure interaction of the health care system in such communities with other services having implications for health including education, welfare, employment, recreation, and corrections.
f. To eliminate the financial barrier to the receipt of comprehensive health services for all medically needy (by 1975).[19]

The intermediate health status goal was to eliminate the mortality and disability differentials between the poor and other income groups within fifteen years. The objectives related to this goal were:

a. To reduce disability among the poor in [poverty] communities (as measured by days of limited activity, working days lost, etc.).
b. To reduce the mortality differentials (as exemplified by cancer of the cervix, maternal and infant mortality, pneumonia, and influenza), between the poor and other income groups.
c. To reduce the differential in incidence of communicable diseases (as exemplified by tuberculosis and measles).
d. To reduce the number of untreated health conditions occurring in the poor.[20]

Details on the services provided under Medicaid for thirty states and territories are given in table 16.9. Twenty-three states provide inpatient hospital service. The nineteen services available are considered state by state.

In the first four years of Medicaid operations many states experienced drains on their treasuries, and subsequently reduced their services, eligibility levels, and funds. California and Maryland (under then-Governor Spiro Agnew) were early sites of Medicaid cuts. In mid-1968, the Maryland Dental Association withdrew from the state's program because Agnew had allocated only $650,000 for dental care. A month later the governor dropped 22,000 persons from Medicaid coverage by lowering the eligibility level for the categorically linked medically needy.

In 1969, Massachusetts dropped 40,000 medically needy families from Medicaid, cut the fees paid, and issued new and longer billing

TABLE 16.9 Medicaid Services Provided by State, 1967

Service Provided	California	Connecticut	Delaware	Guam	Hawaii*	Idaho	Illinois	Kansas*	Kentucky	Louisiana	Maine	Maryland*	Massachusetts	Michigan	Minnesota	Nebraska	New Mexico	New York*	North Dakota	Ohio	Oklahoma	Pennsylvania*	Puerto Rico	Rhode Island	Utah	Vermont	Virgin Islands*	Washington*	West Virginia	Wisconsin	I	—	Total
Inpatient hospital	—	—	—	—	—	I	—	—	—	I	I	—	—	—	—	—	I	—	—	I	—	—	—	—	—	I	—	—	I		7	23	30
Outpatient hospital	—	—	—	—	—	I	—	—	—	I	I	—	—	—	—	—	I	—	—	I	—	I	—	I	—	I	—	—	I		9	21	30
Skilled nursing home	—	—	—	—	—	I	—	—	—	I	I	—	—	—	—	—	I	—	—	I	—	—	—	—	—	I	—	—	I		7	22	29
Physicians	—	—	—	—	—	I	—	—	—	I	I	—	—	—	—	—	I	—	—	I	—	I	—	—	—	I	—	—	I		8	21	29
Transportation or ambulance	—	—	—	—	—	—	—	—	—	I	—	—	—	—	—	—	I	—	—	I	—	I	—	I	—	I	—	—	I	I	8	18	26
Prescribed drugs and pharmaceuticals	—	—	—	—	—	—	—	—	I	I	—	—	—	—	—	—	I	—	—	I	—	—	—	—	—	—	—	—	I		6	19	25
Prosthetic devices and appliances	—	—	—	—	—	—	—	—	I	I	—	—	—	—	—	—	I	—	—	I	—	I	—	—	—	I	—	—	I	I	8	17	25
Home health care	—	—	—	—	—	—	—	—	—	I	—	—	—	—	—	—	I	—	—	I	—	—	—	I	—	—	—	—	I		5	19	24
Dental	—	—	—	—	—	—	—	—	I	—	—	—	—	—	—	—	I	—	—	I	—	—	—	—	—	—	—	—	I		5	19	24
Laboratory and X-ray work	—	—	—	—	—	—	—	—	I	I	—	—	—	—	—	—	I	—	—	I	—	I	—	—	—	I	—	—	I		6	17	23
Eyeglasses	—	—	—	—	—	—	—	—	I	—	—	—	—	—	—	—	I	—	—	—	—	I	I	—	—	—	—	—	I	I	5	13	18
Physical therapy and related services	—	—	—	—	—	—	—	—	—	—	—	—	—	—	—	—	I	—	—	—	—	—	—	—	—	I	—	I	I		3	12	15
Private duty nursing	—	—	—	—	—	—	—	—	—	—	—	—	—	—	—	—	I	—	—	I	—	—	—	—	—	—	—	I	I		3	7	10
Podiatrists	—	—	—	—	I	—	—	—	—	—	—	—	—	—	—	—	I	—	—	I	—	I	—	I	—	—	—	—		I	5	5	10
Clinic	—	—	—	—	—	—	I	—	—	—	—	—	—	—	—	—	I	—	—	I	—	—	—	—	—	—	—	—			0	7	7
Audiology or speech	—	—	—	—	—	—	—	—	—	—	—	—	I	—	—	—	—	I	—	—	—	—	—	—	—	I	—	I	I		3	4	7
Chiropractors, naturopaths, other sectarian practitioners	—	—	—	—	I	—	—	—	—	—	—	—	—	—	—	—	—	I	—	—	—	I	—	—	—	—	—	—		I	3	3	6
Hearing aids	—	—	—	—	—	—	—	—	—	—	—	—	—	—	—	—	—	—	—	—	—	—	—	—	—	—	—	—	—		0	5	5
Other diagnostic, screening, preventive, rehabilitative	—	—	—	—	—	I	—	—	I	—	—	—	—	—	—	—	I	—	—	—	—	—	—	—	—	I	—	—		I	5	12	17

Source: HEW, Human Investment Programs, *Delivery of Health Services for the Poor* (December 1967), p. 38.

I Categorically needy only

— Categorically needy and categorically related medically needy

*States that also provide services to the non-categorically-related medically needy, ages 21-64, without federal financial participation. Details as to types of services provided are not available.

forms to be filled out after each visit. The New Mexico legislature voted to cancel its Medicaid plan and replace it with the narrowest possible program that would still receive federal funds. This action was vetoed by HEW as a violation of the Medicaid law. Other states to cut the number of persons covered and reduce the services were Louisiana, Oklahoma, Utah, Kansas, and North Carolina.

Medicare

A second program under the Social Security Act is Health Insurance for the Aged (Title XVIII), known as Medicare. This covers hospital and related costs and offers voluntary supplementary medical insurance to cover part of the cost of physicians' and other medical services. It is estimated that 40 percent of the medical costs incurred by the aged are potentially reimbursable under Medicare. Of the 19.2 million people covered in this program about 7.3 million fall under the low-income index.

The Comprehensive Health Center Program

Another program under this legislation is the Comprehensive Health Center or Neighborhood Health Center program. The objective of comprehensive health centers is to

offer comprehensive care which may be defined as a system of person-and-family-centered service rendered by a well-balanced, well-organized core of professional, technical and vocational personnel who, by using facilities and equipment that are physically and functionally related, can deliver effective preventive, diagnostic, therapeutic, advisory, rehabilitative service at a cost that is economically compatible with individual, family, community, and national resources.[21]

Comprehensive health centers are also subject to constraints. How can they overcome the fragmentary crisis-oriented care now given to lower socioeconomic groups? Possibilities include improvement in outpatient clinics, providing ancillary personnel to group practices, and supporting rural projects.[22] Especially helpful would be increasing the productivity of scarce manpower.

The centers need to be located in areas of concentrated low-income population. Approximately 53 percent of the 45 million low-income people live outside metropolitan areas. "The present metropolitan area universe of need for CHC then is about 10.6 million low-income people. . . . Thus, the total universe of need for CHC appears to be a minimum of 16.6 million (10.6 million metropolitan, 6.0 million nonmetropolitan)."[23] These figures are reduced to some extent by migrations from rural areas and reduction of the poor population.[24]

Appendix to Chapter 16

An excellent report by the Task Force on Medicaid and Related Programs (Walter J. McNerney, Chairman) was released in June 1970. It started from the premise that "health must remain high on the scale of social, economic and political priorities—not only because the health of the nation is basic to the growth and productivity of the economy, but also because human compassion insists that essential individual health needs should be met."[25] The Task Force argued that

access to basic medical care shall be a right or entitlement of all citizens. It is the position of the Task Force that the right of entitlement is not fulfilled when millions in the population do not know or cannot get to the places where [services] are available or when the millions who do get to such places are given a kind of service that is woefully inferior by every standard known to man and doctor.[26]

Only about one-third of the 30 million to 40 million indigent and medically indigent people who could potentially be covered by Title XIX of the Social Security Act (Medicaid) will in fact receive service. The legislative promise that some care would be available for all has not been realized. "That the cost of covering less than one-third has exceeded earlier estimates of the cost of covering the whole medically deprived population is due to a combination of factors, including inflation. It also suggests how badly the expenditures have been controlled or how badly the program costs were estimated or both."[27]

There are some 5 million poor women who want and need family planning services and almost 20 million poor children. Medicaid reached only a small fraction of them. Yet even without needed extensions of eligibility and coverage, the program could, through normal growth, outstrip state tax resources at present levels within the next five to ten years.

The Task Force advocated federal management that would "guide, not direct; motivate, not demand; assist not provide; and evaluate, not ordain."[28] It felt:

The system must be oriented towards encouraging people to stay well, towards health maintenance instead of only towards getting well. . . . The health field needs not *only* a strong infusion of money and effectiveness, it also needs a sounder philosophic framework and reevaluation of goals.

Increased participation of and influence of consumer interests is in the views of the Task Force absolutely essential. Consumers should express preferences and needs and yet resist the eroding process of institutionalization.[29]

On the issue of timing reform measures, the Task Force was concerned that patchwork improvements "might reduce the incentive to take a broader view but the conclusion was that persons without adequate purchasing power need help now, not at some indeterminate future date, and that it should be possible to fashion short-run recommendations not incompatible with long-term steps.[30]

There are wide variations among states in the programs provided. As of June 1970, only twenty-eight states had extended Medicaid coverage to medically needy who are not in need of cash.[31] The Task Force warns:

If the nation is serious about commitment to a basic floor of health care for all citizens, a considerable expansion of financing and a larger investment of manpower and facilities resources are required. By a simple extension of the $5 billion cost of providing services for 10 million people, for example, one can approximate the cost of providing the same service for 25 million.[32]

The Task Force recommends converting Medicaid to a program with uniform minimum levels of health benefits financed 100 percent by federal funds plus federal matching funds for certain types of supplementary benefits provided by states and for state payments to individuals not covered under the minimum plan.[33] "The commitment to provide comprehensive care to substantially all needy and medically needy should be reaffirmed."[34]

Innovative facilities such as neighborhood health centers, community health centers, group-practice organizations, and outpatient services of hospitals that provide neighborhood comprehensive ambulatory care, need to be used for provision of medical care.[35]

For twenty-five years, financial programs for medical care "have served largely to provide financial underpinning for conventional ways of providing services. . . . Instead of encouraging change, the programs have been rewarding traditional methods and old inefficiencies. The revolution of rising expectations in medical care brings more informed and expensive tastes."

Comprehensive services and continuity of care, contractual services for definable population groups, integrated fiscal and managerial responsibilities, and risk-sharing through prepayment should, in the view of the Task Force, be elements of the health care system.

Legislation should make as much as 5 percent of the federal Medicaid appropriation available each year for the development and improvement of health care services and resources. The Task Force emphasizes using this money as front-end money in localities with a high proportion of low-income people. It could be used to provide substitutes for expensive hospital inpatient services and improvements in the utilization, efficiency, and quality of existing health care services. These funds can also be used to reward states that successfully develop and use innovative programs, services, and payment methods such as contract payments to prepaid group-practice plans.[36] Federal funding should be "encouraged to give high priority to development, support and demonstrations of model health care delivery systems."[37]

The Task Force strongly supports the growth of health maintenance organizations, and it

endorses the innovative approach of the Administration's HMO proposal. [The members] support the principle of providing an option for Medicare and Medicaid beneficiaries that would permit them to elect to receive health services through a single organization in a coordinated manner, financed through prepaid capitation. The Task Force suggests financing methods, benefits to be covered, enrollment methods and charges in relation to costs.

Unfortunately, the Task Force does not offer any explanation for the slow rate of growth of health maintenance organizations.[38]

Reimbursement to providers of services under Medicare and Medicaid should be on a prospective instead of a retrospective basis. The payment of "reasonable" fees to physicians and suppliers without effective limitation is an invitation to escalate charges. "To be reasonable and fair, as well as governable, reimbursement must tie its recognition of increases in fees to some accepted index."

Medicaid should be amended to permit varying benefits for different population groups or areas within a state.[39]

There must be a closer relationship among claims review, cost control, cost effectiveness, program planning and professional input. . . . No state has yet established an effective system of reviewing and controlling utilization from the standpoint of appropriateness, quality or timeliness of services. . . .

Without minimum Federal requirements mandatory on all states uniformly— states will probably retain their own policies and procedures which can vary widely.[40]

Failure to coordinate federal and state programs has brought confusion, duplication of effort, and inadequate surveillance of quality. States should have greater flexibility in requiring periodic medical reviews of skilled nursing homes and mental hospitals. The Task Force feels that reimbursement under Titles V, XVIII, and XIX of the Social Security Act for expenses connected with capital expenditures for plant and equipment must be related to state planning activities for health services and facilities.[41]

The Task Force would like the federal government to make a greater contribution to leadership in the health field by taking "responsibility for developing, financing, influencing, evaluating and regulating an efficient and responsive health system." This country has made only "partial progress towards measuring the status of our health system and the measures that exist usually center around gross measures of health status rather than cost, accessibility, and quality of care." The Secretary of Health, Education, and Welfare should take immediate steps to redefine the authority of advisory councils "with the purpose of placing decision making authority with publicly accountable officers . . . . and substantially increasing public and consumer representation on these councils." The Task Force found several sources of trouble: weak organization and lack of manpower; passive operations by the Medical Service Administration; and fragmentation of policy direction over health service programs.[42]

Consumers have had little influence in policy making. The Task Force recommends that "any Board or group set up to advise policy making officials at any level of government . . . provide for consumer representation to protect and present the interest and needs of the consumer." Consumer training is required if consumers are to assume larger responsibilities. "Federal agencies involved in planning, delivering, and purchasing health services must make provisions in budgets for special orientation programs . . . including consumer representation in such groups."[43]

The Task Force further feels that

State Medicaid Programs should be required to undertake educational efforts designed to: improve recipients' use of the Medicaid program; improve the health of Medicaid recipients through preventive education; improve providers' use of the program; and provide for greater participation by provider and consumer in the planning, implementation, and evaluation of the program.[44]

Comprehensive health planning receives much attention from the Task Force. The total financial requirements for 250 to 300 local planning agencies to cover the whole country are estimated at $100 million per year.[45]

Long-term care is another concern on the agenda of the Task Force. In 1968-69, over $2.4 billion was spent on nursing home care, with three-quarters financed from public funds. Nearly one out of every three Medicaid dollars goes for skilled nursing home care. Long-term care in an institutional setting is becoming an inevitable burden of later life, in part owing to the breakdown of family life. Long-term care is often neglected, and as a result this area is underdeveloped. Medicare and Medicaid do not treat the problem well. The Task Force "therefore recommends that HEW develop a policy which addresses directly the need for long-term services."[46] When the Medicare legislation was drafted, long-term care was not covered under the statute, because of a preoccupation with preventing overutilization of high-cost hospital beds. Instead, a special "extended care" benefit was developed as part of the hospital insurance program, and efforts were made to encourage the growth of special extended care facilities. However, most extended care services are still provided in nursing homes.[47]

The Task Force noted that

great disparities existed and continue to exist in access to and utilization of health services, with related disparities in health and status among different income, racial and ethnic groups among geographic areas. . . .

Maldistribution of resources, shortages and inefficiencies in the delivery of services, combined with inflation and steadily increasing consumer demand have resulted in a rapid escalation of prices, threatening both the public capacity to finance health services to eligible groups and the private capacity of individuals to pay for care. . . . Medicare today shares fully all the stresses and difficulties to which other health-care mechanisms are exposed. . . .

Only as orderly financing for the provision of these expensive services to citizens throughout the land becomes a matter of high political activity do we realize that the delivery of care, its pricing and its prepayment must be made more orderly, more economical and more generally satisfactory to the public at large.[48]

Key problems are the effects of financing programs on utilization and costs, the wide variations in manpower per patient day among comparable hospitals, and the wide variations in numbers of beds per thousand population. In the opinion of the Task Force, they all indicate the need for greater purchasing power by individuals as an instrument of change.[49]

Notes

1. For more information on the medically indigent, see "Turning Point for Public Hospitals," *Health/PAC Bulletin* no. 51, April 1973.

2. R. S. Duff and A. B. Hollingshead, *Sickness and Society* (1968), especially pp. 153, 165, 177-78, 204-5, 213, 248, 269, 280, 306, 329-30, 356, 359, 367, 381.

3. P. Devise et al., *Slum Medicine: Chicago's Apartheid Health System* (January 1969).

4. Ibid., pp. iv, 17-24, 33-34, 41-48, 51, 54.

5. Ibid., pp. 46-47.

6. Ibid., p. 51.

7. M. H. Lepper et al., "An Approach to Reconciling the Poor and the System," *Inquiry*, March 1968, pp. 37-38.

8. J. T. English, "Office of Economic Opportunity Health Programs," *Inquiry*, March 1968, pp. 46-47.

9. Ibid., pp. 43-44.

10. See especially J. R. Storey, "Public Income Transfer Programs," A Study for the Subcommittee on Fiscal Policy of the Joint Economic Committee of Congress, *Studies in Public Welfare*, Paper no. 1.

11. Ibid., p. 1.

12. Ibid., p. 19.

13. Ibid., p. 24.

14. U.S. Department of Labor, *Statistics on Manpower, A Supplement to the Manpower Report of the President* (March 1969), table E-11, p. 85.

15. HEW, Human Investment Programs, *Delivery of Health Services for the Poor* (December 1967), pp. 31-33.

16. Ibid., pp. 36-47.

17. Ibid., p. 35.

18. Ibid., p. 49.

19. Ibid., p. 46.

20. Ibid., p. 47.

21. Ibid., p. 53.

22. Ibid., pp. 49-50.

23. Ibid., p. 51.

24. Ibid., p. 52.

25. *Report of the Task Force on Medicaid and Related Programs* (June 1970), pp. 1-2.

26. Ibid., p. 2.

27. Ibid.

28. Ibid., p. 3.

29. Ibid., pp. 4-5.

30. Ibid., p. 6.

31. Ibid., pp. 9-12.

32. Ibid., p. 13.

33. Ibid., pp. 14-15.

34. Ibid., p. 15.

35. Ibid., p. 22.

36. Ibid., pp. 27-29.

37. Ibid., p. 30.

38. Ibid., pp. 33-36.

39. Ibid., pp. 37-39.

40. Ibid., pp. 41-43.

41. Ibid., pp. 45-50.

42. Ibid., pp. 55-63.

43. Ibid., pp. 72-73.

44. Ibid., p. 74.

45. Ibid., pp. 79-80.

46. Ibid., pp. 83-84.

47. Ibid., pp. 86-87.

48. Ibid., pp. 7-8.

49. Ibid., p. 9.

17

Medicare

Introduction of the Program

Medicare was introduced in 1966, after Title XIX of the Social Security Act had provided for Medicaid. Medicare involved larger resources, offered larger fees, and hence appealed more to physicians than Medicaid. Whereas Medicare made available to the old the means of financing their hospital and medical needs, Medicaid remained largely an assistance program to all age groups, with the standards of care subject to considerable control by state governments.

The introduction of Medicare contributed greatly to meeting the heavier medical care needs of older people. Those sixty-five and over in 1969-70 accounted for 10 percent of the population but 27 percent of personal health care outlays. In contrast, those under nineteen accounted for 36 percent of the population and only 16 percent of personal health care expenditures. The aged received roughly six times as much care per capita as the young.

In 1969-70 public funds covered 27 percent of the personal health care expenditures of those under nineteen, but 65 percent of the spending for those sixty-five and over. Here again the impact of Medicare is obvious.[1]

Benefits

In 1966-67, seven services were covered by Medicare: under the hospital insurance program—inpatient hospital services, outpatient hospital services, extended care facilities services, and home health agency services; and under the supplemental medical insurance program—physicians' and other medical services, outpatient hospital services, and home health agency services.[2]

A 1971 report from the Office of Research and Statistics of the Social Security Administration describes the benefits available and the use of services by enrollees in 1966 and 1967:

The Health Insurance for the Aged program (Medicare) provides a variety of service benefits. This report describes the combinations of these benefits used in July-December 1966 and 1967 by persons enrolled for Medicare.

In the hospital insurance (HI, or A) part of the Medicare program, the benefits for the period covered by these data were: inpatient hospital services (INP); outpatient diagnostic services (OUT-A); and home health agency services following hospitalization (HHA-A). Beginning with 1967, posthospital care in extended-care facilities (ECF) was added.

Under the supplementary medical insurance (SMI, or B) part of the program, the benefits were: physicians' and other medical services (PHYS); outpatient therapeutic services (OUT-B); and home health agency services (HHA-B). . . .

The statistical system of the Medicare program is designed to assemble all bills for reimbursed services for a 5-percent sample of the enrolled population. These records are linked so as to make it possible to relate the various reimbursed services used by an individual. . . . Counts have been multiplied by 20 to give an estimate of the total number of persons who used benefits under the program. . . .

In 1966, 93 percent of the persons reimbursed under the program used either one or two types of benefits. While the absolute number of such persons almost doubled in 1967 compared with 1966, the percent dropped to 85 in 1967. The decline was partly the result of the introduction of the ECF benefit which, almost by definition, requires a combination of three types of services—inpatient hospital, physicians', and extended-care facilities services. The remainder of the shift into the categories of three or more benefits per person was scattered throughout [various] combinations. . . .

Persons using only one benefit were generally those using nothing but physicians' services or inpatient hospital services. About 40 percent of the total were reimbursed only for physicians' and other medical services in both years. In 1966, 11 percent, and in 1967, 7 percent of the total reimbursed, used inpatient hospital services and no other benefit. Some of these persons may represent hospital admissions without use of a private physician. Some used physicians' services for which the allowed charges did not exceed the SMI deductible—or for which they did not file a claim. There are also a number of persons with Medicare coverage for hospital insurance only. More than 100,000 persons in the HI program and eligible for SMI chose not to enroll in the latter program.

About one-third of the persons reimbursed were hospital inpatients who also had covered expenses under physicians' and other medical services; this was the most frequent two-benefit combination. Other combinations of two benefits brought this group to 39 percent of the total in 1966, and 37 percent in 1967.[3]

Initial Costs

In the first year of Medicare (1966-67), the Social Security amendments as a whole cost $6.46 billion. The basic hospital plan accounted for $2.5 billion and the supplementary medical insurance program $1.1 billion of this total.[4] Expenditures for physicians' services for the aged amounted to $1.6 billion, with Medicare providing 39 percent. But benefits actually paid for medical insurance were only $669 million. The corresponding figures for hospital expenditures were $4.1 billion and 57 percent. By 1970-71, public spending for Medicare had reached $7.9 billion, while Medicaid (covering all ages) was expending another $6.5 billion.

The financing of Medicare involved assessments on employers, employees, general revenues, and beneficiaries (see table 17.1). In the first year (1966-67), claims averaged $481 for inpatient hospitals, $300 for extended care facilities, $62 for home health agencies, and $12 for outpatient diagnosis. Short-stay hospitals dominated the statistics, accounting for 98.0 percent of claims, 95.3 percent of care days, 97.9 percent of charges, and 97.8 percent of reimbursements. The percentage distribution under supplementary medical

TABLE 17.1   Initial Financing of Medicare Programs, 1966

Program	Source of Funds	Schedule
Basic hospital insurance	Employer, employee, and self-employed contributions; general revenues for transitional insured status	Each contributor pays 0.35% of payroll, rising to 0.80% in 1987, on $6,500 earning base
Supplemental medical insurance	Beneficiary and federal government	Each contributor pays $3 monthly

Source: HEW, *Medicare-Social Security Amendments of 1965*, p. 9.

TABLE 17.2   Distribution of Supplementary Medical Insurance by Supplier, 1967

	Bills		
Supplier	Percentage	Average Amount	Charges (Percentage)
Physicians	85.5	$77	93.6
Home health agencies	1.5	59	1.3
Outpatient hospitals	8.2	15	1.8

insurance as of August 4, 1967, is shown in table 17.2. Clearly physicians dominated these charges. Thus, hospital insurance payments were heavily concentrated in short-stay hospitals, while physicians were by far the major beneficiaries of the funds made available under the supplemental medical insurance program.

Per capita benefit payments averaged $132 for hospital insurance and $38 for supplementary medical insurance in 1966-67. The range among states was wide, as table 17.3 indicates.

The percentage of persons enrolled who used reimbursed services was higher for men than for women, for white people than for those of other races, and for the most aged than for those closer to sixty-five. It rose especially rapidly with increasing age. This maldistribution reduced the impact of the total.

Persons reimbursed less than $50 for any type of Medicare service during 1967 accounted for 1.6 percent of the total amount reimbursed. Those reimbursed $2,000 or more accounted for 39 percent of the total funds expended, although they constituted only 7.5 percent of the enrollees who received reimbursements.

TABLE 17.3   Maximum and Minimum Per Capita Benefits by State, 1966-67

	Maximum		Minimum	
Type of Benefit	State	Amount	State	Amount
Hospital insurance	Nevada	$191	Mississippi	$66
Supplementary medical insurance	California	72	Alabama	23

Source: HEW, Office of Research and Statistics, *Variations among States in Per Capita Benefit Payments under Medicare, FY 1967.*

The Hospital Insurance Program

In 1968, 3.9 million people aged sixty-five and over were hospital-ized under the hospital insurance program, for an average of 19.7 days per year. Benefit payments were concentrated on inpatient hospital services, which received 86 percent of approved claims and 96 percent of reimbursements. What is striking in these percentages is the relatively high level of reimbursements in comparison with claims. Reimbursements are lower in relation to approved claims for other types of benefits (see table 17.4): extended care benefits were 5.1 percent of claims and 3.6 percent of reimbursements; outpatient diagnostic services were 6 percent of claims and only 0.2 percent of reimbursements.

In 1968, more than 20 million persons were enrolled in hospital insurance. This constituted 18.6 percent of all persons using covered hospital insurance services. Short-stay hospitals rendered most of the services to enrollees (see table 17.5). The percentage using covered hospital insurance services varied by sex, race, age, and region, with the largest variations by age and race.[5]

Of the 21 million persons enrolled under Medicare for some time during 1967, 5 percent died. Yet 22 percent of all reimbursements were made on behalf of the decedents. About 70 percent of the decedents used some reimbursed services, and they used more than double the proportion used by the Medicare population alive at the end of 1967. The hospitalization rate among decedents (611.4 per thousand) was over four times that of beneficiaries who were alive

TABLE 17.4   Amounts of Approved Hospital Claims, 1966-67

Type of Benefit	Approved Claims		Amounts Reimbursed		
	Number	Percentage	Total (Thousands)	Percentage	Per Claim
Total	5,127,608	100.0	$2,212,248	100.0	—
Inpatient hospital	4,403,797	85.9	2,119,918	95.8	$481
Outpatient diagnostic	305,687	6.0	3,646	.2	12
Extended care facility	263,499	5.1	79,050	3.6	300
Home health	154,625	3.0	9,634	.4	62

Source: Claims for payment under the hospital insurance program approved by inter-mediaries and recorded in the Social Security Administration central records, compiled by the Office of Research and Statistics.

TABLE 17.5 Percentage of Enrollees Using Hospital Insurance Services by Type, 1968

			Hospital				
Characteristic	Number of Enrollees (Thousands)	Percentage Using Covered HI Service	Total	Short-Stay	Other	Extended Care Facility	Home Health Agency
Total	20,641	18.6%	18.5%	18.3%	0.4%	1.9%	0.8%
Sex							
Men	8,769	20.5%	20.4%	20.3%	0.5%	1.8%	0.6%
Women	11,872	17.2%	17.0%	16.8%	0.4%	2.0%	0.9%
Race							
White	19,049	19.1%	18.9%	18.8%	0.5%	2.1%	0.8%
All other	1,592	13.3%	13.3%	13.1%	0.2%	0.5%	0.5%
Age							
65-74	13,225	16.7%	16.7%	16.6%	0.4%	0.9%	0.4%
75-84	6,127	20.6%	20.3%	20.1%	0.5%	2.7%	1.1%
85 and over	1,289	25.1%	24.1%	24.1%	0.7%	6.7%	2.3%
Region							
Northeast	5,439	17.0%	16.8%	16.5%	0.9%	1.9%	1.1%
North Central	6,009	20.8%	20.6%	20.6%	0.3%	1.5%	0.9%
South	6,059	17.8%	17.7%	17.5%	0.3%	1.4%	0.4%
West	3,122	18.9%	18.6%	18.5%	0.1%	3.9%	0.6%

Source: HEW, Office of Research and Statistics, *Current Medicare Survey Report, Persons with Covered Hospital Stays* (1968), p. 7.

at the end of 1967 (149.0 per thousand). Similarly their utilization rate for physicians' and other medical services was 567 per thousand, while for persons alive at the end of 1967 it was 295 per thousand.

The Supplementary Medical Insurance Program

A 1967 study determined the average charge under supplementary medical insurance by deductibles and selected characteristics. In urban communities, the average charge per person served was $172; in rural areas it was $144. Table 17.6 suggests the effect of such characteristics as age, sex, race, health limitations, family income, insurance coverage, welfare status, and region on the proportion an enrollee pays for services. Based on the total number of persons using supplementary medical insurance services, enrollees and their spouses paid 49 percent of the costs, insurance 20 percent, welfare 10 percent, and other combinations or unknown sources 21 percent.

TABLE 17.6   Sources and Percentages of Payment for Supplementary Medical Insurance Services

Characteristic	Enrollees Using Services (Thousands)	Percentage by Source of Payment			
		Self or Spouse	Insurance	Welfare	Other
Total	14,946	49	20	10	21
Age					
65-69	4,448	53	23	7	17
70-74	4,350	51	20	9	20
75 and over	6,148	44	17	12	27
Sex					
Men	6,039	50	20	9	21
Women	8,907	48	20	10	22
Race					
White	13,605	49	21	9	21
All other	1,134	48	7	19	26
Unknown	207	36	14	18	32
Education					
Less than 7 years	3,503	52	10	15	23
7-8 years	3,795	51	23	9	17
9 years and over	5,456	53	25	4	18
Not reported	2,191	29	18	17	36
Health limitations					
Confined to bed or house	825	28	14	17	41
Other limitation	1,931	42	14	15	29
No limitations	10,266	55	22	7	16
Not reported	1,923	30	19	15	36
Marital status					
Nonmarried	6,757	47	18	12	23
Married	6,814	54	23	6	17
Not reported	1,375	29	16	19	36
Living arrangement					
Institution	812	16	10	30	43
Living alone	3,162	50	20	12	18
Living with spouse only	5,274	55	25	4	16
Living with others	3,997	55	16	8	21
Not reported	1,700	29	19	16	36
Household size					
1 person	3,907	43	18	16	23
2 persons	6,670	55	23	5	17
3 or more persons	2,663	53	16	8	23
Not reported	1,704	29	19	16	36

TABLE 17.6   Sources and Percentages of Payment for Supplementary Medical Insurance Services (Continued)

Characteristic	Enrollees Using Services (Thou-sands)	Percentage by Source of Payment			
		Self or Spouse	Insurance	Welfare	Other
Work status					
None	9,914	50	19	10	21
Part time	1,164	60	22	4	14
Full time	1,236	59	24	1	16
Not reported	2,632	34	20	14	32
Family income					
Less than $3,000	4,674	53	14	14	19
3,000-4,999	1,886	51	26	7	16
5,000 or more	2,072	50	23	4	23
Not reported	6,314	44	22	9	25
Private health insurance coverage					
No plan at all	6,210	57	4	20	19
Hospital care only	1,046	57	22	2	19
Hospital and surgical care only	1,611	52	30	1	17
Hospital, surgical, and physicians' care	3,809	42	42	1	15
Other combinations	268	41	36	6	17
Not reported	2,001	30	18	15	37
Welfare status					
No welfare	12,077	55	24	—	21
Some welfare	2,869	20	3	50	27
Region					
Northeast	4,130	43	23	10	24
North Central	4,313	50	26	7	17
South	4,190	56	14	8	22
West	2,313	45	14	17	24
Size of community					
Urban	13,242	47	21	10	22
Rural	1,699	64	13	10	13

Source: "Use of Medical Services under Medicare," *Social Security Bulletin*, March 1971, p. 10.

Note: Small numbers are subject to relatively large sampling variability. They are shown here only to assist the users of data should they wish to form aggregates and not because they possess reliability in and of themselves.

Enrollees confined to bed or house paid only 28 percent of their costs, while those with no health limitations paid 50 percent.[6]

Growth of Medicare

It is estimated that by 1980 there will be approximately 21 percent more families in the over sixty-five age group than in 1965. Average disposable income is expected to rise more than prices, and if this occurs the burden of health care expenses will be reduced.[7]

Admission rates to hospitals under Medicare rose from 278 per thousand enrollees in 1966-67 to 309 per thousand in 1971. But the rate of increase in covered days slowed from 7 percent in 1966-67 and 1967-68 to 1 percent by 1971.

Figure 17.7 shows the rise in enrollees and charges under the supplementary medical insurance program from 1967 to 1970. The latter increased substantially more than the former. Services were largely concentrated on office visits in 1969. The average number of visits per person using specified services was 26.9 for nursing homes and 34.7 for inpatient hospital care.[8]

FIGURE 17.7 Enrollees and Charges under Supplementary Medical Insurance, 1967-70

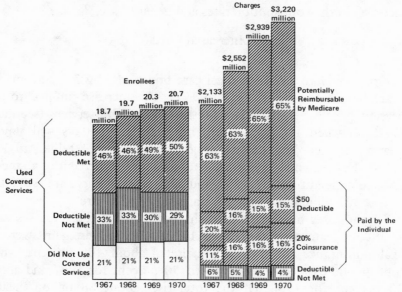

Source: "Five Years of Medicare," *Social Security Bulletin,* December 1971, p. 26.

Trends in the use of Medicare benefits and in enrollments from 1968 to 1971 are shown in table 17.8. Enrollments rose by about 5 percent per year for both hospital and supplementary programs. Amounts reimbursed increased by roughly one-half. Amounts reimbursed rose over one-third more than the number of enrollees.

Since resources rose less than reimbursements, the net impact was inflationary. Among the items that dropped were charges for services in short-stay hospitals, tubercular hospitals, and extended care facilities. The number of extended care facility beds and admissions also dropped.[9]

One estimate of the impact of Medicare put the increase in demand at 30 percent for health services, an estimate based on a regression equation using hospital admissions of aged persons and admissions of aged persons on welfare. Yet, despite these anticipated large gains, a poll showed that only 33 percent of the aged were relieved of worry about medical bills by October 1968.

The large rise in benefits under Medicare induced a number of amendments in 1967, urging experimentation with incentive reimbursement methods, payment under medical insurance for certain ancillary services not payable under hospital insurance, a study of coverage of drug benefits, and additional finance provisions through increases in the contribution rates and benefit base.[10]

Increased Costs

For Medical Care in General

From 1960 to 1967, medical care prices rose by 3.2 percent per year, but in the years 1967 to 1971, the increase jumped to 6.6 percent per year. Inflationary pressures varied by services (see table 17.9). Between 1968 and 1980 hospital care outlays will almost quadruple, according to low projections—from $21 billion to $76 billion. Hospital care is expected to consume 36 percent of all medical care expenditures by 1980, and physicians' services are estimated to cost $29 billion by 1980, 2½ times the 1968 figure.[11]

Expenditures have risen in each program, but the increases vary greatly by categories (see table 17.10). The largest gains were in health insurance for the aged, a rise of about 400 percent, while total public expenditures advanced 50 percent for 1967 and about 20 percent for 1968. Of the total rise, about $8 billion, health insurance for the aged accounted for $4.8 billion and public

TABLE 17.8   Trends in Enrollments, Resources, and Reimbursements under Medicare, 1968-71

Item	1968	1969	1970	1971
Persons enrolled as of January 1				
Hospital insurance (HI)	19,465,411	19,750,572	20,173,819	20,588,456
Supplementary medical insurance				
(SMI)	18,021,125	18,854,607	19,329,363	19,738,504
HI and/or SMI	19,495,512	19,815,300	20,278,398	20,732,693
Amounts reimbursed				
HI total (thousands)	$3,736,322	$4,654,000	$4,804,243	$5,442,971
SMI total (thousands)	$1,389,622	$1,644,842	$1,979,288	$2,034,999
HI amount per enrollee	$192	$236	$240	$264
SMI amount per enrollee	$77	$87	$103	$103
Participating facilities				
Number				
All hospitals	6,865	6,825	6,776	6,745
Short-stay	6,221	6,182	6,153	6,153
Tuberculosis	118	113	105	95
Psychiatric	341	344	341	335
Other long-stay	185	186	177	162
Extended care facilities	4,702	4,849	4,656	4,287
Beds				
All hospitals	1,164,931	1,176,656	1,199,030	1,188,013
Short-stay	781,990	798,652	815,244	834,514
Tuberculosis	23,903	23,263	21,712	18,995
Psychiatric	318,896	313,519	320,709	300,696
Other long-stay	40,142	41,222	41,365	33,808
Extended care facilities	329,621	341,735	333,630	307,548
Beds per 1,000 HI enrollees				
Short-stay hospitals	40.1	40.4	40.4	40.5
Extended care facilities	16.9	17.3	16.7	15.2
Home health agencies	2,093	2,209	2,350	2,284
Independent laboratories	2,566	2,670	2,684	2,751
Admissions (thousands)				
Hospital inpatient	5,780	6,072	6,139	6,230
Extended care facility	443	519	474	417
Admission rate per 1,000 HI enrollees				
Hospital inpatient	297	307	307	305
Extended care facility	23	26	24	20

Source: HEW, Office of Research and Statistics, *Medicare, Fiscal Years 1968-1971, Selected Data* (1972), p. 5.

TABLE 17.9   Rise in Medical Care Prices, 1967-71

Medical Service	Percentage Increase
Total, all services	38.9
Medical care services	46.2
Physicians' fees	39.7
Hospital daily service charges	95.5
Consumer price index	25.1

assistance (vendor medical payments) about $2 billion (doubling over the two years). In contrast, veterans' care rose less than 20 percent.

What stands out is the much larger increase for insurance, which relates to relatively high income groups, than for public assistance. The former gains four times as much proportionally as the latter.

The percentages of private and public expenditures for 1968 are shown in figure 17.11. Private expenditures went mainly for professional personnel, hospital care, and drugs and appliances, while public expenditures were concentrated in hospital care, followed by payments to professional personnel. Nursing home care and medical research received a greater proportion of the total under public expenditures.

In eleven months of 1971 alone, medical care prices rose substantially, as table 17.12 indicates. The most costly item, hospital daily service charges, rose six times as much as drugs and prescriptions. But it is well to note some reservations here. Index numbers do not

TABLE 17.10   Public Expenditures for Health Services and Supplies, 1966-68

Program	Amount (Billions)		
	1966	1967	1968
Total	$10.62	$15.70	$18.7
Health insurance for the aged	1.20	4.74	6.0
Public assistance (vendor medical payments)	1.98	2.83	4.0
Veterans' hospital and medical care	1.21	1.31	1.4

Source: *Social Security Bulletin*, January 1970, pp. 9-11.

FIGURE 17.11 Percentage Distribution of Private and Public Health Expenditures, 1968

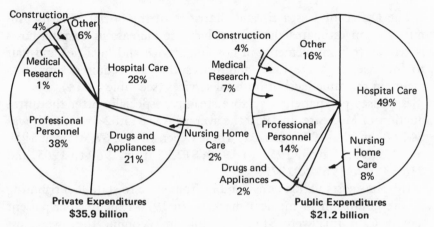

Private Expenditures
$35.9 billion

Public Expenditures
$21.2 billion

Source: *Social Security Bulletin,* January 1970, p. 7.

indicate the varying importance of items covered or not covered. In addition to the amount of fee increases, allowances must be made for the number of fees collected, the percentage of the amounts charged that are collected, and any changes in the quality of services provided.[12] If quality deteriorates, prices are actually rising more than they seem to be.[13]

Hospitals encountered the greatest inflationary pressures. A striking feature was the large increase brought on by the Medicare and

TABLE 17.12 Rise in Medical Care Prices, 1971

Medical Service	Percentage Increase
Total, all services	4.4
Physicians' fees	5.0
Dentists' fees	6.2
Drugs and prescriptions	1.4
Hospital daily service charges	8.3
Consumer price index	2.9

Medicaid programs (see table 17.13). The hospital daily service charge and hospital expense per patient day move similarly. Both rose substantially more from 1965 to 1970 than from 1956 to 1965.[14]

The Office of Research and Statistics of the Social Security Administration estimates that about half the increase in hospital costs is related to improvements in hospital service and facilities and half to increases in wage rates and prices that are required simply to maintain the same level of hospital services (see table 17.14).

Expenses per patient day rose steadily, especially after the introduction of Medicare. In 1950 the average was $15.62; by 1965 it was $44.48; and by 1970, $81.01. These expenses rose $7.50 from 1950 to 1955; $9.11 from 1955 to 1960; $12.25 from 1960 to 1965; and $36.53 from 1965 to 1970.

Hospital costs varied considerably from state to state, contributing to the confusion in medical markets. In 1970 expenses per patient day in California were $111.77, while in Wyoming they were less than half—$53.34.[15]

Increases in Medicare Costs

Medicare costs have greatly exceeded estimates. For the hospital insurance program, income in 1966-67 was about 15 percent higher and benefit payments 21 percent higher than anticipated, while administrative expenditures were double the estimate.

The program's financial problems were aggravated as costs increased more than the flow of personnel, facilities, and services generally. From 1965 to 1970, the cost per medical service rose sharply. Supplementary medical insurance charges rose by 19 percent in 1968 although the proportion of the population incurring charges for covered medical services was almost identical to that in 1967.

TABLE 17.13   Average Annual Increases in Hospital Costs and Charges, 1956-70

Period	Average Annual Percentage Increase	
	Hospital Daily Service Charges	Hospital Expenses per Patient Day
1956-65	6.4	7.0
1965-70	13.4	12.7

TABLE 17.14   Average Annual Increase by Type of Hospital Cost, 1955-70

Type of Cost	Percentage Increase		
	1955-60	1960-66	1966-70
Total	6.9	6.9	13.9
Wage rates and prices	3.8	3.1	7.8
Improvements in services	3.1	3.8	6.1

Source: Adapted from HEW, Office of Research and Statistics, *Medical Care Costs and Prices: Background Book* (January 1972), p. 25.

The increase in covered charges was accompanied by an upward shift in the dollar distribution of charges. Again in 1969 charges for the medical insurance sample rose by a third of a billion dollars, or about 10 percent. But the rise in numbers of visits and persons using services was modest indeed.

In 1969, monthly per capita reimbursement for hospital insurance and supplementary medical insurance combined was $25.98, compared with $22.24 in 1968. The increase of reimbursements for hospital coverage alone averaged 20.5 percent; under the supplementary program it was 7.4 percent. These increases marked a decelerating trend, however. Between the first eighteen months of Medicare and 1968, per capita payments rose 44 percent under hospital insurance and 66 percent under supplementary medical insurance.

The relative stability of the output of services is suggested by several statistics. From September 1966 to the end of December 1967, the covered days of care per discharge from hospitals was remarkably uniform. From July 1966 to June 1967, estimated monthly enrollment in the medical insurance program rose by only 1 percent; the number of enrollees using covered services rose by 6 percent.[16]

Another indication of inflationary pressures is suggested by the modest rise in hospital admissions. In 1967-68, 1968-69, and 1969-70, hospital admissions rose 11.3 percent, 3.7 percent, and 0 percent respectively. These are small increases compared with an annual increase in hospital daily service charges of 12.7 percent from 1965 to 1970.[17]

From July 1966 to March 1969, the Medicare premium rate

was about 7 percent lower than the combined benefits and administrative expenses accrued during this period. The slightly unfavorable experience during this period resulted primarily from an increase of approximately 13 percent in the average fees charged by physicians between July 1965 (when the premium rate was determined) and July 1967 (the approximate mid-point of the period in which the benefits were paid) as compared with the 6 percent increase assumed for this period.[18]

The accumulated surplus of the supplementary medical insurance program was significantly depleted from 1966 to 1968, and this was clearly related to the rise in the average fee charged by physicians. But the full inflationary impact of physicians' charges went even further.

The actuarial state of the supplementary program is related to both its assumptions about inflation and the extent to which inflation is reflected proportionately by physicians' fees. Also relevant is the assumption by program administrators that benefit payments would continue to be the same proportion of physicians' charges as in the past.[19]

From 1969 to 1971 the rise in services provided was disappointing. In fact, doctor visits dropped by 10 percent, and home visits by 75 percent. The hospital insurance services increased relatively more than supplementary medical, although one of the Medicare objectives was to increase medical care rather than hospital care. The charge for nursing home care dropped 30 percent, another change inconsistent with Medicare goals.

The government's absolute and relative contribution to the program increased greatly in the late 1960s. One important result has been substantial pressure on Blue Cross, Blue Shield, and other private insurance interests to liberalize their benefit programs.[20] In light of the failure of services to keep up with increased demand in the years 1969-71, it is not surprising that the government took direct measures to depress prices.

Beneficiaries had problems financing deductibles and coinsurance. To alleviate their difficulties, a new technique, the "buy-in" procedure, was introduced, whereby state governments agreed to provide financing for these costs. By 1969, negotiations had been completed with forty states, involving 11 percent of all supplementary medical insurance beneficiaries. The beneficiaries of the buy-in program were primarily (85 percent) recipients of aid to the aged. They were persons eligible for Medicare benefits and enrolled in the supplementary insurance program.

Another program designed to attack the financial problems was the federal supplementary security income procedure. Payments under this program were based on the needs of recipients and related to the incomes of beneficiaries. Most buy-in recipients were either public assistance recipients or categorically needy persons eligible for medical care under Medicaid. The mean amount of payments received varied among beneficiaries, depending on living arrangements, type of pay, and marital status.

Hospital admissions per thousand enrollees and average monthly reimbursement per enrollee in Medicare's hospital insurance program changed very little in 1970, but, contrary to the Medicare objectives, extended care facilities charges per thousand enrollees dropped by 15.7 percent.

Payments to Physicians

Physicians' fees rose more than the cost of living. From 1965 to 1967 the annual increase in physicians' fees was 7 percent compared to an average hourly wage increase of 4.5 percent and a cost-of-living rise of 2.8 percent.

Physicians' incomes rose much more than the prices of services. From 1966 to 1971, total expenditures for physicians' services rose from $8,865 million to $14,245 million, more than 60 percent. This was a large factor in inducing inflation.

In 1970-71, expenditures for medical care amounted to $75 billion. The major items were $29.6 billion for hospital care, $14.2 billion for physicians' services, $7.5 billion for drugs and sundries, and $4.7 billion for dentists' services. Thus, physicians accounted for almost one-fifth of the total. The effect of their increase in income was multiplied for various reasons. First, an increasing amount of their payment was made by third parties, who were not oversolicitous about verifying the value of purchases made. Secondly, the minority of doctors making excessive incomes aroused the resentment of the public against the profession as a whole. In the third place, even in 1971, physicians' incomes were largely funded out of private resources (75 percent privately funded, whereas 62 percent of *all* expenditures were financed privately). And finally, the *rate* of increase of physicians' net incomes aroused much public criticism. The median net income of physicians under sixty-five almost doubled from 1959 to 1969. The annual percentage increases from 1965 to 1969 were

2.0 percent, 11 percent, 8 percent, 8 percent, and 8 percent respectively. The 1966 rise of 11 percent was especially affected by the 1965 legislation.[21]

Reimbursement under medical insurance is required by law to be based on reasonable charges. A special adaptation of this provision is applied to group-practice prepayment plans that elect to have their services to members reimbursed on a reasonable cost basis.

The reasonable charge, except in unusual circumstances, is the lowest of the following: (1) the actual charge of the physician rendering the service, (2) the charge customarily made by the physician for a similar service, (3) the prevailing charges in the locality for similar services, or (4) the charge on which the carrier bases payment to its own subscribers for similar services under comparable circumstances.

Increases in the customary charges of individual physicians and in the charges prevailing among physicians in a locality were originally recognized under Medicare if there was adequate evidence that the increases had been in effect for a period of time. In December 1970, the Secretary of Health, Education, and Welfare announced that carriers in each fiscal year were to recognize charges that fell within the seventy-fifth percentile of the customary charges.

Provider-based physicians required special reimbursement measures. Many providers retain physicians on a full-time basis—for example, in pathology and radiology. These physicians may be engaged in many activities. Under Medicare it is necessary to distinguish between services rendered by a physician to an individual patient, which are reimbursable on a reasonable *charge* basis, and provider services (including services to a hospital), which are reimbursable on a reasonable *cost* basis. The regulations by and large are intended to make the Medicare reimbursement to provider-based physicians equal to the compensation they would receive from a provider if they were salaried or on a similar compensation basis. The 1967 amendments to the Social Security Act permitted consolidated billings by the hospital for inpatient radiology and pathology services. Under these charging arrangements, however, an excessive burden may be put on Medicare.

Medicare compensates attending physicians who supervise interns and residents in a teaching setting only if the physician renders or directs a required medical service. A reasonable charge will be paid if the supervising doctor's services to the patient are those he renders to his other paying patients.[22]

An exchange of letters between the Associated Physicians of Cook County Hospital and the General Accounting Office revealed that after examining the medical charts and records in seventy-five cases, the GAO generally found no documentation of identifiable services rendered by the relevant physicians. The Social Security Administration estimated that $1,109,000 had been overpaid to the Cook County Hospital doctors, and demanded a $300,000 repayment immediately, with repayment of the balance over time.

Group-practice prepayment plans eliminate the fee-for-service pricing concept in favor of a prepayment mechanism. Thus, there is no established "customary charge" for each service furnished by the plan or physician to a plan member. The customary charge of the plan is a charge for enrollment, regardless of services furnished. It is an amount calculated to cover the cost of services plus a markup intended to meet the plan's needs for capital expansion. Medicare allows an organization that furnishes medical services on a prepayment basis to be paid 80 percent of its reasonable *costs* for those services in lieu of reasonable *charges*. Costs that are necessary, proper, and essential for furnishing medical care are considered appropriate; both direct and indirect costs required to develop, maintain, and operate patient care facilities and activities may be included. Expenses, such as costs of sales promotion, that are not related to patient care are excluded.

A congressional committee noted that excessive charges by physicians could have a serious impact on the program, since these costs accounted for 25 percent of the Medicare budget. The committee stressed the need for cost-control methods. Only reasonable charges should be accepted.

The chairman of the Senate Finance Committee raised several questions concerning physicians' charges:

What is proposed is not a limit on what a physician may charge under the Medicare program, but rather a limit on what the program will recognize as the prevailing fee in the locality. Thus a limitation would be imposed only where a physician's charges are significantly higher than the usual or prevailing charge in the locality for the same service, or where a physician raises his customary charge significantly above former levels.

... The objective is to move toward a system of determining reasonable charges which will be related to the general state of the economy. Indexes will be developed to give recognition to such things as the cost of producing medical services, cost of living and earnings of other professional people.[23]

Carriers paying physicians' charges under Medicare varied widely in taking responsibility for evaluating the medical necessity and appropriateness of the services rendered. The Senate committee labored the point that only doctors can determine whether services ordered by other doctors are necessary: "The Committee is aware of increasing instances of criticism directed at the use of insurance company personnel and government employees in reviewing the medical necessity of services." The medical profession is the proper group to advise physicians of overutilization or overtreatment of patients.[24]

The assignment of Medicare bills has a tendency to keep fees within reasonable bounds. An allowed charge for services may be paid to the *patient* under the supplementary medical insurance program "or the patient may assign the bill for collection to the physician or other supplier of the service if he is willing to accept assignment." When a doctor or supplier accepts assignment, he agrees that his total charge will not exceed the reasonable charge allowed under Medicare. The patient must pay the $50 deductible, if this has not yet been paid, and 20 percent of the balance of reasonable charges (the coinsurance).

If either the patient or the doctor does not want to use the assignment method, the medical insurance payment is made directly to the patient. The patient submits an itemized bill to the carrier and is reimbursed. "When the payment is made directly to the physician (or supplier) on assignment the allowed or reasonable charge determined by the carrier is the total charge."[25]

To illustrate the effect of using or not using assignment, assume that an ophthalmologist's bill for a cataract operation amounts to $700, and the fiscal intermediary finds that this exceeds the usual and customary charge by $150. If the doctor accepts the assignment, the intermediary pays the doctor 80 percent of $550 (the usual and customary charge), which is $440. The patient pays the doctor 20 per cent of $550 (assuming he has paid the $50 annual deductible), which is $110. The total paid to the ophthalmologist is $550.

If there is no assignment, the doctor sends the bill to the patient, who pays $700 to the doctor and then forwards the bill to the fiscal intermediary for reimbursement. The intermediary pays the patient $440 (80 percent of the usual and customary charge of $550). The patient remains unreimbursed for the balance, $260. The total paid to the doctor is still $700, however.[26]

Attempts to Control Costs

A comparison of trends reveals much larger rises of prices, incomes, and expenditures from 1965 to 1970 than from 1960 to 1965. Medicare, Medicaid, and the growth of private insurance largely explain the difference.

In the late 1960s benefits under the supplementary medical insurance provisions increased more than under the hospital insurance provisions, and outlays under insurance increased much more than under assistance, although the needs were greater in assistance. This is explained in part by the greater ease of controlling reimbursements under hospital insurance than under supplementary medical insurance. Large rises of benefits resulted in part from the failure to achieve an effective utilization review program.

Enrollments in hospitals and in less costly services, such as extended care facilities, suggest that there was less substitution of economical services than had been hoped for. But the 1969 statistics point to relatively large gains compared to 1968.

Medicare authorities tried to treat inflationary pressures in numerous ways by tying charges to those imposed by carriers on their own customers, by limiting increases in fees, by introducing incentive reimbursement methods, and by setting limits on fees with the seventy-fifth percentile.

Unsatisfactory improvements in productivity were reflected in inflation in medical markets. By seeking to improve the quality of services, the government contained rising prices to some extent. But excessive pressures for high quality interfered with the availability of needed services.

Greater relative recourse to preventive medicine was also seen as a way to raise output vis-a-vis input. But there are many obstacles to reallocating resources to emphasize preventive care. The effective use of Professional Standards Review Organizations was strongly urged as a weapon to induce increased productivity. Improved methods of choosing intermediaries and carriers and better scrutiny of their performance would also raise productivity.

The Senate Finance Committee noted that the large rise in costs was due partly to a higher cost per service and partly to an increase in services rendered. This committee was particularly concerned about the weakness of utilization reviews. A survey of 1968 revealed that

10 percent of the hospitals were not conducting reviews of extended-stay cases; 47 percent were not reviewing any sample of admissions as required by statute; and 42 percent did not even maintain medical records that could provide a basis for evaluating utilization.[27]

Financial problems plagued the administrators of the Medicare programs, and they tried to solve these problems by putting part of the burden on the beneficiaries. Various approaches were used. They raised payroll taxes, increased the base to be taxed, and increased the premium shared by the government for financing supplementary medical insurance. The use of deductibles, coinsurance, and ceilings on benefits reduced the relief provided for the old.

Continuing Burden on the Aged

In some respects the financing of Medicare has raised serious problems. Even in 1968, couples enrolled in the supplementary medical insurance program paid a $96 contribution. On top of this they had to pay a deductible of $50 per year under Medicare hospital insurance, a coinsurance requirement of 20 percent of the bill (exclusive of the deductible), and any part of the bill held nonreimbursable on the grounds of not satisfying the reasonable charge criterion. A large proportion of doctors, perhaps half, refuse to accept assignments (which limit them to reasonable charges), and this further increases costs to the aged. Obviously doctors generally choose the payment alternative that will yield them the larger income. Despite all the help given under Medicare, those aged sixty-five or over in 1967-68 were paying an average of $170 for medical care each year, compared with an average of $153 paid by persons under sixty-five. This disproportion is especially unwelcome because the older group is much less able to pay for medical bills. The problem is complicated by the fact that the old have health needs about three times as great as the rest of the population. Despite its large contribution, Medicare financed only 45 percent of the medical bill for the aged. Undoubtedly the burden on the old has grown since 1968. The increasing number of people aged sixty-five and over and the rising percentage of the old among women aggravate the problem. In the years ahead, growth will be especially large for the segment of the aged population with the toughest problems—those eighty-five and over—which may nearly double from 1960 to 1985 while the entire population sixty-five and over is expected to increase 50 percent.[28]

In 1969, the medical insurance sample for 16 million Medicare enrollees using services revealed the following financial sources for payments: 85 percent depended on themselves or their spouses; 9 percent on their families; 28 percent on private insurance companies; and 15 percent on welfare. Individual participation (as the source of funds) rose as charges increased: with charges of $10 or less, 69 percent relied on themselves or their spouses; at $50 or more, 87 percent. The amounts of charges incurred vary, depending on a variety of factors. Thus 1 percent of families had charges under $10, and 12 percent had charges of $50 or more.[29]

Successes and Failures of the Program

On the whole, Medicare has been a successful program. It provided $7 billion to $8 billion in funds for health care in 1970-71 where the needs were especially great and the benefits had been modest. As early as 1966-67, President Lyndon Johnson commented: "The success of the Medicare program in its first year has surpassed even the expectations of some of its staunchest supporters. The program is fulfilling the promise that older Americans and their families will be free of major financial hardship because of illness."

But this does not mean that there have not been disappointments. Prices and expenditures escalated way beyond anticipated levels, far exceeding the rise of services. In 1963, the government actuary planning the program estimated costs at $1 billion. By 1970-71, Medicare expenditures were around $8 billion. Failure to introduce incentive reimbursement, the lack of utilization reviews, the excessive incomes of providers, and a disappointing lag in productivity contributed to the inflation. Third-party responsibility for expenditures became increasingly important, but intermediaries and carriers have failed to check overuse of services and to protest adequately against deterioration in quality. Large cost burdens are still imposed on the aged, because of deductibles, coinsurance provisions, premium payments, exclusions of needed services from coverage, and unwillingness of many physicians to accept assignments. Only slight progress has been made in shifting from high-cost hospital services to less costly alternatives.

Under Medicare, concentration of both hospital and supplementary medical benefits among a relatively small percentage of enrollees has occurred. This unfortunate concentration is aggravated by the maldistribution of services from state to state.

An important advance under Medicare has been its payments based on indexes of reasonable, customary, and usual charges instead of extensive dependence on public assistance and welfare payments, as in pre-Medicare days. The subsidy element in payments has been greatly reduced.

Physicians' incomes have risen in response to Medicare and Medicaid. One estimate stated that physicians' incomes rose 60 percent in five years and about 100 percent from 1959 to 1969. These increases were costly, in part because productivity did not advance as rapidly. A study of hospitals showed that the rise of expenditures was accounted for equally by inflation of prices and wages and by real gains in output.

Why has the rise of physicians' services been so costly? First, this is because of heavy price inflation. Rising prices and costs create price movements rather than genuine gains. Secondly, physicians' bills are financed disproportionately out of private resources, which are difficult to come by. Thirdly, there is a rising dependence on third-party operations, which are costly. Third-party arrangements have been growing at an unprecedented rate in the market for physicians' services. Intervention by third parties brings high prices and deterioration of services.

It was hoped that Medicare would improve the distribution of medical services. But here, too, the results are disappointing. The underfinancing of long hospital stays has not been corrected. Nor has the investment in outpatient services been spectacular. The goal of expanding services by extended care facilities and home treatments has not been fully achieved.

The Medicare experience from 1966 to 1971 was reassuring in some respects and disappointing in others. The program made vast additional sums available, which contributed to inflation as the flow of real resources and the delivery systems lagged behind the flood of dollars. Some disappointing results stemmed from abuses, such as fraud by providers; excess payments for work done under teaching conditions; fixed premium and coinsurance payments irrespective of income levels; expansion of private insurance, which greatly increased inflationary pressures in the markets for physicians and other professionals; failure to control fees and to monitor the reasonableness of charges; and increases in the number of fees per procedure. There were special difficulties involved in the large growth of physicians' services and the recent growth of third-party operations for financing physicians' services. Despite the large contribution of the Hill-Burton Act to improving and expanding facilities, and some shifts to low-cost outpatient services, inflation rose much beyond the expected level. The continued increase in the aged population, which has the greatest medical need, further induced inflation. Despite the Blue Shield practice of reimbursing services under a usual, customary, and reasonable pricing policy, which tends to contain demand, inflation continued in medical markets, reaching levels much higher than might be inferred from an index of fees.

Though the evidence supports the view that expansion of less costly services was disappointing in the late 1960s, reimbursements to extended care facilities rose almost six times as much in 1969 (8.5 percent) as in 1968 (1.5 percent). Reimbursements are related to numerous characteristics, including age, sex, dependence on welfare, and location.

Medicare apparently strengthened the financial position of hospitals and extended care facilities, judging from their overall profit and income figures. But large costs of depreciation, increasing service requirements by the aged, bad debts, and excessive demands of doctors in medical school settings were unfavorable factors. The situation is clarified by table 17.15.

Medicare provides large additional resources for medical services, especially for the old. It has brought improved distribution, has increased interest in planning and organization, has made hospitals more viable, and has increased the proportion of services financed by public resources. The financial position of physicians and other professionals reflects the rising flow of funds from Medicare. Greater use of incentive reimbursement methods to providers has been

TABLE 17.15   Rise in Expenditures for Health Services and Supplies, 1966-68

Item	Amount of Increase (Billions)	Proportion of Increase
Total expenditures	$8	—
Health insurance for the aged	4.8	400%
Public assistance (vendor medical payments)	2.0	100%

achieved, and the performance of intermediaries and carriers has come under increased scrutiny.

But there have emerged numerous complaints about the inadequacies of Medicare. The response of extended care facilities and home health agencies was disappointing. Many services, such as outpatient drugs, are not covered or are covered inadequately. The requirement of a three-day hospital stay as a prerequisite to coverage for patient care at an extended care facility was widely criticized. Overutilization and excessive admissions concerned many. The large dependence on deductions, coinsurance payments, premiums, and payroll taxes greatly increased the financial burden on the aged and reduced the gains they received under Medicare. The favored position offered to the elderly raised some questions about benefits for those under sixty-five and spurred demands for enrollment of all permanently disabled persons. The failure to provide an adequate definition and use of the "reasonable" cost criterion also concerned many. Quality standards were supervised most inadequately, and outpatient benefits were insufficient. Medicare was not well integrated with Medicaid, in part because the states were primarily responsible for Medicaid although the federal government provided a substantial part of the financing.

Once Medicare was in operation, it became necessary to complement it with other programs. A survey of the over-sixty-five group revealed the following proposals for supplements: 35 percent favored a $25,000 reserve plan to pay for services not covered by Medicare or incurred after Medicare benefits were used up; 23 percent preferred a cost-indemnity plan; 21 percent wanted financing for out-of-hospital costs such as drugs; and 14 percent asked for a gap-filling program of the type offered by Blue Cross.[30]

Recommendations for Improvements

Since 1956, the Advisory Council to the Department of Health, Education, and Welfare has issued a report every four years. In its April 4, 1971, report, the council made twenty-five specific recommendations.[31] Several of these recommendations concerned Medicare. The council expressed the view that Medicare coverage should be extended to Social Security disability beneficiaries. Benefits should include coverage of out-of-hospital prescription drugs, with beneficiaries paying a flat coinsurance amount of $2 for each new prescription and $1 for each prescription refill.

The council made recommendations for revising the financing of Medicare. Supplementary medical insurance, which is now financed through premiums and general revenues, should be combined with the hospital insurance program of Medicare, as enlarged under the council's recommendations, and the entire package should be financed by equal one-third contributions from employees, employers, and general revenues. Thus, people would pay in advance during their working years toward supplementary medical insurance as they do toward hospital insurance.

The council felt that the number of lifetime reserve days of hospital care and extended care for which inpatient benefits are paid should be increased from 60 to 120. The daily rate of coinsurance, now applicable to such lifetime reserve days, should be one-fourth (rather than the present one-half) of the inpatient hospital deductibles.

The council found that adequate provision has been made in the law to meet all the costs of the cash benefits program, both in the short run and over the long range. But, unless income is increased, it estimated that the hospital insurance trust fund would be exhausted in 1973.

Even though the operations of the Social Security trust funds and other federal trust fund programs are combined with the general operations of the federal government in a unified budget, policy decisions affecting the Social Security program should be based on the objectives of the program rather than on any effect that such decisions might have on the federal budget, the council asserted. The actuarial cost estimates for the cash benefits program should be based— as the estimates for the hospital insurance program now are—on the assumption that earning levels will rise, that the contribution and benefit base will increase as earning levels rise, and that benefit payments will increase as prices rise.

Notes

1. "Medical Care Outlays for Three Age Groups," *Social Security Bulletin*, May 1971, pp. 3-8.

2. "Five Years of Medicare, A Statistical Review," *Social Security Bulletin*, December 1971, pp. 22-25.

3. HEW, Office of Research and Statistics, *Use of Benefits Under Medicare, 1966 and 1967* (April 8, 1971), pp. 1-2.

4. For details see HEW, *Medicare-Social Security Amendments of 1965*, p. 3.

5. HEW, Office of Research and Statistics, *Current Medicare Survey Report, Persons with Covered Hospital Stays* (1968).

6. "Use of Medical Services under Medicare," *Social Security Bulletin*, March 1971, pp. 4-14. Use of and charges for drugs under supplementary medical insurance are included.

7. HEW, Office of Research and Statistics, *The Impact of Medicare* (1970), pp. 53-55.

8. HEW, Office of Research and Statistics, *Current Medicare Survey Report* (1969), charts 2 and 3.

9. For this section, sources were the following, all by HEW, Office of Research and Statistics: *Health Insurance for the Aged: Monthly Reimbursements for Persons by State, 1971* (1973); Ibid., *1970; Supplemental Security Income: A Preliminary Look at the Aged Eligible* (1973); *Health Insurance for the Aged: Hospital and Extended Care Admissions by State Fiscal Year 1971* (1973); *Medicare, Number of Persons Using Reimbursed Services in 1968* (1973); *Medicare Reimbursed for Services in 1967 by Age, Race, and Sex* (1973); *Utilization and Reimbursements under Medicare for Persons Who Died in 1967 and 1968* (1973); *Medicare, Fiscal Years 1968-1971, Selected State Data* (1972).

10. See especially Letter from the Secretary of HEW, *First Annual Report on Medicare*, House Document no. 331 (June 24, 1968), pp. v-viii, 86-93.

11. HEW, Office of Research and Statistics, *Medical Care Costs and Prices: Background Book* (January 1972), pp. 3-5; *Projections of National Health Expenditures, 1975 and 1980*, Senate Report no. 91-710 (October 30, 1970), p. 4.

12. HEW, Office of Research and Statistics, *Medical Care Costs and Prices: Background Book* (January 1972), pp. 5, 9.

13. Ibid., pp. 19-21.

14. Ibid., p. 23.

15. Cf. ibid., pp. 26, 31.

16. Material based on HEW, Office of Research and Statistics, *Current Medicare Survey Reports*, various years.

17. HEW, Office of Research and Statistics, *Health Insurance for the Aged* (September 9, 1971), p. 4.

18. *Annual Report of the Federal Supplementary Medical Insurance Trust Fund*, House Document no. 91-47 (January 16, 1969).

19. Ibid., pp. 7-13.

20. HEW, Office of Research and Statistics, *The Impact of Medicare* (1970), p. 32.

21. HEW, Office of Research and Statistics, *Medical Care Costs and Prices: Background Book* (January 1972), pp. 39, 43, 88.

22. On the issue of compensation of physicians in a teaching setting, see U.S. Senate, Committee on Finance, *Hearings on Medicare and Medicaid, 1969*, App. A, part 2 (1970), pp. 47-78, 597-612; HEW, Office of Research and Statistics, *Medical Care Costs and Prices: Background Book* (January 1972), pp. 127-28.

23. Social Security Amendments of 1970, H.R. 17550, *Opening Statement of Senate Debate* (December 14, 1970), pp. 25-26.

24. U.S. Senate, Committee on Finance, *Report to Accompany H.R. 17550, The Social Security Amendments of 1970*, Senate Report no. 91-1431, pp. 3-4.

25. HEW, *Your Medicare Handbook* (January 1971), p. 22.

26. U.S. Senate, *Hearings on the Economics of Aging: Towards a Full Share of Abundance*, Senate Report no. 91-1 (1969), p. 712.

27. Excerpt from U.S. Senate, Committee on Finance, *Report to Accompany H.R. 17550, The Social Security Amendments of 1970*, Senate Report no. 91-1431, especially pp. 1-3.

28. U.S. Senate, Advisory Committee on Aging, *Health Aspects of the Economics of Aging* (1969), pp. 1-15.

29. HEW, Office of Research and Statistics, *Current Medicare Survey, Medical Insurance Sample, January-December 1969*, table 5.

30. See HEW, Office of Research and Statistics, *The Impact of Medicare* (1970), pp. 8, 32-35, 40, 50-54; *Report of the Advisory Council on Health Insurance for the Disabled under Social Security* (1969); U.S. Senate, Committee on Finance, *Social Security Amendments of 1967* (1967); U.S. Senate, Special Committee on Aging, *Impact of Medicare* (1968), chap. 3, part I; Hospital Review of Planning Council of Southern New York, *Impact of Medicare on the Demand and Financing of Health Facilities and Services in Southern New York* (August 1965); U.S. Senate, Special Committee on Aging, *Developments in Aging*, Senate Report no. 91-875 (February 1970); HEW, *Social Security Amendments of 1965*.

31. HEW, Advisory Council, *Summary of Major Findings*, release of April 4, 1971.

18

Medicaid

History of the Program

Medicaid is one of a series of federal health insurance programs that started in 1950. That year Congress initiated a program giving states very limited matching funds to pay for the care of welfare recipients. Twenty states participated. Ten years later Congress enacted the Kerr-Mills amendment to the Old Age Assistance welfare program, increasing federal matching funds for elderly welfare recipients. Called Medical Assistance for the Aged, it granted funds for the first time to some older persons who were not eligible for welfare. Unfortunately, this program was not widespread, helping only 148,000 older people in its third year of operation. In 1965, Congress replaced the program with Medicare for the elderly and developed Medicaid for low-income people.

Medicaid, enacted as Title XIX of the Social Security Act, expanded the inadequate Kerr-Mills program to include the remaining federally funded welfare categories established by the Social Security Act of 1935: Aid to the Blind, Aid to the Permanently and Totally Disabled, and Aid to Families with Dependent Children.

Medicaid was a departure from previous federally financed plans.

It substituted a single medical assistance program for the four categorical assistance programs. It provided for uniformity in administration, standardized eligibility standards, listing of medical services offered, and federal-state cost-sharing. The federal contribution exceeded the funds that had been made available under the four categorical programs (see table 18.1). States also had the option to provide assistance to people who were *medically* needy although not receiving other public assistance, and they were encouraged to do so by the offer of federal cost-sharing. The federal contribution under Medicaid ranged from 50 percent to 83 percent of the cost of programs, varying inversely with per capita income in the state. Medicaid's ultimate goal was the extension of medical assistance to all people who were found to be needy according to state standards of eligibility. The program hoped to be furnishing comprehensive care and services to substantially all needy or medically needy Americans by July 1, 1975.

In practice, this ambitious goal had to be circumscribed. State governments, slated to carry all nonfederal costs, were generally in financial trouble and could not afford to fulfill these promises. Many critics thought the program's dependence on government funding was excessive. Even the federal government had to retract initial statements and protect its fiscal position by new legislation in 1967. The 1975 objective was not implemented by Congress or the executive branch, and the date was pushed forward to 1977 at the earliest.

Rising medical costs forced the retrenchment. Some states did not

TABLE 18.1   Federal, State, and Local Vendor Medical Payments under Medicaid, 1965-68

	Amount (Millions)	
	1965	1967-68
Total	$1,358	$4,184
Federal	756	2,040
State and local	602	2,145

Source: Advisory Commission on Intergovernmental Relations, *Intergovernmental Problems in Medicaid* (September 1968), p. 56.

Note: Thirteen states authorized medical care only for the categorically needy and the categorically related needy.

join the system, and others did not comply with the benefit structure specified. Frightened by the large influx of medically indigent enrollees, the federal government excluded payments to those with incomes over 133 percent of the maximum payment under Aid to Families with Dependent Children. This technique disqualified those with relatively high incomes from the medically indigent group.

Provisions

Each state decides how to administer its Medicaid program, which services to give, who is eligible to receive services, and how to pay providers. Medicaid required states to consolidate some previous programs, while it increased federal matching funds for aid to the medically needy, the blind, the disabled, dependent children and their families, and the aged. It required state programs to offer benefits for outpatient and inpatient care at hospitals, X-ray and other laboratory work, skilled nursing home care, and physicians' services. But all benefits were, of course, subject to the availability of facilities and services.[1]

A state may extend its coverage to people who fit the description of any of the welfare categories but whose incomes or assets are too large for them to receive welfare. These people are known as the "categorically linked medically needy." Another important concept is "spend-down." A categorically linked family (or individual) at any income level may become eligible for Medicaid if it incurs so many medical bills that, after subtracting them, its income is "spent down" to the eligibility level.

A crucial issue was what income level should be the cutoff point for eligibility of the medically needy. Individuals were considered needy if the income they had or could obtain from other sources was less than the minimum living assistance standard set by their states. All people on welfare were automatically eligible for Medicaid. Others were eligible for Medicaid in 1968 if they had an income of $5,000 or less (for a family of four), but by 1970 the maximum had been reduced to $4,500. At the peak of the program, 2.5 million people were eligible for Medicaid in New York City. When families earning more than 133 percent of the income level for Aid to Families with Dependent Children were excluded from the program, this greatly reduced the number eligible for help under Medicaid.[2] The decline in the number eligible resulted in pressure to move patients from private hospitals and private physicians to clinics and municipal hospitals.

Costs

The amount of funding available for Medicaid depends in part on the amount provided through all welfare programs. The public welfare bill rose from around $52 billion in 1959-60 to $128 billion in 1968-69 and $145 billion in 1969-70. Health and medical programs accounted for $9.6 billion in 1969-70. In addition, $1.8 billion was spent under veterans' programs and $1.56 billion went for research.[3]

During 1968, $4.1 billion was expended from public assistance funds for medical care. Of this amount, $3.8 billion went to Medicaid, $237 million went to medical care under the other federally aided public assistance programs, and $76 million was expended under state and local general assistance programs in which the federal government did not participate financially.

In that year, the average number provided medical assistance was 5.4 million people. The average monthly amount paid for medical bills to money-payment recipients was $55.55. For those receiving services for which money payments were made to the vendors, the monthly average in 1968 was $118.35.

In many states, medical assistance expenditures tended to exceed income maintenance expenditures. Thus, in 1968, twenty-four states spent more for medical care of the aged than for maintenance care of the aged.[4] The nation as a whole spent $8.55 per capita for medical assistance for aged persons and only $8.25 per capita for maintenance payments to the elderly.[5]

From 1965 to 1968, increases occurred in public assistance expenditures for all types of medical services, particularly those by institutions. Inpatient hospital care rose $818 million, or 140 percent, while nursing home care rose $618 million, or 137 percent.[6] Inpatient hospital and nursing home expenditures account for at least 70 percent of all spending for health care since 1962. Shortages of nursing homes and personnel were especially disturbing.[7] Expenditures for other services also increased from 1965 to 1968. Dental expenditures rose by five times, other practitioners' services rose by three times, and physicians' services rose by more than two times.[8]

Rising costs were associated especially with the increase in hospital charges and physicians' fees, which rose an average 6.3 percent and

2.8 percent, respectively, from 1960 to 1965 but rose 16.5 percent and 7.8 percent, respectively, from December 1965 to December 1966. These large rises reflect increases in both prices and the number of services. Pressure for use of facilities was marked in nursing homes, where the rise of demand outpaced available facilities and personnel. Inpatient hospital and nursing home care have accounted for at least 70 percent of all expenditures for medical services since 1961-62.

Monopoly elements raised the costs of medical care. Interference, for example, by Blue Shield, that acts to increase doctors' incomes contributes a monopoly element, as does the conflict of interests that ensues when physicians buy into extended care facilities and pharmacies. Physicians cooperating with nursing homes are responsible in part for the fragmentation of medical care and such unacceptable practices as gang visits. The overcapitalization of assets through excessive turnover of plants also introduces rising costs.[9]

Medicare's relatively high standards for care for the aged tended to push up Medicaid benefits and costs also, although the government sought to discourage the assumption of the standards of one program by the companion program. To some extent, Medicaid financed Medicare, since elderly people insured under the supplementary medical insurance program of Medicare were often unable to finance the $50 deductible and the 20 percent coinsurance provisions. Medicaid resources could be used for these amounts and through the buy-in programs initiated after Medicaid went into operation.

Projections tend to greatly underestimate expenditures. For example, in 1969, the estimate for public assistance and medical assistance was $521 million; for 1975, it was $1,024 million (with the federal government paying about half). In 1968-69, actual medical assistance payments were $381 million for New York and $450 million for California, totaling $831 million, or 82 percent of the 1975 total.[10] These trends may well attest to uneven distribution as well as underestimates of spending. By 1968-69, annual expenditures for medical care assistance were exceeding $4 billion. When outlays on Medicare and Medicaid greatly exceeded estimates, the federal government retreated. New York State was confronted with a $41 million cut in the federal contribution from the first year of Medicaid and an estimated $61 million from the second year, stemming from withdrawals of federal aid. The eligibility of 600,000 people was terminated, and the 133 percent limit on income for eligibility was introduced. In addition, a 2 percent payment to cover unidentifiable costs was revoked. Other restraints on increased payments to purveyors also became popular.[11]

Four years after enactment of medical assistance for the aged, the percentage of all medical assistance that went to medical care for the aged had risen by 186 percent. Four years after enactment of Medicaid in 1965, the increase in medical expenditutes for *all* recipients was 223 percent.[12]

The *New York Times* noted that Medicaid expenditures by government at all levels rose by 20 percent from 1969 to 1970, reaching $5.6 billion. New York's current Medicaid budget of $1.2 billion is exceeded only by California's $1.6 billion program. Both New York and California cut back their Medicaid programs in the spring of 1970.

Variations among States

State obligations grew at uneven rates, and the obligation of the federal government depended on such decisions as whether a state chose to provide medical assistance payments to the medically needy and the categorically needy; whether it decided to include noncategorically related persons in the medically needy group; what the definition of medically needy was in relation to income and resources; the scope and level of services provided to both categorically needy and medically needy; and the division of cost-sharing between state and local governments.[13]

States were required to finance at least 40 percent of the nonfederal share of Medicaid expenditures, and, beginning in 1969-70, they were to take full responsibility for the nonfederal funds. Of thirty-seven states reporting Medicaid expenditures, fifteen shared the nonfederal burden with local governments. The state providing the highest proportion was North Dakota, giving 86 percent from state funds, and the minimum state share was 47 percent, contributed by Nevada. On the whole, few states responded to Medicaid by introducing new taxes.[14] State fiscal ability was not always matched by expenditures for assistance by state and local governments (see figure 18.2).

In 1968, New York alone spent more than one-fourth of the $4.1 billion in public assistance that went to medical care. New York, California, and Massachusetts together spent about one-half. These three, plus Michigan, Wisconsin, Minnesota, three New England states, and Oklahoma constituted the top ten, which accounted for three-quarters of the expenditures.[15] These statistics illustrate the unevenness of the distribution of Medicaid. Even as late as 1969, five states, relatively poor ones, were not covered at all. The ten states with the highest per capita expenditures were New York, California, Massachusetts, Michigan, Wisconsin, Minnesota, Oklahoma, Connecticut, Rhode Island, and Vermont.[16]

In the first years of implementation, Medicaid had varying effects on the numbers of people receiving public assistance medical care: in four states, the number declined, but in five (Connecticut, Delaware, Michigan, Montana, and Oklahoma) coverage more than doubled.[17]

The number of services covered by states under Medicaid for thirty-eight states, as of July 1968, varied from twenty services in California and Connecticut, to five services in Wyoming. Seven states offered fewer than ten services, and twenty-one states provided fifteen or more services.

The most critical factor in determining medical need is the amount of annual income that is presumed sufficient to meet normal maintenance requirements. Despite the program's emphasis on uniformity, states varied greatly in their eligibility ceilings on income and resources. The range of income levels for the medically needy from state to state, on June 1, 1968, was substantial. A single person earning from $1,200 to $1,399 was eligible in one state, whereas in others the income level was $2,200 or $2,900. The low range for a family of four was $2,400 to $2,799, while the high range was $4,800 to $6,200.[18]

The contribution of the federal government tended to rise. Yet in a recent year only 7.4 million of the 34 million people in poverty received public assistance. And the federal government then was not funding care for the medically needy who were aged twenty-one to sixty-five.[19]

In the 1967 amendments to Title XIX of the Social Security Act, some efforts were made to protect the federal government against excessive obligations under Medicaid. In particular, one amendment prohibited "Federal sharing in expenditures for medically needy families whose income is more than 133-1/3 percent of the highest amount ordinarily paid under its AFDC program to a family of the same size and without any income or resources."[20]

FIGURE 18.2 Comparison of State Fiscal Ability and Public Welfare Spending, 1964

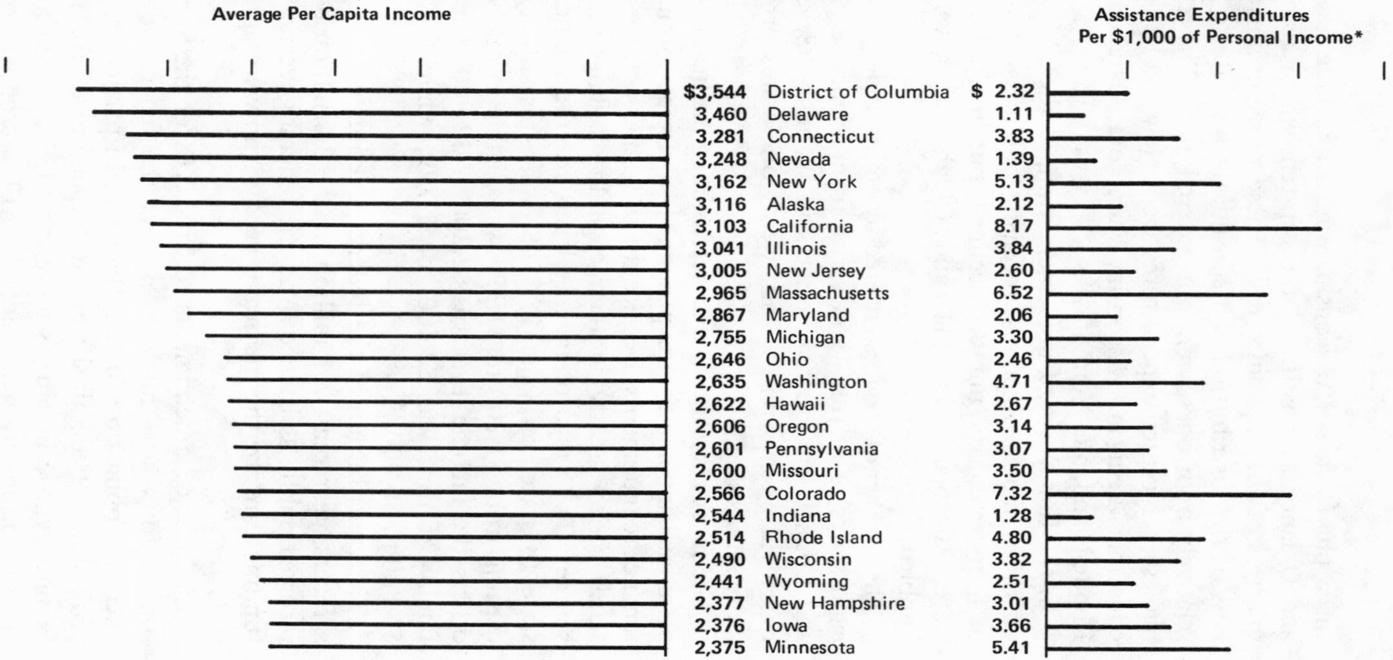

	Average Per Capita Income	State and Local Assistance Expenditures Per $1,000 of Personal Income*
District of Columbia	$3,544	$ 2.32
Delaware	3,460	1.11
Connecticut	3,281	3.83
Nevada	3,248	1.39
New York	3,162	5.13
Alaska	3,116	2.12
California	3,103	8.17
Illinois	3,041	3.84
New Jersey	3,005	2.60
Massachusetts	2,965	6.52
Maryland	2,867	2.06
Michigan	2,755	3.30
Ohio	2,646	2.46
Washington	2,635	4.71
Hawaii	2,622	2.67
Oregon	2,606	3.14
Pennsylvania	2,601	3.07
Missouri	2,600	3.50
Colorado	2,566	7.32
Indiana	2,544	1.28
Rhode Island	2,514	4.80
Wisconsin	2,490	3.82
Wyoming	2,441	2.51
New Hampshire	2,377	3.01
Iowa	2,376	3.66
Minnesota	2,375	5.41

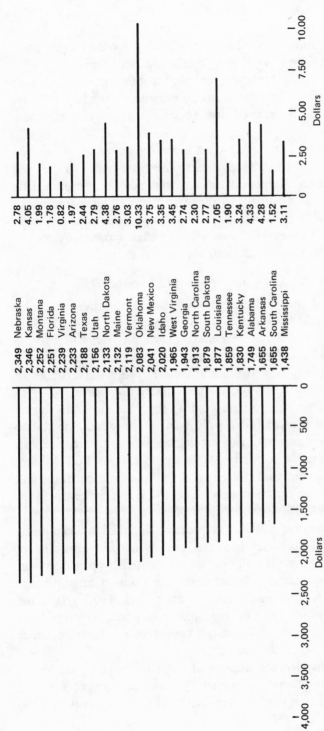

	Dollars
2,349 Nebraska	2.78
2,346 Kansas	4.05
2,252 Montana	1.99
2,251 Florida	1.78
2,239 Virginia	0.82
2,233 Arizona	1.97
2,188 Texas	2.44
2,156 Utah	2.79
2,133 North Dakota	4.38
2,132 Maine	2.76
2,119 Vermont	3.03
2,083 Oklahoma	10.33
2,041 New Mexico	3.75
2,020 Idaho	3.35
1,965 West Virginia	3.45
1,943 Georgia	2.74
1,913 North Carolina	2.30
1,879 South Dakota	2.77
1,877 Louisiana	7.05
1,859 Tennessee	1.90
1,830 Kentucky	3.24
1,749 Alabama	4.33
1,655 Arkansas	4.28
1,655 South Carolina	1.52
1,438 Mississippi	3.11

Dollars

Source: HEW, "National Blueprint for Public Welfare," *Indicators*, November 1966, p. 10.

*Excludes general assistance.

After the amendments, a state that included a broad segment of noncategorically related needy and medically needy people got no federal matching funds for these people although it was receiving Medicaid for categorically related needy persons.[21] Inadequate state standards for the needy carried over to standards for the medically needy.[22]

Medicaid demand was reduced when increased coverage of benefits for the aged was enacted by Medicare.[23] The costs of aid to the aged were especially large. "Expenditures for the aged composed a little more than 40% of all medical assistance and 30% of all maintenance assistance. . . . In Massachusetts, expenditures per inpatient for medical care of the aged alone—$22—were larger than inpatient expenditures for medical care for all recipients in the 46 states."[24]

The Goal of Comprehensive Coverage

The 1975 goal of the Medicaid program was comprehensive coverage of all needy and medically needy persons. In 1966-67, $2.5 billion was spent by thirty-seven states with programs of varying comprehensiveness in numbers covered and services offered. The Department of Health, Education, and Welfare projected a total outlay of $4.1 billion for 1968-69, with six states not participating in the program at all and six others coming into the program during that fiscal year and thus included only part of the year. The thirty-eight others had programs with varying degrees of comprehensiveness.

The estimated outlay for fifty states by 1975 was $6.7 billion, based on an assumption that present conditions would continue and costs would rise 5 percent annually. The 1975 comprehensive program is set by section 1903(e) of Title XIX.

To implement section 1903(e) requires a financial underpinning that is not there. A broader financial base is needed—possibly an employee-employer payroll program supplemented by private insurance cooperation in financing benefits for the poor. Rising coverage and escalating costs have made attainment of the 1975 goal most difficult, especially in light of the inadequacy of personnel and facilities. The pressure on government resources is excessive; other sources of finance need to be found.

In general, judging by the actions of the House Ways and Means Committee and the Senate Finance Committee, Congress is not taking the 1975 goal seriously. In fact, it seemed disposed in 1966 and 1967 to retreat from federal programs, and it gave little encouragement to the states to expand their programs. Little progress had been made by 1968.[25] Recently the 1975 goal was moved forward to 1977.

Any implementation of section 1903(e) will depend on what the states do. The prospects are not too bright. Thus, in 1966, almost 30 million people were below the poverty level, but only 8 million were receiving public assistance. The 21 million excluded "were denied, refused, or decided not to avail themselves of the opportunity to get assistance."

Shortcomings of the Program

The achievements of Medicaid after three years of operation have been disappointing. By 1969 coverage was only one-third the figure estimated in 1965. Possession of a Medicaid card does not mean a person can find a doctor. Because of the maldistribution of doctors geographically and among specialties, poor people have a hard time finding doctors. Those who can get an appointment usually have to wait weeks. Medicaid also shows how the private sector responds to public money. A New York grand jury reported that Medicaid in that state had wasted $1 billion in nursing home bills for dead patients, pharmacy claims for nonexistent prescriptions, and kickbacks among providers. In California, testimony before a state legislative committee told of doctors collecting $50 for each referral to home health agencies. And although a goal of the program was to encourage preventive care, hospitals have been the largest consumers of Medicaid money, taking 40 percent of the program's budget, for inpatient care.

Neighborhood health care centers are spreading, but the choice of location is determined too often by the convenience of the physicians, and the funds allocated to them are inadequate. Because of the great pressures for more personnel and facilities, emanating from Medicare and Medicaid, it is difficult for new institutions to mobilize required resources.[26]

Attempts to contain the high demand for medical care are often too effective, bringing underutilization of health services. Thus Dr. John Knowles has noted the heavy cash outlays required under Medicare, which have unfortunate results in deterring patients from seeking care.[27] Supplementary medical insurance payments for an aged couple are $96, drugs cost $50 to $60, and coinsurance and deductibles run between $50 and $100, for an annual total out-of-pocket expenditure of $196 to $256. Moreover, the cost of drugs may rise as high as $500 in cases of chronic diseases.

Uneven distribution of hospital beds is also a troublesome area. The variations from one region to another are much greater for long-term facilities than for short-term hospitals (see table 18.3).

Maldistribution of physicians is another problem. To reduce medical care costs, a potent medicine is abandonment of fee-for-service reimbursement. But in a market where the supply of physicians is much smaller than the demand, the poor are squeezed out, as doctors will elect to practice under fee-for-service arrangements, instead of the less lucrative capitation or salary reimbursement programs.[28] The strong bargaining position of physicians is suggested by the fact that their income of $1,291 million constituted 25 percent of payments under Medicare.[29]

The Reagan administration in California estimated that the coverage of all patients under Medi-Cal, California's Medicaid program, through prepaid health care plans, instead of the traditional fee-for-service system, would save the state's taxpayers $150 million to $300 million. But the gains were not to be made at the expense of the state's medically indigent, numbering between 2 million and 4 million. By January 1973, the state had negotiated twenty-five prepaid contracts, covering approximately 150,000 patients and having an ultimate capacity of 500,000 patients.

Patients dropped out of programs at a rate of 34 percent a year, however, indicating violations of and dissatisfaction with the contracts. Yet, as quality controls are achieved, costs increase, and savings are reduced. In theory, the prepaid programs have a financial incentive to keep their patients well. But they may also cut corners.[30]

Much difficulty arises from a reimbursement system under which

TABLE 18.3   Geographic Variations in Hospital Bed Distribution

Type of Facility	Beds per 1,000 Population	
	Lowest Area	Highest Area
Short-stay hospital	36.6	46.7
Long-stay hospital	0.4	3.8
Extended care facility	11.1	33.8

Medicaid will pay all the costs of both an efficiently run hospital that provides high quality care and an inefficiently operated hospital that provides lower quality care. Because there is no distinction in reimbursement for higher quality care or more efficient operation, there is obviously little financial incentive for improvement.

Recommendations for Improvement

To increase efficiency and economy in the provision of health services, the Advisory Commission on Intergovernmental Relations offered several proposals:

Pursuant to Sections 237 and 402 of the 1967 amendments to the Social Security Act, the States [should] move vigorously to experiment with methods of increasing the efficiency and economy of health services under the Medicaid program. Such experiments should include (a) reimbursing hospitals contingent on their operating under an acceptable standard of management efficiency, (b) expanding prior authorization for elective surgical procedures, (c) payment for physicians' services on a basis other than usual and customary charges, (d) use of copayments for the purchase of specified health care services, and (e) improved techniques of utilization review.[32]

The commission felt that divorcing Medicaid from Medicare's inpatient hospital reimbursement formula would go a long way toward removing the cost-plus factor, which does not encourage hospitals to hold costs down. Rates could then be related to overall economic trends and to costs of services and facilities in comparable hospitals. Hospitals could receive more favorable rates, for example, if they centralized blood banks and laundry facilities.[33] The National Conference on Medical Costs suggested that incentives for reducing costs could be explored for hospitals that

—provide efficient and measurably effective use of the utilization review process.

—develop weekend utilization more comparable with weekday use.

—engage in shared activities with others—laboratories, computers, laundries, etc.

—use formularies and generic drugs.

—maintain high-caliber cost records and develop use of effective cost-control systems.

—use professional advisory and consultant talent for more efficient use of hospital services.

—use social and other services to plan for the discharge and next steps for patients.

—devise working departmental incentive programs which lower supply consumption and increase productivity.[34]

The advisory commission added:

Another form of utilization control deserving exploration is prior authorization for elective medical and surgical procedures. Objections are sometimes made that prior authorization interferes with the practice of medicine. It is generally acknowledged, however, that certain procedures have been abused in private practice and are thus likely to occur in State Medicaid programs. Singled out are tonsillectomies and hysterectomies. It may also be contended that physicians' decisions are already reviewed post-operatively by hospitals' medical staffs, thus checking any tendency to undertake surgical procedures unnecessarily. In such a review, however, the staff committee is aware that a physician's professional reputation is more affected by a criticism of his decision after a surgery has been performed than by a withholding of authorization in advance, and therefore the committee is likely to be less rigorous in its interpretation of the "necessity" of a surgical procedure than a prior authorization review body.[35]

The commission would also remove barriers to prepaid group health care practice. Twenty states apparently have serious restrictions on group practice in their laws.[36]

According to the advisory commission, the reimbursement standards and practices followed under Medicare should not be applied to Medicaid. The commission also recommended against spreading high-cost hospital charges among all patients, by averaging per diem costs, for example, instead of charging only the beneficiaries of these services.

Title 19 provides that State Medicaid programs must pay for inpatient hospital services on the basis of "the reasonable cost (as determined in accordance with standards approved by the Secretary and included in the plan) . . . ." HEW implementing regulations provide that, for each hospital also participating in the Medicare program, the State agency must apply the same standards, principles, and method of computing payments that are provided under Medicare. The Medicare formula is a Ratio of Costs to Charges (RCC) formula. It is designed to charge a patient for all costs incurred for him, and to avoid attributing any part of his allowable cost to the cost of another patient's care or to another program. It is distinguished, for example, from a system using the average per diem rate, which involves spreading the expenses of certain high cost services to all patients, rather than to only those receiving those services.[37]

The advisory commission noted the adverse effects of Title XIX on state finance and reflected on the relationship of this to the failure of twelve states to join the program. There is need for a study of the impact of Medicaid on state and local governments.[38] According to the commission, federal criteria for evaluating state resources and limitations also need further study. For a family of four, the cash asset limitation among twenty-three states ranged from $450 in Washington to $6,200 in Rhode Island.[39]

The commission recommended federal matching for noncategorically related needy and medically needy persons, and open-ended appropriations rather than fixed sums. Open-ended funding excludes limitations on the amount appropriated to any state. Indeed, this approach puts a great burden on the federal government.

Notes

1. U.S. Senate, Committee on Finance, *Staff Report: Medicare and Medicaid, Problems, Issues and Alternatives* (February 1970), pp. 41-42.

2. Ibid., p. 42.

3. A. M. Skolnik and S. R. Dales, "Social Welfare Expenditures, 1968-69," *Social Security Bulletin,* December 1969, p. 5.

4. HEW, National Center for Social Statistics, *Medicaid, Selected Statistics, 1951-69,* p. 11.

5. Ibid.

6. Ibid., p. 12.

7. Ibid., pp. 12-13.

8. Ibid., p. 12.

9. See, for example, U.S. Senate, Committee on Finance, *Staff Report: Medicare and Medicaid, Problems, Issues and Alternatives* (February 1970), pp. 5-25.

10. See HEW, *Report of the State-Federal Task Force on Costs of Medical Assistance and Public Assistance* (1968), especially pp. 38-39, 52-53, 121; HEW, National Center for Social Statistics, *Medicaid, Selected Statistics, 1951-69,* p. 55.

11. *Medical Care in America,* vol. 1, pp. 428-29.

12. Statistics from HEW, National Center for Social Statistics, *Medicaid, Selected Statistics, 1951-69,* pp. 1-5.

13. Advisory Commission on Intergovernmental Relations, *Intergovernmental Problems in Medicaid* (September 1968), p. 26.

14. Ibid., p. 36.

15. HEW, National Center for Social Statistics, *Medicaid, Selected Statistics, 1951-69,* p. 7.

16. Ibid.

17. Advisory Commission on Intergovernmental Relations, *Intergovernmental Problems in Medicaid* (September 1968), p. 30.

18. Ibid., p. 33.

19. HEW, "National Blueprint for Public Welfare," *Indicators,* November 1966, pp. 3-14; for details of the history of the federal government's rising share in financing medical assistance, see U.S. Senate, Committee on Finance, *Staff Report: Medicare and Medicaid, Problems, Issues and Alternatives* (February 1970), especially pp. 91-92.

20. Ibid., p. 25.

21. Ibid., p. 28.

22. Ibid., p. 41.

23. Ibid., pp. 38-40.

24. HEW, National Center for Social Statistics, *Medicaid, Selected Statistics, 1951-69,* p. 11.

25. Advisory Commission on Intergovernmental Relations, *Intergovernmental Problems in Medicaid* (September 1968), pp. 40-41.

26. "A Panel Discussion," *Inquiry,* March 1968, pp. 57-64.

27. U.S. Senate, Special Committee on Aging, Subcommittee on Health of the Elderly, *Hearings on the Economics of Aging: Towards a Full Share of Abundance,* Senate Report no. 91-1 (1969), vol. 3, p. 578.

28. *Medical Care for America,* vol. 2, pp. 655, 754-68; "A Panel Discussion," *Inquiry,* March 1968, pp. 57-61.

29. U.S. Senate, *Hearings on the Economics of Aging: Towards a Full Share of Abundance,* Senate Report no. 91-1 (1969), p. 722.

30. *Los Angeles Times,* January 29, 1973; see also HEW, National Center for Social Statistics, *Programs: Facts on Federally Aided Public Assistance Income Maintenance Programs* (1970).

31. Advisory Commission on Intergovernmental Relations, *Intergovernmental Problems in Medicaid* (September 1968), p. 79.

32. Ibid., p. 75

33. Ibid., p. 76.

34. Ibid., p. 77.

35. Ibid., p. 78.

36. Ibid., pp. 72-73.

37. Ibid., p. 73.

38. Ibid., pp. 68-69.

39. Ibid., p. 70.

Index